How to Perform Ultrasonography in Endometriosis

Stefano Guerriero
George Condous • Juan Luis Alcázar
Editors

How to Perform Ultrasonography in Endometriosis

Springer

Editors
Stefano Guerriero
Department of Obstetrics and Gynecology
University of Cagliari
Cagliari
Italy

Juan Luis Alcázar
Obstetrics and Gynecology Department
University of Navarra
Pamplona
Spain

George Condous
Acute Gynaecology, Early Pregnancy and Advanced Endosurgery Unit
Sydney Medical School Nepean
University of Sydney
Nepean Hospital
Sydney, Australia

ISBN 978-3-030-10019-3 ISBN 978-3-319-71138-6 (eBook)
https://doi.org/10.1007/978-3-319-71138-6

Printed on acid-free paper

This Springer imprint is published by the registered company Springer Nature Switzerland AG
The registered company address is: Gewerbestrasse 11, 6330 Cham, Switzerland

Preface

How to Perform Ultrasonography in Endometriosis is an international collaborative which brings together experts in the different fields of endometriosis, with a special focus on imaging. This book primarily aims to give sonologists, radiologists and sonographers a blueprint which enables them to understand not only the different phenotypes and anatomical locations of endometriosis but also the steps involved when performing an ultrasound-based evaluation in a woman with potential underlying endometriosis.

Before the recent 2016 publication on the systematic approach to ultrasound in women with suspected endometriosis by the International Deep Endometriosis Analysis (IDEA) group, there was significant heterogeneity in the scientific literature in nomenclature, definitions and components of this particular type of ultrasound scan. The dynamic ultrasound-based evaluation of the pelvis in women with potential endometriosis is divided into four distinctive systematic steps as defined by the IDEA group. In this book, we have taken each of the four steps and dissected every aspect of the ultrasound evaluation so that the reader is clearly guided and gets a clear understanding of what is involved. The format of each chapter includes a 'short update', 'how we do it', 'technical tips' and 'future perspectives' to thoroughly assist the reader in the intricacies of all aspects of the patient evaluation. We have also included where relevant pictorials, images and videos to illustrate different aspects of the specific imaging evaluation being discussed.

Step one of the IDEA approach includes both assessment of the uterus and ovaries. In this 'how-to', we go into great detail examining and explaining the methodology behind uterine and myometrial evaluation as adopted by the Morphological Uterus Sonographic Assessment (MUSA) group. We also elaborate on the classification of ovarian endometrioma according to the International Ovarian Tumor Analysis (IOTA) group.

Step two of the IDEA approach evaluates 'soft markers' including ovarian mobility and site-specific tenderness. Again in this 'how-to', great insight is given to this important dynamic aspect of the ultrasound-based evaluation.

Step three of the IDEA approach evaluates the status of the pouch of Douglas (POD). This is explained in the 'how-to' with implementation of the 'sliding sign' which is also a dynamic part of the ultrasound-based evaluation.

Step four of the IDEA approach evaluates the anterior and posterior compartments of the pelvis for the presence or absence of deep endometriosis. We have allocated separate and detailed chapters in the 'how–to' on the ultrasound evaluation of specific deep endometriosis anatomical locations, including the bladder and ureters, the uterosacral ligaments, the posterior vaginal fornix and the rectum–rectosigmoid–sigmoid.

We have also outlined extra-pelvic sites for endometriosis and discussed other modified ultrasonographic techniques as well as additional radiological techniques including magnetic resonance imaging.

In broadening the content of this 'how-to' book, we believed it was important to include chapters on the clinical and anatomical considerations of endometriosis, an up-to-date overview on medical and surgical management strategies and currently available biomarkers being used and evaluated in endometriosis. These evidence-based chapters give an update in these key areas of the disease.

We hope that when reading this book you become well versed in the detail involved in assessing women with endometriosis. The incredibly relevant experience shared by the different co-authors throughout this 'how-to' commentary should educate and expand your knowledge in this rapidly evolving field of endometriosis imaging. The simplification of the IDEA approach through pictorials, images and videos should empower you in your endeavours to improve your diagnostic performance in endometriosis ultrasound. In turn, this will enable you to not only map disease location but more importantly convey important information about the extent of disease. Enjoy.

Cagliari, Italy — Stefano Guerriero
Sydney, New South Wales, Australia — George Condous
Pamplona, Spain — Juan Luis Alcazar

Contents

1 **Endomitriosis: Clinical and Anatomical Considerations** 1
Sukhbir S. Singh

2 **Medical and Surgical Management of Endometriosis** 13
Errico Zupi, Lucia Lazzeri, and Caterina Exacoustos

3 **Standardized Ultrasonographic Diagnostic Protocol to Diagnose Endometriosis Based on the International Deep Endometriosis Analysis (IDEA) Consensus Statement** 27
Mathew Leonardi and George Condous

4 **Uterine Evaluation Using a Diagnostic Protocol Based on MUSA** 37
Thierry Van den Bosch

5 **Ovarian Endometriosis** 47
Juan Luis Alcázar

6 **Soft Marker Evaluation** 57
Shannon Reid

7 **Ultrasound in the Evaluation of Pouch of Douglas Obliteration** 63
Shannon Reid

8 **Anterior Compartment Including Ureter** 67
Luca Savelli and Maria Cristina Scifo

9 **Uterosacral Ligament Endometriosis** 77
Francesco Paolo Giuseppe Leone

10 **Forniceal-Vaginal Deep Endometriosis** 89
Stefano Guerriero, Gil Cohen, Silvia Ajossa, Ornella Comparetto, Camilla Ronchetti, Bruno Piras, Alba Piras, and Valerio Mais

11 **Rectovaginal Septum Endometriosis** 97
Gernot Hudelist and Kristine Aas-Eng

12 **Rectum, Rectosigmoid, and Sigmoid Endometriosis** 103
Manoel Orlando Goncalves, Leandro Accardo de Mattos, and Mauricio S. Abrao

13 Other Locations of Deep Endometriosis 121
Stefano Guerriero, Silvia Ajossa, Ornella Comparetto, Camilla Ronchetti, Virginia Zanda, Bruno Piras, Alba Piras, and Valerio Mais

14 Modified Ultrasonographic Techniques 133
Simone Ferrero, Umberto Leone Roberti Maggiore, Fabio Barra, and Carolina Scala

15 Additional Radiological Techniques (MRI) 147
Federica Schirru, Stefano Guerriero, and Luca Saba

16 Biomarkers in Endometriosis 169
Vicki Nisenblat and M. Louise Hull

17 Clinical Cases and Videos 185
Mauricio León, Hugo Sovino, and Juan Luis Alcazar

Index 191

List of Videos

Video 1.1 Scar endometriosis—An example of a post cesarean section incisional endometriosis nodule resulting in cyclical left lower quadrant pain and a palpable mass. (Courtesy of Dr. S. Singh)

Video 1.2 Excision of superficial endometriosis—An educational video. (Courtesy of Dr. M. Suen)

Video 1.3 Surgical approach to endometriosis of the posterior cul-de-sac. (Courtesy of Dr. D. Evans and M. Suen)

Video 1.4 Video demonstrating excision of an invasive bladder nodule. (Courtesy of Dr. S. Singh)

Video 5.1 In this video, acoustic streaming in a case of ovarian endometrioma can be observed. Note the movement of the cyst's particles

Video 5.2 In this case, the adhesion of the ovary to the uterus is clearly noted when moving the transvaginal probe back and forth

Video 5.3 In this case, the ovarian endometrioma is not attached to the uterus, and we can observe the sliding of the cyst against the cervix

Video 5.4 This video corresponds to a case of endometrioma decidualization during pregnancy. A highly vascularized cystic solid mass can be seen. The cyst was surgically removed, and histologic analysis proved it was a decidualized endometrioma

Video 6.1 Transvaginal ultrasound is used to demonstrate a mobile right ovary (RO) along the right pelvic sidewall (RPSW) in the transverse plane. *EIV* external iliac vessel

Video 6.2 Transvaginal ultrasound is used to demonstrate ovarian (O) mobility along the lateral uterus (U), as well as the right pelvic sidewall (PSW), in the transverse plane

Video 6.3 Transvaginal ultrasound is used to demonstrate fixation of the left ovary (LO) to both the posterior uterus (U) and left pelvic sidewall (LPSW), in the sagittal plane

Video 6.4 Transvaginal ultrasound is used to demonstrate fixation between the left ovary (O) and the posterior uterine cervix (C), in the sagittal plane

Video 7.1 (**a**) Transvaginal ultrasound is used to demonstrate a positive "sliding sign" between the anterior rectum and posterior uterine cervix/retro-cervix (C) in the sagittal plane. *POD* pouch of Douglas. (**b**) Transvaginal ultrasound is used to demonstrate a positive "sliding sign" between the rectosigmoid bowel and posterior uterine fundus (U) in the sagittal plane

Video 7.2 (**a**) Transvaginal ultrasound is used to demonstrate a negative "sliding sign" between the anterior rectum (R) and posterior uterine cervix/retro-cervix (C) in the sagittal plane. (**b**) Transvaginal ultrasound is used to demonstrate a negative "sliding sign" between the rectosigmoid bowel (RS) and posterior uterine fundus (U) in the sagittal plane
Video 7.3 (**a**, **b**) Transvaginal ultrasound is used to demonstrate a positive "sliding sign" for a retroverted uterus, at both the posterior uterine fundus and anterior lower uterine segment, respectively (sagittal plane). In Video (**a**), the anterior rectum glides freely over the posterior uterine fundus. In Video (**b**), the rectosigmoid bowel glides freely over the anterior lower uterine segment. *U* uterus
Video 8.1 Normal anterior pelvic compartment. Note the sliding of the bladder and uterus. The bladder wall has normal shape and morphology
Video 8.2 Normal posterior pelvic compartment. Note the sliding of the rectum and uterus. The vaginal wall, uterosacral ligaments, and anterior rectal wall appear normal and the sliding sign is positive
Video 8.3 Transvaginal sagittal scan of the bladder showing a ureteral jet
Video 10.1 Tenderness-guided evaluation of a forniceal nodule
Video 10.2 Tenderness-guided evaluation of a diabolo-like nodule
Video 10.3 A forniceal nodule evaluated without sonovaginography
Video 10.4 The same nodule evaluated using sonovaginography
Video 13.1 An ultrasonographic evaluation of a scar endometriosis in a 32-year-old woman with a cesarean section 6 years before with uncorrect focalization
Video 13.2 An ultrasonographic evaluation of a scar endometriosis in the same patient of Video 13.1 but with a better focalization
Video 13.3 A color Doppler scan of the same nodule of Videos 13.1 and 13.2
Video 13.4 An ultrasonographic evaluation of two nodules of scar endometriosis in a 39-year-old woman with a previous cesarean section 6 years before
Video 13.5 An ultrasonographic evaluation of two nodules of scar endometriosis in a 39-year-old woman with a previous cesarean section 6 years before
Video 13.6 An ultrasonographic evaluation of Villar's nodule in a 33-year-old woman without previous abdominal surgery
Video 13.7 An ultrasonographic color Doppler evaluation of Villar's nodule in a 33-year-old woman without previous abdominal surgery
Video 13.8 An ultrasonographic evaluation of a rectus abdominis endometriosis in a 30-year-old woman with one previous cesarean section 4 years before
Video 13.9 An ultrasonographic color Doppler evaluation of a rectus abdominis endometriosis in a 30-years-old woman with one previous cesarean section 4 years before

Video 13.10 Sonographic features of right inguinal endometriosis presenting as a cystic mass with internal septa (few color Doppler spots peripherally) and hypoechoic content located in inguinal area

Video 14.1 RWC-TVS shows a mild stenosis (≥50%) of the rectal lumen due to endometriosis. The endometriotic nodule is hypoechoic and has blurred margins. A thinner section ("tail") is noted at one end. During surgery, nodule shaving was performed

Video 14.2 RWC-TVS shows a significant intestinal stenosis (≥50%) of the rectal lumen due to endometriosis. The endometriotic nodule, located on the anterior rectum, causes a thickening of the hypoechoic muscularis propria. The nodule is hypoechoic and has blurred margins. A thinner section ("tail") is noted at one end. The nodule infiltrates the rectal submucosa and mucosa. The patient was treated by segmental resection (Fig. 14.13)

Video 14.3 Sonovaginography with gel. An assistant holds the bottle of gel with its mouth facing downward. The syringe is introduced into the lower part of the inverted bottle. The plunger is held steady in position, and the barrel (outer sleeve) is slowly pushed farther up into the inverted bottle of gel to fill the syringe with 20 mL of gel [6]

Video 17.1 Complete septate uterus, rectovaginal nodule with involvement of vaginal posterior wall, uterosacral ligaments, and anterior rectum wall (diabolo-like nodule)

Video 17.2 Presence of negative sliding sign in the anterior compartment (obliteration of uterovesical region). Also can be observed a uterovesical region nodule of 12 × 10 × 12 mm. In the posterior compartment, it is possible to observe a nodule of 16 × 9 × 12 mm with involvement of left uterosacral ligament insertion

Video 17.3 Presence of fixed ovaries, right atypical endometrioma with solid component without vascularization. Corpus luteum in the left ovary and presence of two anterior rectal wall nodules of 12 × 11 × 8 mm and 13 × 7 × 9 mm, respectively (multifocal lesions). Also, it can be observed another lesion of 14 × 10 × 11 mm in between both rectal lesions. Negative sliding sign in the posterior compartment

Video 17.4 Multifocal compromise of rectosigmoid with anterior rectal wall nodules with complete septate uterus. In addition, you can observe another lesion with compromise of the left uterosacral ligament and posterior vaginal wall

Video 17.5 The measurement of anterior rectal wall nodule was 22 × 9 × 14 mm, without involvement of submucosa. Another lesion of 14 × 9 × 10 mm, fixed to the previous one, involving the uterosacral ligaments was found

Video 17.6 Bladder dome nodule of 10 × 7 × 10 mm. Ureteral intravesical segment nodule (extrinsic compromise) of 18 × 9 × 10 mm

Video 17.7 Bladder base intramural nodule of 19 × 20 × 21 mm, without compromise of intravesical ureters. Also can be observed a right uterosacral ligament nodule of 9 × 6 × 7 mm, fixed to the posterior vaginal wall

Video 17.8 A rectosigmoid anterior rectal wall nodule of 43 × 13 × 14 mm with involvement of vagina and uterosacral ligament. In addition, you can observe another lesion of 16 × 16 × 11 mm

Video 17.9 At seven centimeters from the anal verge, it can be seen a rectosigmoid anterior rectal wall nodule with involvement of vagina and uterosacral ligaments of 42 × 7 × 19 mm. Also you can observe vaginal lesion of 17 × 8 × 12 mm

Video 17.10 Retroverted uterus. A rectosigmoid anterior rectal wall nodule with transmural compromise with involvement of submucosa of 30 × 10 × 22 mm. It can be observed a lesion involving the uterosacral ligaments with superficial vaginal involvement

---

Electronic supplementary material is available in the online version of the related chapter on Springer Link: http://link.springer.com/

Endometriosis: Clinical and Anatomical Considerations

1

Sukhbir S. Singh

1.1 Introduction

Endometriosis is one of the most challenging diseases to diagnose and manage in gynecology today. It is a common condition and has been reported to have an overall prevalence of 5–10% in the general population [1, 2]. In females with pelvic pain and infertility, endometriosis is known to have a higher prevalence of 50% and 25–40%, respectively [3, 4].

Endometriosis is defined as "endometrium-like tissue that is found outside of the uterine cavity." Its underlying etiology remains elusive and likely involves multiple mechanisms rather than one simplistic explanation [5]. Furthermore, the clinical presentation of this complex disease can vary from completely asymptomatic in some to significant pelvic pain in others. Anatomical distortion, inflammation, and impaired endometrial receptivity may lead to infertility in some but not all.

Electronic Supplementary Material The online version of this chapter (https://doi.org/10.1007/978-3-319-71138-6_1) contains supplementary material, which is available to authorized users.

S. S. Singh
University of Ottawa, Ottawa, ON, Canada

Shirley E. Greenberg Women's Health Centre, The Ottawa Hospital, Ottawa, ON, Canada

Ottawa Hospital Research Institute, Ottawa, ON, Canada
e-mail: susingh@toh.ca

One of the key challenges for the individual who presents with symptoms of chronic pelvic pain and/or infertility due to endometriosis is accessing a timely diagnosis and management plan. Delayed diagnosis of endometriosis-associated pelvic pain is a recognized global challenge with an average delay of 7–10 years in reported surveys [6]. As a result, there is a need for guidance and education to help assess and evaluate those with suspected endometriosis-related sequelae.

The diagnosis of endometriosis has traditionally relied on histology from surgical specimens. This "gold standard" approach, when performed by laparoscopy, in experienced surgical settings, offers both diagnostic and therapeutic benefits [7]. Surgical management of endometriosis-associated pelvic pain has shown to improve pain and, in cases of mild to moderate disease, may improve fertility as well. However, endometriosis is recognized as a chronic relapsing condition, which requires a long-term care plan.

Surgical diagnosis and management has its limitations including access to experienced surgeons, inherent risks of surgery itself, and the possibility of missing disease on laparoscopic evaluation. In addition, chronic pelvic pain is seldom due to one condition alone, and while surgery may assist in managing the pathology (endometriosis lesions), it may not address the other comorbid pain conditions or improve

S. Guerriero et al. (eds.), *How to Perform Ultrasonography in Endometriosis*,
https://doi.org/10.1007/978-3-319-71138-6_1

symptoms in those who have developed central sensitization [8].

Because of the identified need for an earlier diagnosis and understanding that surgery has its limitations, there is growing support to provide health-care providers with the tools necessary to help make a clinical diagnosis of endometriosis. When endometriosis is part of the differential diagnosis, a thorough history, physical examination, and targeted imaging are key to guiding management [9, 10]. Proper evaluation allows for earlier targeted interventions including medical, surgical, and/or fertility therapies.

1.2 How We Do It?

1.2.1 History

On history, it is important to assess all aspects of the presenting complaint, related systemic issues, past medical and surgical history, habits, and family history. A review of pain symptoms with a focus on the four "D"s (dysmenorrhea, dyspareunia, dyschezia, and dysuria) is important. If a patient has more than one of these symptoms, there is a greater likelihood of endometriosis [11].

While cyclic (catamenial) symptoms of pain prompt us to consider endometriosis, nonmenstrual pelvic pain (NMPP) should also be evaluated through history. A classic history of pain that began as cyclic in nature earlier in reproductive life may turn into daily pelvic or abdominal pain with catamenial exacerbation. This finding may represent a shift from nociceptive pain (pain due to inflammation and local tissue damage) to centralized pain.

Systemic complaints in women with endometriosis are also commonly described. Gastrointestinal or urinary tract symptoms including bloating, constipation, nausea, or dysuria may be seen in women with endometriosis-associated pain. However, systemic complaints may also require evaluation of comorbid conditions such as irritable or inflammatory bowel disease and painful bladder syndrome [12].

Extrapelvic endometriosis is a less common variation of the disease but often seen in high-volume referral centers. Endometriosis implants and invasive disease may be found throughout the body with corresponding signs and symptoms as noted below:

Site of disease	Potential symptoms
Lung/pleural cavity	Catamenial pneumothorax or hemothorax
Diaphragm (Fig. 1.1a, b)	Catamenial shoulder tip pain
Nerves (i.e., sciatic)	Catamenial or non-menstrual-related nerve irritation (i.e., sciatica)
Past surgical incisions (i.e., Pfannenstiel for cesarean section or laparoscopy site) Video 1.1: Scar Endometriosis	Catamenial swelling, pain localized to incision site
Bowel	Intermittent obstruction, hematochezia

A past surgical history confirming endometriosis is helpful; however the quality of the surgical evaluation, documentation of the findings, and images (if available) should be reviewed. Misclassification of disease in inexperienced hands may mislead clinicians, and as a result, current history and examinations should help guide next steps for evaluation.

Family history is important as endometriosis has a genetic component as shown in twin and family studies [12]. However, assessment for risk for ovarian or breast cancer should also be considered as treatment options may change in high-risk patients.

1.2.2 Key Historical Points

Consider endometriosis in females with:

- Chronic pelvic pain (pain that persists for greater than 3 months)
- Catamenial (cyclic)-related pain symptoms including:
  - Dysmenorrhea
  - Dyspareunia
  - Dysuria
  - Dyschezia

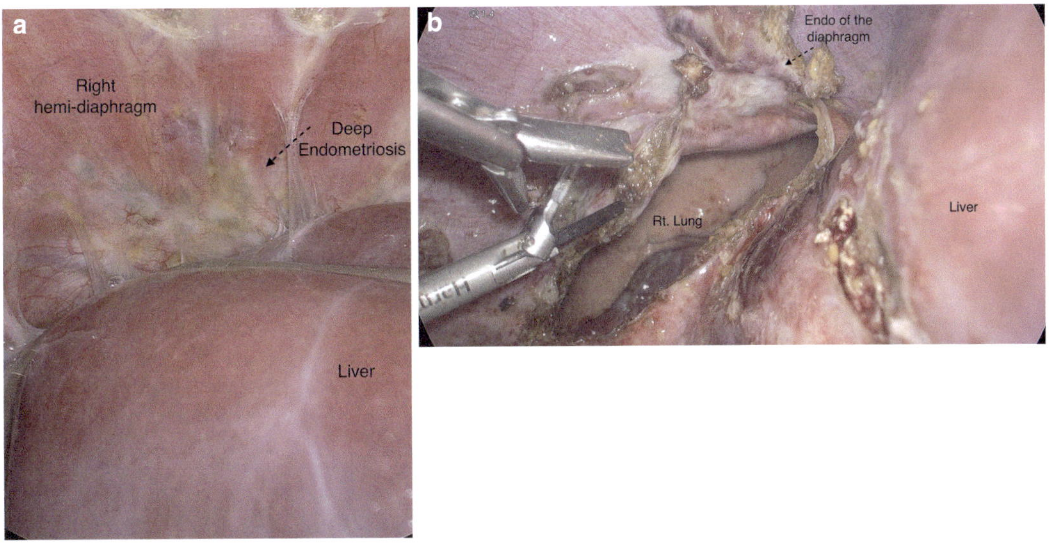

Fig. 1.1 (**a**) Right diaphragm endometriosis lesions causing catamenial right shoulder tip pain for greater than 10 years. (**b**) Post resection of deep endometriosis of the diaphragm. (Courtesy of Dr. S. Singh)

- Infertility and pelvic pain
- Catamenial symptoms in other systems (extrapelvic)

1.3 Examination

An appropriate and targeted abdominal/pelvic examination will help evaluate the patient with suspected endometriosis-related pelvic pain. Many with endometriosis may be asymptomatic, and examination findings may be incidental. Females with infertility may or may not have pelvic pain. Rectal (or pelvi-rectal) examination may be required in cases of suspected rectal pathology or rectovaginal deep endometriosis (DE).

Upon bimanual examination, the clinician should attempt to distinguish the axis of the resting uterus (anteverted, retroverted), palpate for nodularity, and map out regions of pain. Figure 1.2 demonstrates a posterior vaginal fornix nodule palpated and visualized on pelvic examination.

An important consideration is to approach the examination of a patient with "pain" in a stepwise manner that begins with light touch externally and subsequently evaluating each aspect of the patient's experience. Pain that is elicited with light touch only is termed allodynia, and pain with deeper palpation but not in keeping with the expected response is termed hyperalgesia. Allodynia and hyperalgesia are signs of central sensitization or neuropathic pain and should be documented separately.

Further evaluation of the pelvic floor and abdominal wall muscles is also extremely important during the evaluation of the chronic pain patient. Severe pelvic floor tension (hypertonicity) is also a common finding among those who have suffered with long-standing pelvic pain, as a protective adaptive response, and should be documented and discussed. Physiotherapy is often an important adjunct to treatment in these patients.

The importance of identifying allodynia, hyperalgesia, and pelvic floor hypertonicity is key to effective multimodal treatment and also should be documented for and by the imaging expert who will be proceeding with transvaginal ultrasound. Patients with extreme vulvodynia and pelvic floor hypertonicity may not tolerate or may refuse transvaginal examination.

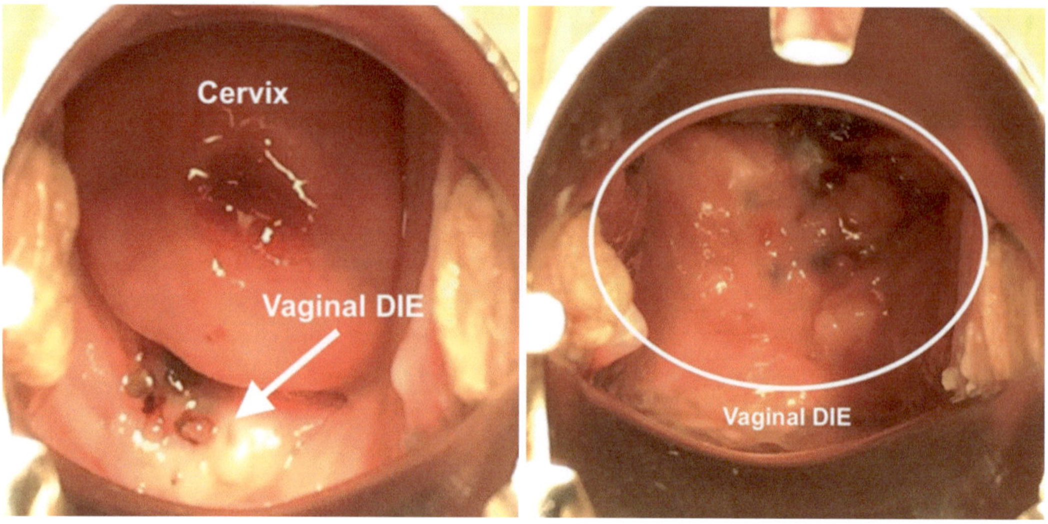

Fig. 1.2 Vaginal nodule (confirmed endometriosis) detected on physical examination. (Courtesy of Drs. S. Singh and H. Stone)

1.3.1 Key Examination Tips

- An abdominal and pelvic exam should assess for sites of pain and identify:
  - Masses
  - Allodynia or hyperalgesia
  - Muscle tone and tenderness (pelvic floor and abdominal wall)
  - Previous scars or injury
  - Nodularity along the vaginal fornices or cul-de-sac
  - Uterine mobility and axis
  - Neurological patterns of pain or sensory deficits
- Pelvi-rectal examination may help identify rectovaginal fullness or nodularity.
- Speculum exam may help identify vaginal lesions of endometriosis.

1.4 Clinical Assessment to Guide Diagnosis, Management, and Triage

The goal of the clinical assessment to help diagnose endometriosis in those with chronic pelvic pain and/or infertility is ultimately to help direct care. Empirical medical management for suspected or clinically diagnosed endometriosis has been widely described in international guidance statements [9, 10]. In individuals with pain, a trial of medical therapies including combined hormonal contraceptives, progestogens, gonadotropin analogues, or intrauterine progestins have all been proposed as potential options. This may help delay or avoid surgery in patients who respond.

Surgery plays an important role in the diagnosis and treatment of endometriosis and has shown to benefit those with pain and infertility. However, the disease has a variable anatomical presentation with three general phenotypes described: superficial, ovarian endometrioma, and deep infiltrating disease (Figs. 1.3a, b, 1.4a, b, and 1.5). The various forms have significant implications for surgical management and require an advanced skill set and interdisciplinary care for deep disease (Video 1.2: Approach to Excision of Endometriosis). As a result, another role for appropriate diagnosis is to help triage patients who would be better served by referral to a center experienced in managing more complex cases of endometriosis.

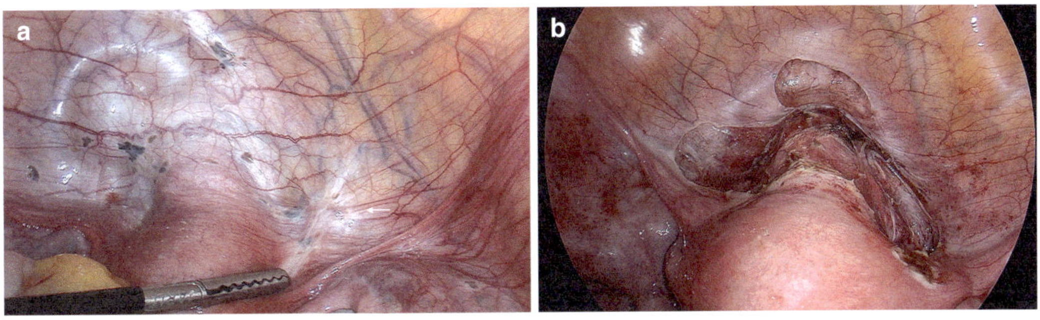

Fig. 1.3 (**a**) An example of superficial endometriosis (black deposits) along the vesicouterine peritoneum. (**b**) Post excision of endometriosis and surrounding peritoneum. (Courtesy of Dr. S. Singh)

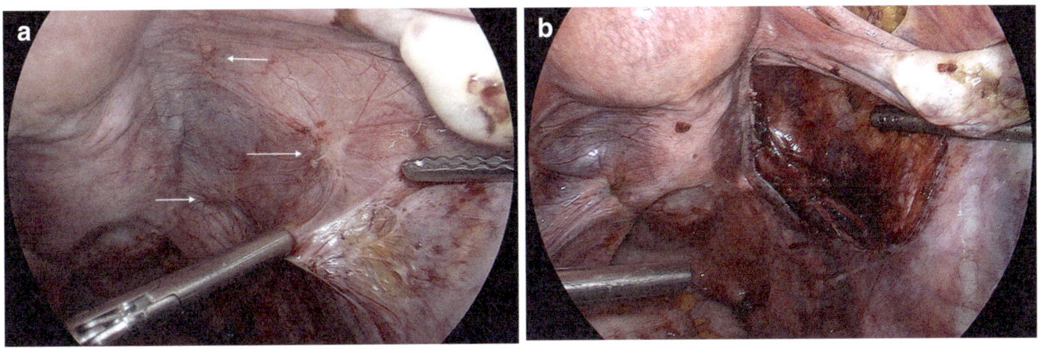

Fig. 1.4 (**a**) Right pelvic sidewall superficial endometriosis deposits (white arrows). (**b**) Post peritoneum excision of superficial disease. (Courtesy of Dr. S. Singh)

Fig. 1.5 Complex pelvis disease: Often there are multiple pathologies in the same patient that require management. In this case the patient had an "obliterated cul-de-sac," fibroids, right ovarian endometrioma, and deep invasion with rectovaginal nodular disease (not seen here). (Courtesy of Dr. S. Singh)

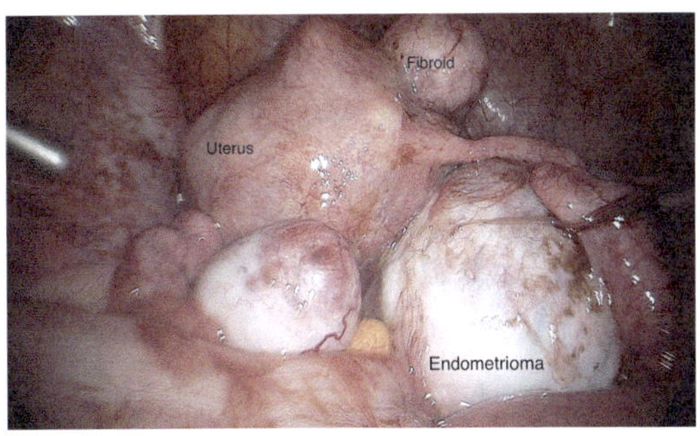

1.5 Role of Clinical Diagnosis

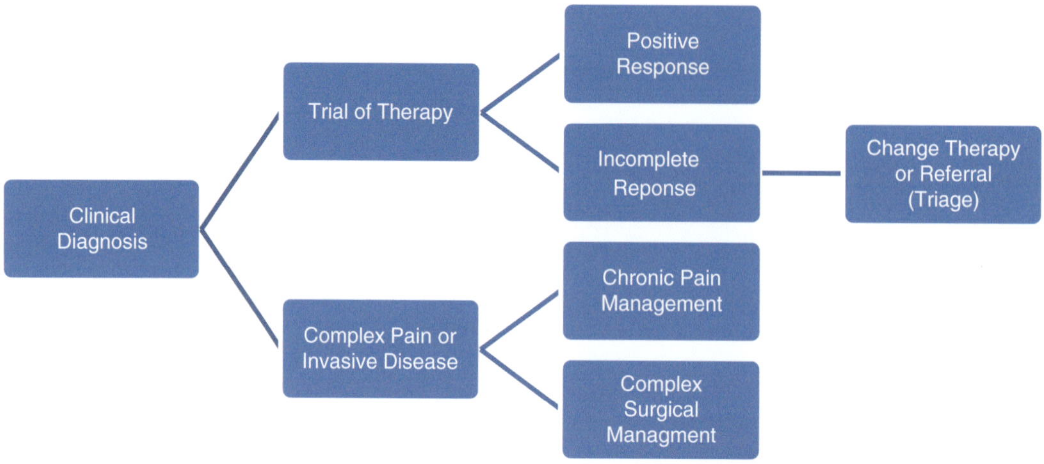

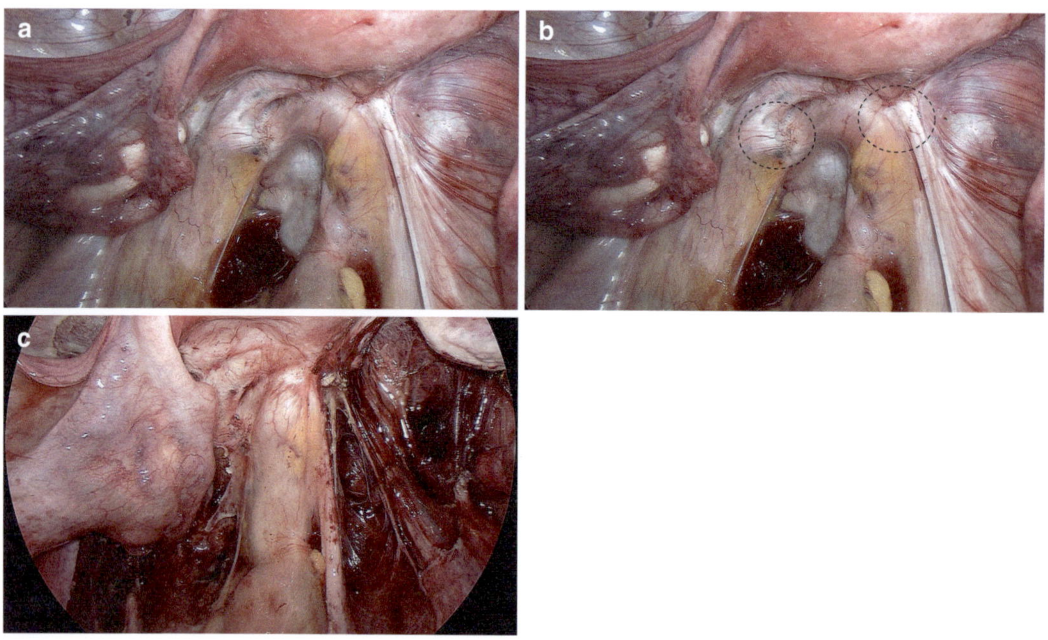

Fig. 1.6 “Hidden disease.” While the cul-de-sac is reported as “open” on traditional imaging (**a**), there is deep invasive disease and anatomical distortion with nodular disease (**b**) identified preoperatively on expert-guided ultrasound. (**c**) Illustrates the level of dissection required (mid-surgery) to help excise the disease. (Courtesy of Dr. S. Singh)

1.6 Imaging in Endometriosis Care

The need for quality imaging for endometriosis care can be demonstrated by the need for a nonsurgical diagnosis of DE. This should be done to help with surgical planning and in certain circumstances to allow for follow-up of response to medical therapies [13].

Traditional imaging that is general or nonspecific may not identify endometriosis [14]. While superficial endometriosis is not identifiable on imaging, ovarian endometriomas and DE often can be visualized. Diagnosis of endometriosis validates the patient experiences and also helps direct therapy (Fig. 1.6a–c).

Reasons for improving imaging for endometriosis care include:

- Identify ovarian and deep endometriosis
- Triage care to appropriate care plan and possibly referral
- Plan for optimal surgical intervention
- Rule out concomitant or alternative conditions

1.7 Anatomical Considerations for Pelvic Endometriosis

The approach to endometriosis evaluation and management should consider the relevant anatomical relationships of the normal pelvic structures that may assist with navigating the distorted pelvic anatomy. The pelvis may be considered in three anatomical compartments to assist with approach to endometriosis involvement: anterior, middle, and posterior compartment.

The anterior compartment includes the bladder and vesicouterine peritoneum. Endometriosis of this area may be present as superficial or deep (Figs. 1.3a and 1.7).

The middle compartment would include the ovaries, fallopian tubes, and uterus itself. Endometriosis of this compartment is the most expected and described forms of the disease including ovarian endometriomas and peritubal adhesions.

The posterior compartment describes the posterior cul-de-sac including the rectum, pararectal spaces, and presacral anatomy. Often, the DE lesions are found here and often involving the rectum (Fig. 1.8).

1.7.1 Pelvic Spaces

From a surgical perspective, there are eight potential *avascular pelvic spaces*. A description of these spaces is provided below:

- *Retropubic/Prevesical Space*
- The retropubic space, also known as the space of Retzius, is a potential space lying immediately posterior to the pubic symphysis, with the urethra and urethrovesical junction forming the floor and the obliterated umbilical arteries forming the lateral boundaries.
- *Paravesical Space*
- The prevesical space is contiguous with the right and left paravesical spaces, with the obliterated umbilical arteries serving as the boundaries. Each paravesical space is bounded laterally by the obturator internus muscle

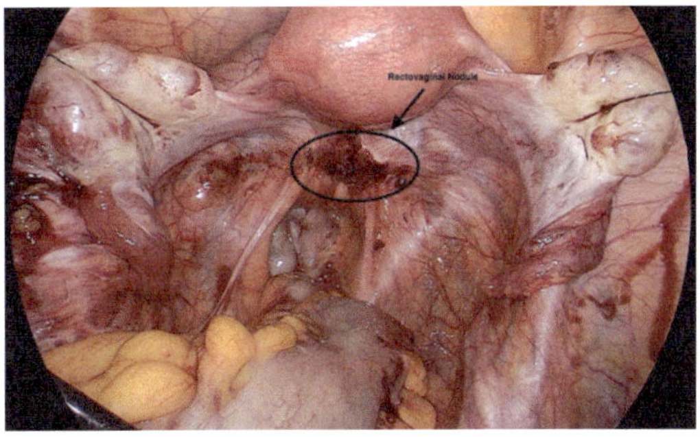

Fig. 1.8 A deep endometriosis nodule obliterates the rectovaginal space. (Courtesy of Drs. S. Singh & H. Stone)

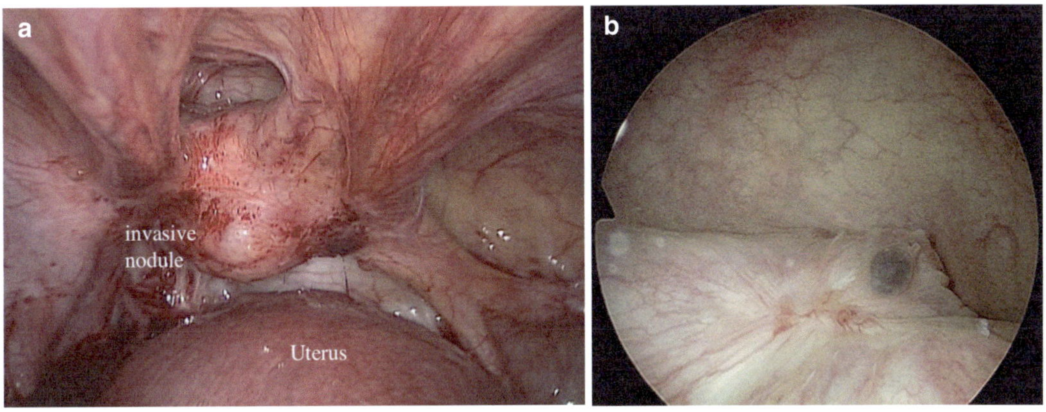

Fig. 1.7 A deep endometriosis nodule invading the bladder at laparoscopy. (**b**) Endometriosis invading the bladder mucosa at cystoscopy. (Courtesy of Dr. S. Singh)

along with the obturator nerve and vessels and posteriorly by the endopelvic fascial sheath that encompasses the internal iliac artery, vein, and its anterior branches.

- *Vesicovaginal Space*
- This is an avascular potential space that exists between the bladder and the vagina.
- *Rectovaginal Space* (Fig. 1.8)
- The rectovaginal space is a potential space between the vagina anteriorly and rectum posteriorly.
- *Pararectal Space* (Fig. 1.9 and Video 1.3)
- The pararectal spaces are also avascular potential spaces located posterior to the crossing of the ureter with the uterine artery. They are bounded by the rectum (medially) and the internal iliac vessels (laterally). Further delineation of a lateral (Latzko's space) and medial (Okabayashi's space) pararectal space divided by the uterosacral ligament has been described to assist with the surgical approach to the rectovaginal nodule [15].
- *Presacral Space/Retrorectal Space*
- While not often accessed during endometriosis surgery, this space may be entered during low anterior segmental bowel resection. The space is an area of areolar connective tissue between the rectum anteriorly, the sacrum and upper coccyx posteriorly, the peritoneal reflection superiorly, the levator ani and coccygeal muscle inferiorly, and the ureter and iliac vessels laterally.

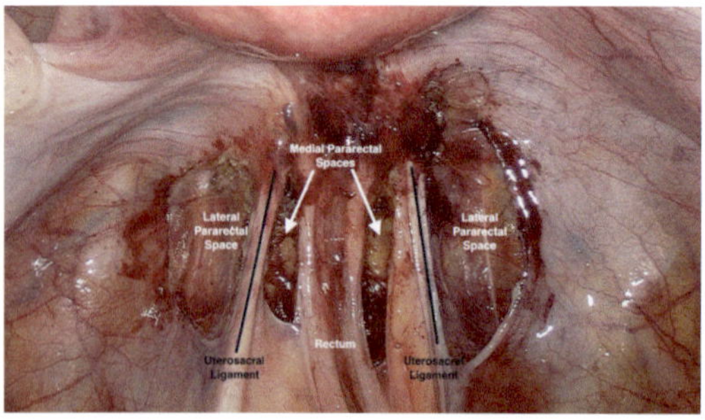

Fig. 1.9 The posterior compartment spaces during dissection for excision of a rectovaginal endometriosis nodule. (Courtesy of Drs. S. Singh & H. Stone)

1.7.2 Relevant Pelvic Sidewall Anatomy

In superficial, ovarian, or deep endometriosis, the disease often involves the pelvic sidewall due to adhesions or infiltrating nodules. As a result, if surgery is required, the sidewall anatomy is an important area to "navigate" to prevent complications and facilitate excision.

The "surgical layers" of the pelvic sidewall caudal to the bifurcation of the common iliac vessels are often taught as follows (Fig. 1.10a, b):

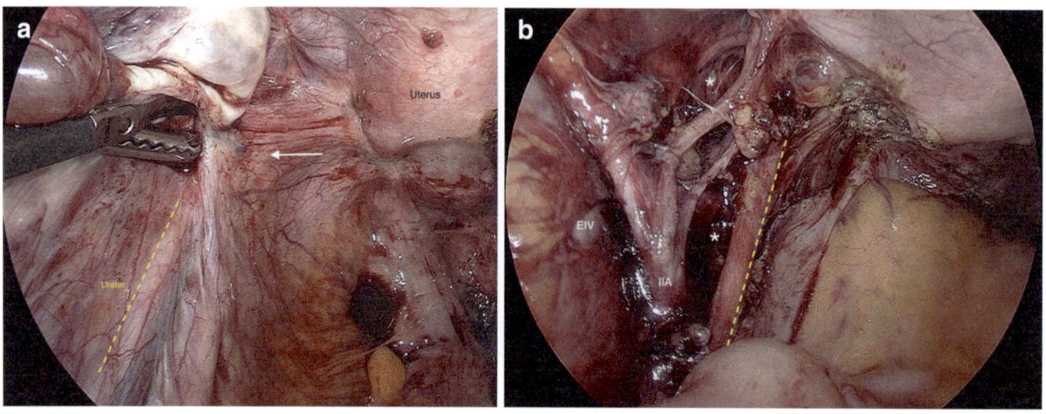

Fig. 1.10 (**a**) Deposit of endometriosis along left pelvic sidewall peritoneum (white arrow) with underlying ureter (yellow line). (**b**) Post excision demonstrating the "surgical" layers of the left sidewall beginning with the ureter (yellow line) with overlying peritoneum excised, avascular spaces (*), and the internal iliac vessels (IIA) and the external iliac vein (EIV). (Courtesy of Dr. S. Singh)

- 1st layer—ureter and overlying peritoneum
- 2nd layer—internal iliac vessels and their branches
- 3rd layer—pelvic sidewall musculature with overlying obturator nerve and external iliac vessels

Between each surgical layer lies a potential avascular space to facilitate dissection.

Disease that involves the sidewall often involves the ureter. Ureteric involvement may be either superficial or in severe cases it can lead to obstruction. Recent reports suggest that over half of patients presenting with DE may have some type of urinary tract endometriosis [16]. As a result, in DE, urinary tract evaluation presurgery should be performed (Figs. 1.11a, b, 1.12, and Video 1.4: Excision of Bladder Endometriosis).

1.7.3 Bowel Endometriosis

Endometriosis may also affect the gastrointestinal tract. Superficial disease may result in adhesions between the bowel and pelvic structures, and ovarian endometriomas may be adherent to the bowel. However, DE of the bowel is estimated to occur in 8–12% of females with endometriosis [17]. These complex patients require experienced care providers and often a multidisciplinary approach [17, 18].

Any part of the bowel may be involved including the appendix and small bowel [19] (Fig. 1.13a–c). However, the large bowel and especially the

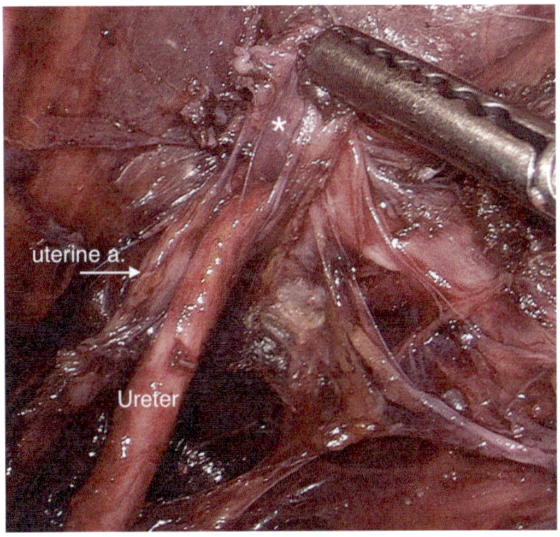

Fig. 1.12 Left ureterolysis required to excise endometriosis plaque (*). (Courtesy of Dr. S. Singh)

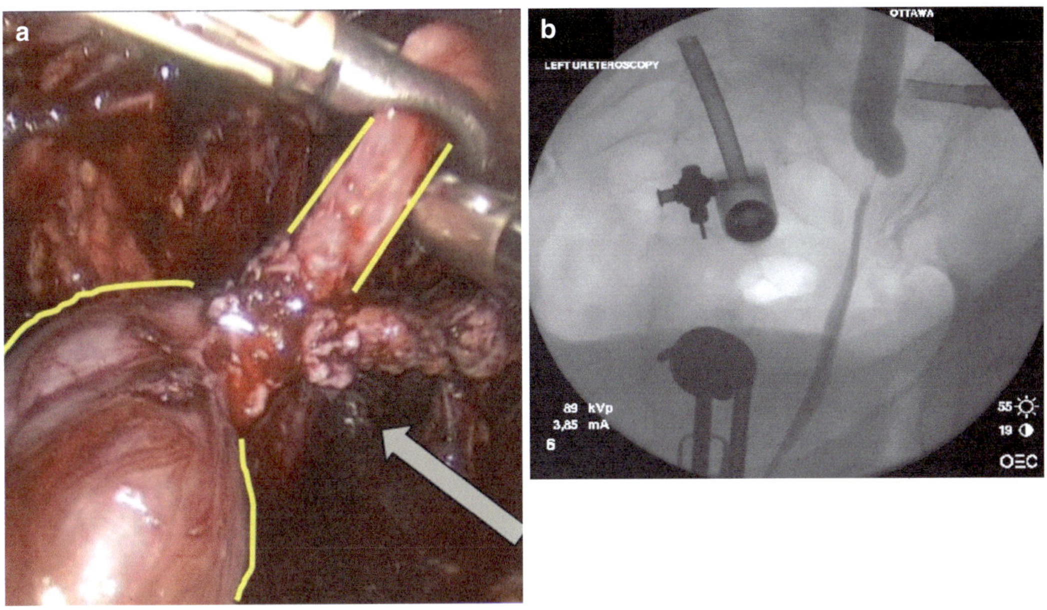

Fig. 1.11 (a) Left ureteric nodule (arrow) that resulted in severe obstruction and left renal dysfunction. (b) Intraoperative fluoroscopy with ureteroscopy confirming external ureteric obstruction. (Courtesy of Dr. S. Singh)

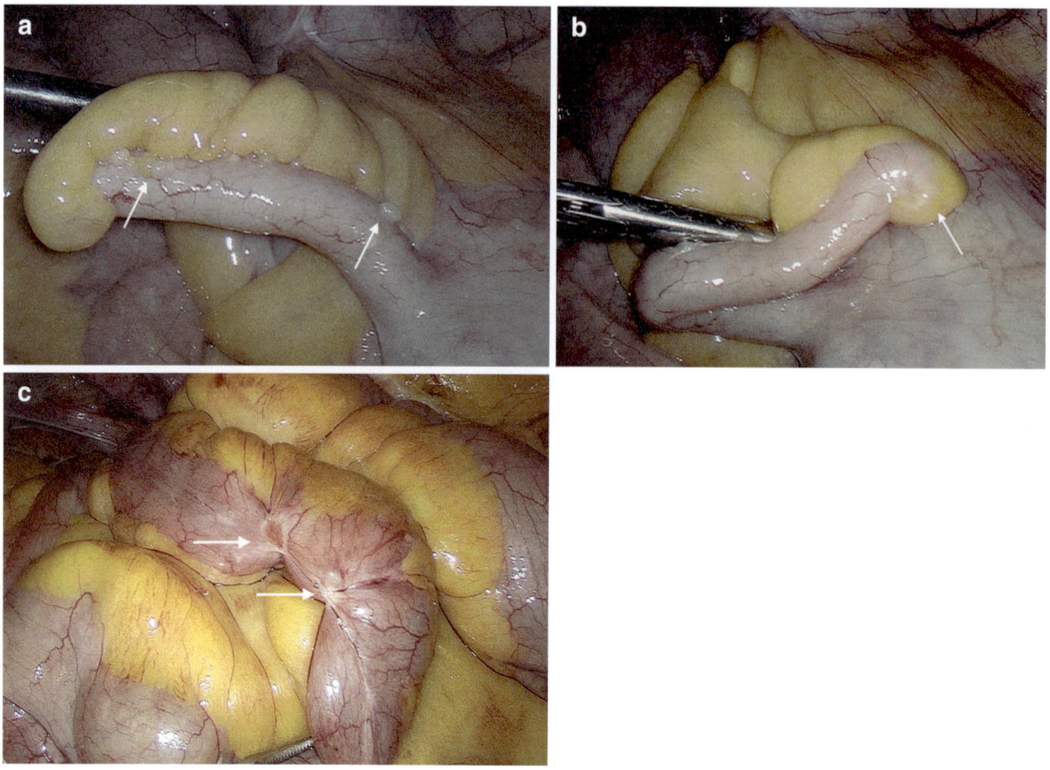

Fig. 1.13 (**a**) Superficial vesicles of endometriosis over the surface (arrow) of the appendix. (**b**) Classic "hockey stick" sign (arrow) at tip of appendix associated with endometriosis invasion. (**c**) Small bowel surface endometriosis deposits (arrows). (Courtesy of Dr. S. Singh)

rectosigmoid colon are most often involved. The disease is seldom isolated, and hence a thorough evaluation is required preoperatively.

One of the key considerations is that colonoscopy may not detect disease of the colon unless it is invading through the mucosa (Fig. 1.14a–c). As a result, imaging is again necessary in the evaluation to enhance appropriate management.

1.8 Summary

Endometriosis is a common and debilitating disease affecting millions of women worldwide. Many of those affected are often struggling with pelvic pain and/or infertility. However, the diagnosis is often delayed likely due to the variable presentation of symptoms and disease states. Thorough clinical evaluation, including focused expert imaging, may help with a timely diagnosis and appropriate referral for treatment in many of these patients.

Acknowledgments Dr. S. Singh would like to acknowledge his local team for making it possible to provide great multidisciplinary care that includes nursing support, expert imaging, and great surgical care. Drs. Margaret Fraser, Shauna Duigenan, and Vincent Della Zazzera provide local expert imaging for complex endometriosis cases. Our fellows Drs. Michael Suen, Cici Zhu, and Maris Yap-Garcia provide surgical and clinical care. Our residents, Drs. Heather Stone and Devon Evans, worked on educational material to help advance our teaching of surgical approaches. Shannen McDonald, Karen Deme, Kelly Lacombe, Monique Newman, and Ottawa Hospital staff help support our patients through their journey. Our surgical team includes Drs. Kristina Arendas, Innie Chen, Karine Lortie, and Hassan Shenassa. Our interdisciplinary team of surgeons includes Drs. S. Gilbert (Thoracics), S. Tadros (General Surgery), and The Ottawa Hospital Urology and Colorectal Services. Finally, our research team including Dr. Teresa Flaxman, Ms. Erica Nichols, Carly Cooke, Suzanah Wojcik, and Cairina Frank help with our endometriosis research program.

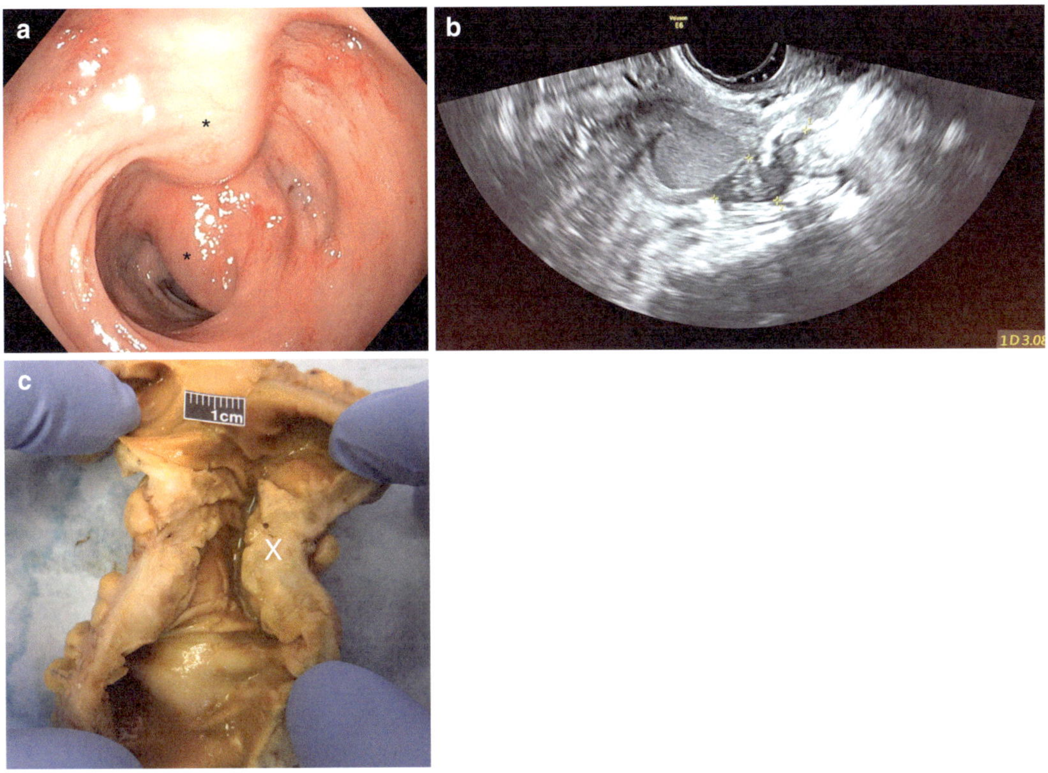

Fig. 1.14 (**a**) Intraoperative colonoscopy is suggestive of a mass effect but not diagnostic of endometriosis (*). (**b**) Transvaginal expert-guided ultrasound completed preoperatively identified a rectal nodule measuring 3 × 1.4cm to aid in surgical planning (Image Courtesy of Dr. V. Della Zazzera, Ottawa Hospital). (**c**) An example of pathology specimen with an invasive intramural nodule (X) of endometriosis from a low anterior resection of the rectosigmoid colon. (Courtesy of Dr. S. Singh)

References

1. Vercellini P, Vigano P, Somigliana E, Fedele L. Endometriosis: pathogenesis and treatment. Nat Rev Endocrinol. 2014;10(5):261–75.
2. Viganò P, Parazzini F, Somigliana E, Vercellini P. Endometriosis: epidemiology and aetiological factors. Best Pract Res Clin Obstet Gynaecol. 2004;18(2):177–200.
3. Giudice LC. Clinical practice. Endometriosis. N Engl J Med. 2010;362(25):2389–98.
4. Somigliana E, Vigano P, Benaglia L, Busnelli A, Berlanda N, Vercellini P. Management of endometriosis in the infertile patient. Semin Reprod Med. 2017;35(1):31–7.
5. Bulun SE. Endometriosis. N Engl J Med. 2009;360(3):268–79.
6. Nnoaham KE, Hummelshoj L, Webster P, d'Hooghe T, de Cicco NF, de Cicco NC, et al. Impact of endometriosis on quality of life and work productivity: a multicenter study across ten countries. Fertil Steril. 2011;96(2):366–73. e8
7. Singh SS, Suen MW. Surgery for endometriosis: beyond medical therapies. Fertil Steril. 2017;107(3):549–54.
8. Aredo JV, Heyrana KJ, Karp BI, Shah JP, Stratton P. Relating chronic pelvic pain and endometriosis to signs of sensitization and myofascial pain and dysfunction. Semin Reprod Med. 2017;35(1):88–97.
9. Kuznetsov L, Dworzynski K, Davies M, Overton C, Committee G. Diagnosis and management of endometriosis: summary of NICE guidance. BMJ. 2017;358:j3935.
10. Dunselman GA, Vermeulen N, Becker C, Calhaz-Jorge C, D'Hooghe T, De Bie B, et al. ESHRE guideline: management of women with endometriosis. Hum Reprod. 2014;29(3):400–12.
11. Sinaii N, Plumb K, Cotton L, Lambert A, Kennedy S, Zondervan K, et al. Differences in characteristics among 1,000 women with endometriosis based on extent of disease. Fertil Steril. 2008;89(3):538–45.
12. Parazzini F, Esposito G, Tozzi L, Noli S, Bianchi S. Epidemiology of endometriosis and its comorbidities. Eur J Obstet Gynecol Reprod Biol. 2017;209:3–7.

13. Guerriero S, Condous G, van den Bosch T, Valentin L, Leone FP, Van Schoubroeck D, et al. Systematic approach to sonographic evaluation of the pelvis in women with suspected endometriosis, including terms, definitions and measurements: a consensus opinion from the International Deep Endometriosis Analysis (IDEA) group. Ultrasound Obstet Gynecol. 2016;48(3):318–32.
14. Fraser MA, Agarwal S, Chen I, Singh SS. Routine vs. expert-guided transvaginal ultrasound in the diagnosis of endometriosis: a retrospective review. Abdom Imaging. 2015;40(3):587–94.
15. Ceccaroni M, Clarizia R, Alboni C, Ruffo G, Bruni F, Roviglione G, et al. Laparoscopic nerve-sparing transperitoneal approach for endometriosis infiltrating the pelvic wall and somatic nerves: anatomical considerations and surgical technique. Surg Radiol Anat. 2010;32(6):601–4.
16. Knabben L, Imboden S, Fellmann B, Nirgianakis K, Kuhn A, Mueller MD. Urinary tract endometriosis in patients with deep infiltrating endometriosis: prevalence, symptoms, management, and proposal for a new clinical classification. Fertil Steril. 2015;103(1):147–52.
17. Abrao MS. Pillars for surgical treatment of bowel endometriosis. J Minim Invasive Gynecol. 2016;23(4):461–2.
18. Abrão MS, Petraglia F, Falcone T, Keckstein J, Osuga Y, Chapron C. Deep endometriosis infiltrating the recto-sigmoid: critical factors to consider before management. Hum Reprod Update. 2015;21(3):329–39.
19. Parr G, Leyland N. The hockey stick sign in appendiceal endometriosis. J Obstet Gynaecol Can. 2010; 32(5):421.

Medical and Surgical Management of Endometriosis

2

Errico Zupi, Lucia Lazzeri, and Caterina Exacoustos

2.1 Introduction

Endometriosis is a chronic, multifactorial disease, affecting predominantly healthy young women with a negative impact on quality of life [1]. It is associated mostly with pelvic pain, dyspareunia, and intestinal disorders and can lead to infertility. Treatment of deep endometriosis (DE) can be either hormonal, aiming at inducing a hypoestrogenic state, atrophy or quiescence of endometriotic lesions, and a reduction of the chronic peritoneal inflammatory status, [2] or surgical, aiming at restoring the normal anatomy by removing endometriotic lesions. In order to plan an appropriate medical or surgical treatment of this condition, imaging (ultrasonography and magnetic resonance imaging (MRI)) is useful for assessing the number, size, and anatomical localization of the endometriotic nodules [3, 4].

Available data suggest that medical treatment and surgical excision are similarly effective in improving pain symptoms associated with DE [5]. Ideally, medications for endometriosis should be curative rather than suppressive. In addition, they should effectively treat pain and have an acceptable side-effect profile. Long-term use should be safe and affordable. Moreover, they should not be contraceptive and not interfere with spontaneous ovulation and normal implantation of the endometrium. Furthermore, they should have no teratogenic potential in case of inadvertent use during the first trimester of a pregnancy. They should suppress the growth of already existing lesions, prevent the development of new ones to limit the need for repeat surgery, and prevent the complications associated with advanced endometriosis. Finally, they should be efficacious for all disease phenotypes, including superficial disease, ovarian endometriomas, DE, extrapelvic disease, and adenomyosis [6].

Currently available medical therapies for endometriosis do not meet all these aforementioned requirements. For the most part, they do not definitively cure the disease but rather are directed at symptomatic relief, typically utilizing the hormone responsiveness of endometriotic tissue to induce lesion atrophy. Pain relapse after treatment suspension is a common event. Even though treatment with pharmacological therapies for endometriosis should be viewed in terms of years, agents that need to be withdrawn after a few months due to poor tolerability or severe metabolic side effects do not greatly benefit women with symptomatic endometriosis.

Laparoscopy still remains the gold standard for the treatment of endometriosis especially in

E. Zupi · C. Exacoustos (✉)
Department of Biomedicine and Prevention Obstetrics and Gynecological Clinic, University of Rome "Tor Vergata", Rome, Italy

L. Lazzeri
Department of Molecular and Developmental Medicine, Obstetrics and Gynecological Clinic, University of Siena, Siena, Italy

S. Guerriero et al. (eds.), *How to Perform Ultrasonography in Endometriosis*,
https://doi.org/10.1007/978-3-319-71138-6_2

very young or premenopausal patients [7]. Laparoscopic management of endometriosis should be individualized, maintaining an approach toward the disease which maximizes surgical cytoreduction while preserving and safeguarding function of pelvic structures [8]. Surgical excision of DE nodules is necessary when they cause bowel stenosis associated with subocclusive symptoms and ureteral stenosis causing hydronephrosis or in cases of symptomatic bladder DE nodules. In addition, surgery is necessary in approximately one in three women in whom hormonal treatments fail [9].

The choice of medical versus surgical treatment of DE must be shared between the physician and the woman, after she has been adequately informed of the risks and benefits associated with both options. Each woman must have a clear understanding that DE lesions are benign and usually not progressive [10], and therefore the choice of treatment should focus on her symptoms and expectations rather than the eradication of the disease. The information about the likelihood of pain relief after surgery or medical therapy should be as detailed as possible, and the rates of both international and institutional surgical complications should be provided. Moreover, the woman's age and the desire for pregnancy are two important variables influencing the therapeutic plan.

In women with endometriosis seeking pregnancy, assisted reproductive technologies should be considered because currently available hormonal treatments are all contraceptive. In case of repeated IVFs, surgery is indicated [11]. The goal of clinical management of endometriosis is to individualize the timing of endometriosis treatment, integrating medical and surgical strategies, to avoid repetitive surgery with the aim of improving quality of life.

2.2 Medical Treatment of Endometriosis

In the last decade, the substantial progress of diagnostic imaging has allowed a reliable noninvasive diagnosis of DE, i.e., without the need for surgical and histological confirmation. This has resulted in a shift of first-line treatment of endometriosis from surgery to medical therapy. Hypoestrogenizing drugs induce atrophy of the ectopic endometrium and possibly allow the control of pain symptoms by reducing the intra- and peri-lesional inflammation of endometriotic nodules. This diminishes the production of prostaglandins and cytokines and thus results in less stimulation of pain fibers. However, since the discontinuation of hormonal medications for endometriosis is associated with the recovery of endometrial function under the influence of ovarian steroids and thus with the recurrence of pain symptoms, such medications need to be administered for long periods [12]. Therefore, provided that the efficacy in the control of pain is comparable between all the available hormonal compounds [13, 14], the choice of treatment is primarily based on safety in the long term, side effects, and costs. Based upon such principles, progestins and estroprogestins in the form of oral contraceptives (OC) represent the first-line choice for the medical treatment of endometriosis [14–19]. In cases of endometrioma associated with pain symptoms, medical therapy should be preferred to surgery when reassuring ultrasound features are present. Surgery should be considered only when medical treatment fails in controlling pain symptoms, when the endometriotic cyst undergoes a rapid growth, or if ultrasound features become less reassuring.

2.2.1 Oral Contraceptives

OC and progestins are considered as first-line medical treatment for endometriosis-associated chronic pelvic pain [20, 21]. OC inhibit the production of gonadal estrogen via a negative feedback mechanism. Moreover, by suppressing ovarian activity, they also lead to a reduction in estrogen-induced production of prostaglandins, decreasing the inflammation associated with endometriosis. The uninterrupted use of the oral contraceptive pill appears to be associated with a greater pain score reduction [22]. Furthermore, the continuous administration represents a valid, safe, and economical therapeutic coverage that might be used in patients who have undergone conservative surgery for endometriosis [23, 24]. Moreover, different studies have demonstrated that women with rectovaginal endometriosis-associated pain benefit from treatment with non-oral contraceptives such as the contraceptive vaginal ring and the contraceptive patch [25].

2.2.2 Progestins

Progestins have been used in the treatment of endometriosis for over 30 years. Thanks to central and peripheral mechanisms, the mitogenic action and estrogen-induced proliferation are lacking. Furthermore, the endometrium, firstly, undergoes a secretory transformation and then a decidualization, and, finally, it becomes atrophic, thus creating a pseudopregnancy state [26, 27]. A recent Cochrane review has shown that the use of medroxyprogesterone acetate (MPA) at a dose of 100 mg/day is more effective in controlling pain if compared with placebo, but it is burdened by several side effects (menstrual irregularities, amenorrhea, weight gain, and breast tenderness) [28]. Norethindrone acetate (NETA) and dienogest are the progestins that have been more extensively evaluated for the treatment of endometriosis. Both of them are 19-nortestosterone derivative progestins, and the pharmacological differences between the two compounds are limited: NETA has "strongly effective" progestogenic activity and androgenic activity, whereas dienogest has "effective" progestogenic activity and antiandrogenic activity [29, 30]. The only randomized controlled trial available, evaluating the medical treatment of rectovaginal endometriosis, has compared oral NETA 2.5 mg daily with an oral contraceptive pill containing ethinyl estradiol 0.01 mg and cyproterone 3 mg [31]. In the NETA group, women who were free of symptom at 12-month follow-up ranged between 74% for dyspareunia and 92% for dysmenorrhea. Comparable results were observed in the estrogen-progestin combination group. Another study showed that after 12 months of treatment with NETA, 40 women with rectosigmoid endometriosis, who were still symptomatic following non-radical surgery, experienced significant improvements in diarrhea, intestinal cramping, passage of mucus with stool, and cyclic rectal bleeding [32]. In 2014, a 24-week open-label prospective study suggested that treatment with dienogest might improve pain symptoms in women with rectovaginal endometriosis who had pain persistent after 6 months of NETA therapy [33]. A recent study has shown that dienogest is as effective as NETA in improving pain symptoms in women with rectovaginal endometriosis. Because the two molecules are similar and because all hormonal therapies for endometriosis have been proven effective without significant differences among different drugs [13, 14], this outcome was expected. No major adverse side events were recorded. Minor side effects were experienced by 55% of women in the NETA group and 41% of women in the dienogest group, the most frequent being weight gain, vaginal spotting, and decreased libido. Overall tolerability was significantly better in women using dienogest than in those using NETA. However, the overall effectiveness was higher with NETA, owing to limited compliance with dienogest therapy resulting from the high cost of this drug [34].

It has been suggested that the effectiveness of dienogest in the treatment of endometriosis depends on its ability to create a hypoestrogenic and hyperprogestinic endocrine environment, which, initially, causes the decidualization of ectopic endometrial tissue. Subsequently, for prolonged treatments, dienogest causes an atrophy of the lesions. An open-label extension of this study for up to 53 weeks showed that long-term dienogest has a favorable efficacy and safety profile, with progressive decrease in pain and bleeding irregularities [35]. Furthermore, the decrease of pelvic pain persisted for at least 24 weeks after therapy discontinuation. These effects should be due to the multiple mechanisms of action of the drug that reduces the growth and the neoangiogenesis of the lesions and provides an anti-inflammatory activity [35].

In recent years, the use of the levonorgestrel-releasing intrauterine device (LNG-IUD) has aroused interest. Its use in the treatment of endometriosis of the rectovaginal septum provides a significant reduction in dysmenorrhea, pelvic pain and deep dyspareunia, as well as the size of the endometriotic implants, showing levels of efficacy comparable to gonadotropin-releasing hormone (GnRH) analogues [36, 37]. Furthermore, it appears to be effective in preventing the recurrence of endometriosis after surgical treatment [38]. Clinical trials that compared the use of LNG-IUD and depot medroxyprogesterone acetate (DMPA), administered for a period of 3 years, showed better compliance in patients who used the IUD [39]. Moreover, bone gain was observed with LNG-IUD, whereas bone loss was reported with DMPA [39].

Danazol is a synthetic androgen derivative of 17α-ethinyltestosterone, commercially introduced about 30 years ago with a specific indication for the treatment of endometriosis [40]. It carries out a multifactorial biological action inducing a hypoestrogenic-hyperandrogenic state, which is very hostile to the endometriotic tissue growth. Several studies have demonstrated the efficacy of danazol in reducing the pain associated with endometriosis [41]. However, its oral use is limited by significant side effects such as weight gain, muscle cramps, acne, seborrhea, decreased breast size, hirsutism, and deepening of the voice, all strongly related to the androgenic action [42]. The vaginal administration, through a vaginal ring or gel or intrauterine device extended-release, has been tested in patients with DE with encouraging results [43].

2.2.3 Gonadotropin-Releasing Hormone Analogues

GnRH analogues (GnRH-a) suppress estrogen ovarian production through a downregulation of GnRH receptors at pituitary level, causing a profound hypoestrogenism and consequently amenorrhea and a hypoatrophic regression of the heterotopic endometrium. This effect is readily reversible after stopping GnRH-a administration. They are considered as a second-line treatment in case of failure of therapy with oral contraceptives or progestins or when they are not tolerated or contraindicated. GnRH-a provide a reduction of symptoms in about 50% of cases [44], and their administration after surgical treatment prolongs the pain-free interval [45, 46]. The treatment for 3 months with a GnRH-a may reduce the painful symptoms for about 6 months [45]. Among the limitations of their use, there are the high rate of recurrence of pelvic pain (5 years after withdrawal of therapy is at 75%) and the side effects, such as deterioration in the lipid profile, depression, flushes, urogenital atrophy, loss of libido, and bone mass decrease [47]. The latter may be avoided by an "add-back therapy" that involves the use of hormone replacement treatment (HRT) alone or in combination with biphosphonates or other antiresorptive agents [48].

2.2.4 GnRH Antagonist

The use of GnRH antagonists in the treatment of endometriosis has been recently introduced, with optimistic results [49]. They reduce estrogen levels in order to inhibit the pain symptoms but without triggering side effects as a result of estrogen deprivation. Furthermore, in contrast to GnRH-a, they do not determine the initial stimulation of the pituitary-ovarian axis with the resulting gonadotropic peak [50]. A recent phase 2, randomized, double-blind, placebo-controlled study has shown that a new GnRH antagonist (elagolix) has an acceptable efficacy and safety profile [51]. More clinical trials are required before such agents should be introduced into clinical practice.

2.2.5 Nonsteroidal Anti-inflammatory Drugs

Nonsteroidal anti-inflammatory drugs (NSAIDs) are the most commonly used first-line treatment for endometriosis [20, 21]. However, there is inconclusive evidence to show whether or not they are effective in relieving pain associated with endometriosis [52]. Furthermore, there is no evidence on whether any individual NSAID is more effective than another [52]. NSAIDs interfere with the function of the enzymes COX-1 and COX-2, inhibiting the production of prostaglandins, molecules involved in the genesis of endometriosis-associated pain [53]. Specific inhibitors of COX-2, as rofecoxib, have also the property to block the growth of ectopic cells and induce apoptosis, with equivalent result to one achieved with GnRH-a [54]. To date, there are no sufficient clinical data to prove the NSAIDs are as effective in the treatment of endometriosis-associated pain.

2.2.6 Selective Estrogen Receptor Modulators

Selective estrogen receptor modulators (SERMs) interact with estrogen receptors as agonists or antagonists depending on the target tissue [55]. In patients with endometriosis, the rationale for their use is related to the estrogen-antagonistic activity at endometrial level and estrogen-agonistic activity on bone and plasma lipoproteins [55]. Although studies on animals looked very promising [56, 57], currently available data in humans on SERMs do not support their clinical use. In fact, a double-blind prospective study comparing raloxifene with placebo was halted early because the raloxifene group had statistically significantly earlier pain and necessity of a second surgery [58].

2.2.7 Aromatase Inhibitors

An overexpression of the aromatase enzyme, the main responsible factor for estrogen synthesis in the ectopic endometrium, has been demonstrated in endometrial tissue [59]. Aromatase catalyzes the conversion of the steroidal precursors into estrogens, which stimulate the expression of the enzyme COX-2. The estrogens produced in the endometrial tissue through aromatase promote the growth and invasion of endometrial lesion and favor the onset of pain and prostaglandin-mediated inflammation [60]. The third-generation aromatase inhibitors, including letrozole, anastrozole, and exemestane, are triazole derivatives and have a selective, potent, and reversible action [61]. Their side effects are represented mainly by headache, stiffness or joint pains, nausea, diarrhea, and flushing. The long-term use of these drugs favors the onset of bone fractures, osteopenia, and osteoporosis [62]. The combination of conventional therapy and aromatase inhibitors determines the block of the production of estrogens both in ovarian and extraovarian endometriotic foci, reducing the painful symptoms. They have been used in a pilot study evaluating 12 women with rectovaginal endometriosis, who had pelvic pain resistant to conventional treatments: after 6 months of treatment with letrozole (2.5 mg/day), norethisterone acetate (2.5 mg/day), calcium citrate, and vitamin D, there have been a significant reduction in abdominal-pelvic pain and the disappearance of endometriotic lesions at second-look surgery [63]. A subsequent study, from the same group, showed that the association of letrozole with norethisterone acetate provides pelvic pain control more effectively than norethisterone acetate alone [64].

2.2.8 Immunomodulators

Tumor necrosis factor-a (TNF-a), a proinflammatory cytokine able to initiate inflammatory cascades, is increased in the peritoneal fluid and serum of women with endometriosis. It has been implicated in the pathogenesis of endometriosis [65]. Clinically, a small randomized controlled trial of infliximab, another TNF-a blocker, was shown to have no effect on endometriosis-related pain [66]. In a systematic review, the effectiveness and safety of anti-TNF-a treatment in the management of endometriosis in premenopausal women were evaluated. Only 1 trial of 21 patients was included where infliximab (a monoclonal anti-TNF-a antibody) was compared with placebo. The reviewer concluded that there is not enough evidence to support the use of anti-TNF-a drugs in the management of women with endometriosis for the relief of pelvic pain [66].

2.2.9 Antiangiogenic Agents

Neoangiogenesis is essential for the initiation, growth, invasion, and recurrence of endometriosis. A wide variety of antiangiogenic agents have been evaluated in vitro as potential treatments for endometriosis. Different members of the statin family have been shown to be effective in vitro in reducing angiogenesis and endometriotic implant size in mice [67–69], rats [70], and human cells in vitro [71, 72]. Multiple dopaminergic agonists also exhibit antiangiogenic activities. Cabergoline was shown to decrease VEGF and VEGFR-2 protein expression in cabergoline-treated mice [73]. In addition, cabergoline and quinagolide have an equal effect in reducing endometriotic lesions as antiangiogenic agents [74]. Moreover, cabergoline and bromocriptine were comparable to GnRH agonist in reducing endometriotic lesion size in one human study [75].

2.3 Surgical Management of Endometriosis

2.3.1 Ovarian Endometrioma

Since endometriomas often do not respond to medical therapy, surgical excision is generally considered the treatment of choice in large endometriomas, especially when associated symptoms are present [17–19, 76, 77]. Surgery may be indicated in particular when pain persists despite medical treatment or in case of enlarging or suspect endometriotic cysts. The surgical approach to an ovarian endometrioma can be either complete excision of the cyst wall (the so-called stripping technique, by which the plane of cleavage between the cyst wall and the ovarian parenchyma is developed by traction and countertraction with two atraumatic forceps) or fenestration and subsequent ablation or coagulation of the cyst wall. Three randomized controlled trials [78–80] and a Cochrane meta-analysis [81] demonstrated that laparoscopic excision of the ovarian endometrioma yields better results in terms of subsequent pregnancy rates, pain control rates, and cyst recurrence rates, compared with fenestration and coagulation/ablation of the cyst wall.

Due to concerns that recently emerged on the possibility that surgical excision may damage the ovarian reserve [82], alternative surgical techniques, such as the "three-stage" [83, 84] and the "combined" technique [85, 86], have been proposed. The "three-stage" technique consists of a first operative laparoscopy, where fenestration and drainage of the endometrioma are performed; a second stage, consisting of a 3-month GnRH analogue treatment; and a second laparoscopy, representing the third stage, where CO_2 laser ablation of the cyst wall is performed. In a randomized controlled trial comparing the "three-stage" technique to the conventional stripping technique, better results in terms of ovarian reserve, evaluated both with antral follicle count (AFC) [83] and anti-Mullerian hormone (AMH) [84], have been reported with the "three-stage" technique. The small sample size (ten patients per arm), the higher recurrence rate in the "three-stage" arm (20 vs. 0% in the excision arm), and the higher costs of a repeat surgical procedure do not sufficiently support the "three-stage" technique as a validated alternative to the stripping technique.

The "combined technique" has been recently proposed [85, 86] as an alternative to the stripping technique, in the attempt to combine the advantages of the two standard techniques (stripping and fenestration with coagulation/ablation), avoiding the disadvantages of both. The excision technique is in fact associated with better results in terms of subsequent fertility and pain recurrence, whereas the fenestration with coagulation/ablation technique may be more respectful of the ovarian reserve. In the combined technique, stripping is performed for most of the surgical procedure, whereas the coagulation/ablation technique is performed in the final part near the hilus, to decrease the possible damage to the tissue. However, a recent randomized controlled trial [87], comparing the stripping technique with the combined technique in bilateral endometriomas, did not report significant differences between the two techniques in terms of recurrence rates and ovarian reserve (evaluated with AFC). Ovarian endometrioma ablation using plasma energy appears to be a valuable alternative to cystectomy, because it could spare the underlying ovarian parenchyma. Recent studies [88, 89] reported high spontaneous conception rate after this ablation technique and suggest ovarian endometrioma ablation using plasma energy as a valuable alternative to cystectomy in patients presenting with endometriosis and pregnancy intention.

Other alternative techniques have been reported [90–92], but none has been proven superior to the standard excisional technique in randomized controlled trials. Therefore, there is still insufficient evidence to recommend any alternative technique instead of the stripping technique as the procedure of choice for the surgical treatment of endometriomas. Whichever the technique, surgery should be performed by expert operators, since it has been demonstrated that damage to the ovary is inversely correlated with surgeon's experience [93].

2.3.2 Deep Endometriosis

2.3.2.1 Anterior Compartment

Urinary Tract Endometriosis

Endometriosis of the urinary tract is generally reported as affecting approximately 1% of women with endometriosis; however, the incidence varies between centers and has been reported to be as high as 20% [94, 95]. Of these cases, 85% involve the bladder, 10% ureter, 4% kidney, and 2% urethra [96]. Bladder endometriosis is more commonly associated with other lesions of the pelvis.

Bladder Endometriosis

Bladder endometriosis is defined as the presence of endometrial glands infiltrating the detrusor muscle. It is associated with a myriad of nonspecific urinary symptoms such as urinary frequency, dysuria, urgency, and, rarely, hematuria, which can delay diagnosis. Cyclical pain related to menses may confirm a clinical suspicion of endometriosis [94, 97]. The gold standard for diagnosis of bladder endometriosis is direct visualization of lesions at cystoscopy or laparoscopy. Transvaginal ultrasonography (see Chap. 8) and MRI (see Chap. 15) may be useful in diagnosis; however, small lesions may be missed. Laparoscopic management of bladder endometriosis is dependent on the anatomical position and size of the infiltrative lesion. Careful dissection using a skinning technique removing superficial endometriosis of the bladder peritoneum can be performed, followed by closure of the defect with interrupted 3-0 monofilament suture. Infiltrative lesions with involvement of the bladder mucosa situated in the bladder dome can be managed with partial cystectomy. Closure of the bladder with a single- or double-layer monofilament is recommended, and methylene blue test should be performed to ensure integrity of the suture line. In cases of more complex lesions involving the posterior wall of the bladder or the trigone, cystoscopy and insertion of double J stents may be considered. Adhesions between the anterior uterine wall and the vesicouterine fold should be divided prior to performing partial cystectomy. Removal of double J stents should be delayed by 6–8 weeks postoperatively and a urinary catheter left in situ for a minimum of 7 days. In our practice, a urinary catheter is more often left in place for a minimum of 10 days. Low-pressure cystography can also be performed prior to removal of the catheter to verify adequate repair and healing of the bladder.

Ureteral Endometriosis

Ureteric involvement can be categorized into intrinsic or extrinsic and although rare can cause significant morbidity with silent loss of renal function. Extrinsic disease accounts for 85% of cases and causes infiltration of the overlying peritoneum, which can cause compression of the ureter resulting in hydronephrosis and, if left untreated, renal impairment [96, 98]. Intrinsic disease occurs in 15% of cases leading to fibrosis of the muscularis and, in some instances, the mucosa. Ureteric endometriosis is more prevalent on the left-hand side, which may be attributed to the menstrual reflux theory and anatomical differences of the right and left hemi pelvis [99]. The main aim of surgical treatment is to relieve obstruction, if present, while preserving renal function and preventing recurrence. Surgical treatment options include ureterolysis, ureteral resection with end-to-end anastomosis, or ureteroneocystostomy, and in cases of complete loss of kidney function, ureteronephrectomy can be considered [96, 100]. Placement of a double J stent should be considered in cases of urinary obstruction and hydronephrosis or where significant ureteric stenosis has been diagnosed preoperatively. Due to the inflammatory nature of endometriosis, the double J stent should be left in place for approximately 6 weeks. At laparoscopy, the ureter should be identified above the level of disease. This is more easily done at the level of the pelvic brim where the retroperitoneal space can be opened and the course of the ureter followed. In ureteric endometriosis, ureterolysis should be performed with care taken to avoid devascularization by preserving the adventitial layer and corresponding vascular branches. Fibrosis secondary to endometriosis often leads to medial displacement of the ureter, and care should be taken during its dissection. In cases of critical stenosis of the ureter or intrinsic disease, a ureteral resection with end-to-end anastomosis can be performed. Studies have shown promising results with minimal complications and recurrence rates [98, 101, 102]. Ureteroneocystostomy is recommended when a long ureteric segment requires resection or if the disease is near the level of the ureterovesical junction. Reimplantation of the ureter allows the fibrotic area of disease to be bypassed, minimizing the risk of recurrence [96]. A tension-free anastomosis should always be observed, and if more length is required, a psoas hitch can be considered. Due to the rarity of this condition, there is limited evidence regarding treatment of ureteral endometriosis. Most studies involve observational case series; however, the results are promising and in terms of patient morbidity are comparable to those treated by laparotomy. The overall incidence of complications has been reported as 12% with some studies illustrating no long-term consequences and low recurrence rates [103]. Similarly, recurrence rates have been reported ranging from 5 to 15%.

2.3.2.2 Posterior Compartment

DE commonly affects the posterior compartment, with involvement of the uterosacral ligaments most frequently found. Isolated uterosacral lesions occur in up to 83% of cases [104]. Lateral extension of lesions from the uterosacral ligament can result in infiltration of the cardinal ligament and may lead to ureteric involvement by means of extrinsic compression [105]. In 16.8% of cases, uterosacral disease was associated with additional lesions, most commonly of the vagina, followed by intestinal and lastly bladder lesions [104]. Surgical excision of uterosacral endometriosis has been demonstrated to be effective in the management of pelvic pain symptoms with a 0.8% risk of major intraoperative complications [104]. Surgical strategy for the management of isolated uterosacral lesions typically involves ureterolysis, with dissection medial to the ureter so it can be lateralized. During dissection, care should be taken to avoid damage to the hypogastric nerve, which is closely related to the uterosacral ligaments as it attaches to the posterolateral aspect of the uterus [106].

Bowel Endometriosis

Endometriosis involving the bowel occurs in 3–37% of cases, commonly affecting the rectum, rectosigmoid junction, or sigmoid colon in up to 90% of cases [107]. This type of DE is complex with distortion of pelvic anatomy which often requires a multidisciplinary team approach with involvement of colorectal surgeons. Different surgical techniques exist, ranging from less radical excision by means of "shaving" or discoid resection to more aggressive surgical treatment, namely, bowel segmental resection with some studies reporting no relapses [98]. Shaving, or mucosal skinning, involves careful dissection of the endometriotic nodule freeing it from the bowel wall without breaching the bowel lumen. Areas of exposed mucosa are then sutured to maintain integrity and avoid postoperative perforation. This shaving technique has had promising results with low complication rates. Donnez and Squifflet reported a 1.4% rate of rectal perforation in a series of 500 patients and a recurrence rate of approximately 7% [108]. The overall pregnancy rate was 84%, with a natural conception rate of 78% [108]. Similar studies have reported low complication rates and recurrence rates of approximately 19%. This conservative approach allows preservation of nerves and blood supply, minimizing the risk of postoperative functional bowel and bladder complications.

Discoid excision involves removal of disease with full-thickness resection of the anterior rectal wall and subsequent laparoscopic repair in 1–2 layers or by using a transanal circular stapler [109]. An initial shaving of the nodule may be necessary for debulking purposes. A guide suture is then placed at the level of the nodule and a circular stapler is inserted transanally. This technique is suitable for bowel lesions up to 2–3 cm in size. For larger lesions up to 5 cm, a double discoid technique can be used. Two circular stapling lines are formed, the first above the lesion and the second more distal including the initial suture line from the first firing [110]. Anterior discoid resection has been shown as effective in reducing a patient's symptoms with low complication rates ranging from 0 to 12.5% [109, 111, 112].

Radical excision is unavoidable, specifically in cases where the nodule is greater than 3 cm in length and where there is sigmoid involvement, more than 50% circumferential disease or concurrent bowel stenosis, and multicentric disease [113, 114]. Studies have demonstrated that complete excision of bowel lesions, including segmental resection, are associated with significant improvement in pain symptoms and subsequent quality of life [115, 116]. Surgical excision of bowel and rectovaginal endometriosis can be associated with major complications such as bowel perforation and peritonitis. Segmental bowel resection may be indicated where endometriosis is found to be infiltrating both serosal and mucosal layers. In these cases, we advocate segmental bowel resection to be as economic as possible. The bowel is dissected at the edge of the mesentery respecting all the vascular branches. Once the diseased segment has been adequately dissected, the bowel is divided caudal to the lesion using a linear stapler device. An endoscopic linear stapler is used to resect the bowel above the nodule. A minilaparotomy incision can be used to cut the rectum and place the anvil in the proximal bowel; alternatively, a transvaginal or transanal approach can be used [114]. A circular stapler is inserted through the caudal portion of the rectum and an end-to-end anastomosis performed [117]. Despite a significant improvement in pelvic pain following segmental bowel resection for endometriosis, postoperative digestive symptoms may persist or de novo symptoms may develop. A recent systematic review of outcomes associated with different surgical treatments of bowel endometriosis described an overall complication rate of 13.9% [118] This varied from 2.8% in the shaving group to 29.6% in the resection group [118].

2.4 Future Perspectives

Endometriosis is a benign complex clinical condition, associated with chronic pelvic pain, which can adversely affect women's quality of life, sexual satisfaction, and the possibility to conceive. Future improvements in imaging modalities and their interpretation in the context of endometriosis and pelvic nerve involvement may help in defining preoperative assessment and surgical planning. This approach would not only aid the surgeon but also provide more accurate information for the patient with regard to the length, type of surgery, subsequent recovery, and risk of complications. Nowadays, the surgical approach is progressively changing its direction with the most aggressive procedures being replaced by more conservative surgeries. Maintaining a balance between high success rates of treatment, minimal risk of recurrence, and low complication rates drive the need for a more conservative surgical approach. At the same time, significant research has been focused on new drugs specifically designed for the treatment of endometriosis. Although current medical treatments are helpful for many women with endometriosis, these treatments have limitations that include side effects in some women and contraceptive action for those desiring pregnancy. Emerging medical treatments range from GnRH antagonists, aromatase inhibitors, and immunomodulators to antiangiogenic drugs. More research into local neurogenesis, central sensitization, and the genetics of endometriosis may provide future targets. The role of the physician is to guide the woman through all therapeutic possibilities in order to resolve or minimize the impact of the disease while managing her expectations.

References

1. Giudice LC, Kao L. Endometriosis. Lancet. 2004;364:1789–99.
2. Practice Committee of American Society for Reproductive Medicine. Treatment of pelvic pain associated with endometriosis. Fertil Steril. 2008;90:S260–9.
3. Exacoustos C, Malzoni M, Di Giovanni A, Lazzeri L, Tosti C, Petraglia F, Zupi E. Ultrasound mapping system for the surgical management of deep infiltrating endometriosis. Fertil Steril. 2014;102:143–50.
4. Bazot M, Bharwani N, Huchon C, Kinkel K, Cunha TM, Guerra A, Manganaro L, Buñesch L, Kido A, Togashi K, Thomassin-Naggara I, Rockall AG. European society of urogenital radiology (ESUR) guidelines: MR imaging of pelvic endometriosis. Eur Radiol. 2017;27:2765–75.
5. Berlanda N, Somigliana E, Frattaruolo MP, Buggio L, Dridi D, Vercellini P. Surgery versus hormonal therapy for deep endometriosis: is it a choice of the physician? Eur J Obstet Gynecol Reprod Biol. 2017;209:67–71.
6. Bedaiwy MA, Alfaraj S, Yong P, Casper R. New developments in the medical treatment of endometriosis. Fertil Steril. 2017;107:555–65.
7. Ahmad G, O'Flynn H, Duffy JM, Phillips K, Watson A. Laparoscopic entry techniques. Cochrane Database Syst Rev. 2012;2:CD006583.
8. Zupi E, Lazzeri L, Centini G. Deep endometriosis: less is better. J Endometr Pelvic Pain Disord. 2015;7:2.
9. Vercellini P, Somigliana E, Consonni D, Frattaruolo MP, De Giorgi O, Fedele L. Surgical versus medical treatment for endometriosis-associated severe deep dyspareunia: I. Effect on pain during intercourse and patient satisfaction. Hum Reprod. 2012;27:3450–9.
10. Fedele L, Bianchi S, Zanconato G, Raffaelli R, Berlanda N. Is rectovaginal endometriosis a progressive disease? Am J Obstet Gynecol. 2004;191:1539–42.
11. Abrão MS, Petraglia F, Falcone T, Keckstein J, Osuga Y, Chapron C. Deep endometriosis infiltrating the recto-sigmoid: critical factors to consider before management. Hum Reprod Update. 2015;21:329–39.
12. Vercellini P, Crosignani PG, Somigliana E, Berlanda N, Barbara G, Fedele L. Medical treatment for rectovaginal endometriosis: what is the evidence? Hum Reprod. 2009;24:2504–14.
13. Vercellini P, Giudice L, Evers JL, Abrao MS. Reducing low-value care in endometriosis between limited evidence and unresolved issues: a proposal. Hum Reprod. 2015;30:1996–2004.
14. Practice Committee of the American Society for Reproductive Medicine. Treatment of pelvic pain associated with endometriosis: a committee opinion. Fertil Steril. 2014;101:927–35.
15. Vercellini P, Crosignani P, Somigliana E, Vigano` P, Frattaruolo MP, Fedele L. 'Waiting for Godot': a commonsense approach to the medical treatment of endometriosis. Hum Reprod. 2011;26:3–13.
16. Remorgida V, Abbamonte HL, Ragni N, Fulcheri E, Ferrero S. Letrozole and norethisterone acetate in rectovaginal endometriosis. Fertil Steril. 2007;88:724–6.
17. Muzii L, Tucci CD, Feliciantonio MD, Galati G, Verrelli L, Donato VD, Marchetti C, Panici PB. Management of Endometriomas. Semin Reprod Med. 2017;35:25–30.
18. Dunselman GA, Vermeulen N, Becker C, et al; European Society of Human Reproduction and Embryology. ESHRE guideline: management of women with endometriosis. Hum Reprod. 2014;29: 400–12.
19. Leyland N, Casper R, Laberge P, Singh SS, SOGC. Endometriosis: diagnosis and management. J Obstet Gynaecol Can. 2010;32(7 Suppl 2):S1–S32.
20. Menakaya U, Infante F, Condous G. Consensus on current management of endometriosis. Hum Reprod. 2013;28:3162–3.
21. Harada T, Momoeda M, Taketani Y, Hoshiai H, Terakawa N. Low-dose oral contraceptive pill for dysmenorrhea associated with endometriosis: a placebo-controlled, double-blind, randomized trial. Fertil Steril. 2008;90:1583–8.
22. Vercellini P, Eskenazi B, Consonni D, et al. Oral contraceptives and risk of endometriosis: a systematic review and meta-analysis. Hum Reprod Update. 2011;17:159–70.
23. Vercellini P, de Giorgi O, Mosconi P, Stellato G, Vicentini S, Crosignani PG. Cyproterone acetate versus a continuous monophasic oral contraceptive in the treatment of recurrent pelvic pain after conservative surgery for symptomatic endometriosis. Fertil Steril. 2002;77:52–61.
24. Seracchioli R, Mabrouk M, Manuzzi L, et al. Postoperative use of oral contraceptive pills for prevention of anatomical relapse or symptom-recurrence after conservative surgery for endometriosis. Hum Reprod. 2009;24:2729–35.
25. Vercellini P, Barbara G, Somigliana E, et al. Comparison of contraceptive ring and patch for the treatment of symptomatic endometriosis. Fertil Steril. 2010;93:2150.
26. Kauppila A, Vierikko P, Isotalo H. Cytosol estrogen and progestin receptor concentrations and 17β-hydroxysteroid dehydrogenase activities in the endometrium and endometriotic tissue. Effects of hormonal treatment. Acta Obstet Gynecol Scand. 1984;63:45–9.
27. Vierikko P, Kauppila A, Ronnberg L, Vihko R. Steroidal regulation of endometriosis tissue: lack of induction of 17β-hydroxysteroid dehydrogenase activity by progesterone, medroxyprogesterone acetate, or danazol. Fertil Steril. 1985;43:218–24.

28. Brown J, Kives S, Akhtar M. Progestagens and anti-progestagens for pain associated with endometriosis. Cochrane Database Syst Rev. 2012; 3:CD002122.
29. Hapgood JP, Africander D, Louw R, Ray RM, Rohwer JM. Potency of progestogens used in hormonal therapy: toward understanding differential actions. J Steroid Biochem Mol Biol. 2013;142:39–47.
30. Stanczyk FZ, Hapgood JP, Winer S, Mishell DR Jr. Progestogens used in postmenopausal hormone therapy: differences in their pharmacological properties, intracellular actions, and clinical effects. Endocr Rev 2013;34:171–208.
31. Vercellini P, Pietropaolo G, De Giorgi O, Pasin R, Chiodini A, Crosignani PG. Treatment of symptomatic rectovaginal endometriosis with an estrogen-progestogen combination versus low-dose norethindrone acetate. Fertil Steril. 2005;84(5):1375–87.
32. Ferrero S, Camerini G, Ragni N, et al. Norethisterone acetate in the treatment of colorectal endometriosis: a pilot study. Hum Reprod. 2010;25:94.
33. Morotti M, Sozzi F, Remorgida V, Venturini PL, Ferrero S. Dienogest in women with persistent endometriosis-related pelvic pain during norethisterone acetate treatment. Eur J Obstet Gynecol Reprod Biol. 2014;183:188–92.
34. Vercellini P, Bracco B, Mosconi P, Roberto A, Alberico D, Dhouha D, Somigliana E. Norethindrone acetate or dienogest for the treatment of symptomatic endometriosis: a before and after study. Fertil Steril. 2016;105:734–43.
35. Petraglia F, Hornung D, Seitz C, et al. Reduced pelvic pain in women with endometriosis: efficacy of long-term dienogest treatment. Arch Gynecol Obstet. 2012;285:167–73.
36. Fedele L, Bianchi S, Zanconato G, Portuese A, Raffaelli R. Use of a levonorgestrel-releasing intrauterine device in the treatment of rectovaginal endometriosis. Fertil Steril. 2001;75:485–8.
37. Bayoglu Tekin Y, Dilbaz B, Altinbas SK, Dilbaz S. Postoperative medical treatment of chronic pelvic pain related to severe endometriosis: levonorgestrel-releasing intrauterine system versus gonadotropin-releasing hormone analogue. Fertil Steril. 2011;95:492–6.
38. Abou-Setta AM, Houston B, Al-Inany HG, Farquhar C. Levonorgestrel-releasing intrauterine device (LNG-IUD) for symptomatic endometriosis following surgery. Cochrane Database Syst Rev. 2013;1:CD005072.
39. Wong AY, Tang LC, Chin RK. Levonorgestrel-releasing intrauterine system (Mirena) and Depot medroxyprogesterone acetate (Depoprovera) as long-term maintenance therapy for patients with moderate and severe endometriosis: a randomised controlled trial. Aust N Z J Obstet Gynaecol. 2010;20:273–9.
40. Greenblatt RB, Dmowski WP, Mahesh VB, Scholer HF. Clinical studies with an antigonadotropin-Danazol. Fertil Steril. 1971;22:102–12.
41. Crosignani P, Olive D, Bergqvist A, Luciano A. Advances in the management of endometriosis: an update for clinicians. Hum Reprod Update. 2006;12:179–89.
42. Vercellini P, Somigliana E, Viganò P, Abbiati A, Barbara G, Crosignani PG. Endometriosis: current therapies and new pharmacological developments. Drugs. 2009;69:649–75.
43. Igarashi M, Iizuka M, Abe Y, Ibuki Y. Novel vaginal danazol ring therapy for pelvic endometriosis, in particular deeply infiltrating endometriosis. Hum Reprod. 1998;13:1952–6.
44. Shaw RW. GnRH analogues in the treatment of endometriosis-rationale and efficacy. In: Thomas EJ, Rock JA, editors. Modern approaches to endometriosis. London: Kluwer Academic Publishers; 1990. p. 257–74.
45. Hornstein MD, Yuzpe AA, Burry KA, Heinrichs LR, Buttram VL Jr, Orwoll ES. Prospective randomized double-blind trial of 3 versus 6 months of nafarelin therapy for endometriosis associated pelvic pain. Fertil Steril. 1995;63:955–62.
46. Surrey ES, Hornstein MD. Prolonged GnRH agonist and add-back therapy for symptomatic endometriosis: long-term follow-up. Obstet Gynecol. 2002;99:709–19.
47. Prentice A. Regular review: endometriosis. BMJ. 2001;323:93–5.
48. Surrey ES. Gonadotropin-releasing hormone agonist and add-back therapy: what do the data show? Curr Opin Obstet Gynecol. 2010;22:283–8.
49. Küpker W, Felberbaum RE, Krapp M, Schill T, Malik E, Diedrich K. Use of GnRH antagonists in the treatment of endometriosis. Reprod Biomed Online. 2002;5:12–6.
50. Finas D, Hornung D, Diedrich K, Schultze-Mosgau A. Cetrorelix in the treatment of female infertility and endometriosis. Expert Opin Pharmacother. 2006;7:2155–68.
51. Diamond MP, Carr B, Dmowski WP, et al. Elagolix treatment for endometriosis-associated pain: results from a phase 2, randomized, double-blind, placebo-controlled study. Reprod Sci. 2014;21:363–71.
52. Allen C, Hopewell S, Prentice A, Gregory D. Nonsteroidal anti-inflammatory drugs for pain in women with endometriosis. Cochrane Database Syst Rev. 2009;2:CD004753.
53. Hayes EC, Rock JA. COX-2 inhibitors and their role in gynecology. Obstet Gynecol Surv. 2002;57:768–80.
54. Dogan E, Saygili U, Posaci C, et al. Regression of endometrial explants in rats treated with the cyclooxygenase-2 inhibitor rofecoxib. Fertil Steril. 2004;82:1115–20.
55. Buelke-Sam J, Bryant HU, Francis PC. The selective estrogen receptor modulator, raloxifene: an

overview of nonclinical pharmacology and reproductive and developmental testing. Reprod Toxicol. 1998;12:217–21.
56. Swisher DK, Tague RM, Seyler DE. Effect of the selective estrogen receptor modulator raloxifene on explanted uterine growth in rats. Drug Dev Res. 1995;36:43–5.
57. P. Fanning, T. J. Kuehl, R. Lee et al., Video mapping to assess efficacy of an antiestrogen (raloxifene) on spontaneous endometriosis in the rhesus monkey, Macaca mulatta. In TJ Kuehl, editor. Bunkley Day Proceedings. 1996; pp. 51–6.
58. Stratton P, Sinaii N, Segars J, et al. Return of chronic pelvic pain from endometriosis after raloxifene treatment: a randomized controlled trial. Obstet Gynecol. 2008;111:88–96.
59. Meresman GF, Bilotas M, Abello V, Buquet R, Tesone M, Sueldo C. Effects of aromatase inhibitors on proliferation and apoptosis in eutopic endometrial cell cultures from patients with endometriosis. Fertil Steril. 2005;84:459–63.
60. Velasco I, Rueda J, Acién P. Aromatase expression in endometriotic tissues and cell cultures of patients with endometriosis. Mol Hum Reprod. 2006;12:377–81.
61. Pavone ME, Bulun SE. Aromatase inhibitors for the treatment of endometriosis. Fertil Steril. 2012;98:1370–9.
62. Amsterdam LL, Gentry W, Jobanputra S, Wolf M, Rubin SD, Bulun SE. Anastrazole and oral contraceptives: a novel treatment for endometriosis. Fertil Steril. 2005;84:300–4.
63. Remorgida V, Abbamonte HL, Ragni N, Fulcheri E, Ferrero S. Letrozole and norethisterone acetate in rectovaginal endometriosis. Fertil Steril. 2007;88:724–6.
64. Ferrero S, Camerini G, Seracchioli R, Ragni N, Venturini PL, Remorgida V. Letrozole combined with norethisterone acetate compared with norethisterone acetate alone in the treatment of pain symptoms caused by endometriosis. Hum Reprod. 2009;24:3033–41.
65. Lu D, Song H, Shi G. Anti-TNF-α treatment for pelvic pain associated with endometriosis. Cochrane Database Syst Rev. 2013;3:CD008088.
66. Becker CM, Sampson DA, Short SM, Javaherian K, Folkman J, D'Amato RJ. Short synthetic endostatin peptides inhibit endothelial migration in vitro and endometriosis in a mouse model. Fertil Steril. 2006;85:71–7.
67. Jiang HQ, Li YL, Zou J. Effect of recombinant human endostatin on endometriosis in mice. Chin Med J. 2007;120:1241–6.
68. Dabrosin C, Gyorffy S, Margetts P, Ross C, Gauldie J. Therapeutic effect of angiostatin gene transfer in a murine model of endometriosis. Am J Pathol. 2002;161:909–18.
69. Oktem M, Esinler I, Eroglu D, Haberal N, Bayraktar N, Zeyneloglu HB. High- dose atorvastatin causes regression of endometriotic implants: a rat model. Hum Reprod. 2007;22:1474–80.
70. Esfandiari N, Khazaei M, Ai J, Bielecki R, Gotlieb L, Ryan E, et al. Effect of a statin on an in vitro model of endometriosis. Fertil Steril. 2007;87: 257–62.
71. Sharma I, Dhawan V, Mahajan N, Saha SC, Dhaliwal LK. In vitro effects of atorvastatin on lipopolysaccharide-induced gene expression in endometriotic stromal cells. Fertil Steril. 2010;94:1639–46.e1.
72. Novella-Maestre E, Carda C, Ruiz-Sauri A, Garcia-Velasco JA, Simon C, Pellicer A. Identification and quantification of dopamine receptor 2 inhuman eutopic and ectopic endometrium: a novel molecular target for endometriosis therapy. Biol Reprod. 2010;83:866–73.
73. Delgado-Rosas F, Gomez R, Ferrero H, Gaytan F, Garcia-Velasco J, Simon C, et al. The effects of ergot and non-ergot-derived dopamine agonists in an experimental mouse model of endometriosis. Reproduction. 2011;142:745–55.
74. Ercan CM, Kayaalp O, Cengiz M, Keskin U, Yumusak N, Aydogan U, et al. Comparison of efficacy of bromocriptine and cabergoline to GnRH agonist in a rat endometriosis model. Arch Gynecol Obstet. 2015;291:1103–11.
75. Yap C, Furness S, Farquhar C. Pre and post operative medical therapy for endometriosis surgery. Cochrane Database Syst Rev. 2004;(3):CD003678.
76. Kennedy S, Bergqvist A, Chapron C, et al; ESHRE Special Interest Group for Endometriosis and Endometrium Guideline Development Group. ESHRE guideline for the diagnosis and treatment of endometriosis. Hum Reprod. 2005;20:2698–704.
77. Beretta P, Franchi M, Ghezzi F, Busacca M, Zupi E, Bolis P. Randomized clinical trial of two laparoscopic treatments of endometriomas: cystectomy versus drainage and coagulation. Fertil Steril. 1998;70:1176–80.
78. Alborzi S, Momtahan M, Parsanezhad ME, Dehbashi S, Zolghadri J, Alborzi S. A prospective, randomized study comparing laparoscopic ovarian cystectomy versus fenestration and coagulation in patients with endometriomas. Fertil Steril. 2004;82:1633–7.
79. Carmona F, Martínez-Zamora MA, Rabanal A, Martínez-Román S, Balasch J. Ovarian cystectomy versus laser vaporization in the treatment of ovarian endometriomas: a randomized clinical trial with a five-year follow-up. Fertil Steril. 2011;96:251–4.
80. Hart RJ, Hickey M, Maouris P, Buckett W. Excisional surgery versus ablative surgery for ovarian endometriomata. Cochrane Database Syst Rev. 2008;16:CD004992.
81. Raffi F, Metwally M, Amer S. The impact of excision of ovarian endometrioma on ovarian reserve: a systematic review and meta- analysis. J Clin Endocrinol Metab. 2012;97:3146–54.
82. Pados G, Tsolakidis D, Assimakopoulos E, Athanatos D, Tarlatzis B. Sonographic changes after laparoscopic cystectomy compared with three-stage management in patients with ovarian endometrio-

mas: a prospective randomized study. Hum Reprod. 2010;25:672–7.
83. Tsolakidis D, Pados G, Vavilis D, et al. The impact on ovarian reserve after laparoscopic ovarian cystectomy versus three-stage management in patients with endometriomas: a prospective randomized study. Fertil Steril. 2010;94:71–7.
84. Muzii L, Panici PB. Combined technique of excision and ablation for the surgical treatment of ovarian endometriomas: the way for- ward? Reprod Biomed Online. 2010;20(2):300–2.
85. Donnez J, Lousse JC, Jadoul P, Donnez O, Squifflet J. Laparoscopic management of endometriomas using a combined technique of excisional (cystectomy) and ablative surgery. Fertil Steril. 2010;94:28–32.
86. Muzii L, Achilli C, Bergamini V, et al. Comparison between the stripping technique and the combined excisional/ablative technique for the treatment of bilateral ovarian endometriomas: a multicentre RCT. Hum Reprod. 2016;31:339–44.
87. Mircea O, Puscasiu L, Resch B, Lucas J, Collinet P, von Theobald P, Merviel P, Roman H. Fertility outcomes after ablation using plasma energy versus cystectomy in infertile women with ovarian endometrioma: a multicentric comparative study. J Minim Invasive Gynecol. 2016;23:1138–45.
88. Motte I, Roman H, Clavier B, Jumeau F, Chanavaz-Lacheray I, Letailleur M, Darwish B, Rives N. In vitro fertilization outcomes after ablation of endometriomas using plasma energy: a retrospective case-control study. Gynecol Obstet Fertil. 2016;44:541–7.
89. Roman H, Auber M, Mokdad C, et al. Ovarian endometrioma ablation using plasma energy versus cystectomy: a step toward better preservation of the ovarian parenchyma in women wishing to conceive. Fertil Steril. 2011;96:1396–400.
90. Angioli R, Muzii L, Montera R, et al. Feasibility of the use of novel matrix hemostatic sealant (FloSeal) to achieve hemostasis during laparoscopic excision of endometrioma. J Minim Invasive Gynecol. 2009;16:153–6.
91. Ghafarnejad M, Akrami M, Davari-Tanha F, Adabi K, Nekuie S. Vasopressin effect on operation time and frequency of electro- cauterization during laparoscopic stripping of ovarian endometriomas: a randomized controlled clinical trial. J Reprod Infertil. 2014;15:199–204.
92. Muzii L, Marana R, Angioli R, et al. Histologic analysis of specimens from laparoscopic endometrioma excision performed by different surgeons: does the surgeon matter? Fertil Steril. 2011;95:2116–9.
93. Kovoor E, Nassif J, Miranda-Mendoza I, Wattiez A. Endometriosis of bladder: outcomes after laparoscopic surgery. J Minim Invasive Gynecol. 2010;17:600–4.
94. Yohannes P. Ureteral endometriosis. J Urol. 2003;170:20–5.
95. Berlanda N, Vercellini P, Carmignani L, Aimi G, Amicarelli F, Fedele L. Ureteral and vesical endometriosis. Two different clinical entities sharing the same pathogenesis. Obstet Gynecol Surv. 2009;64:830–42.
96. Maccagnano C, Pellucchi F, Rocchini L, et al. Diagnosis and treatment of bladder endometriosis: state of the art. Urol Int. 2012;89:249–58.
97. Schneider A, Touloupidis S, Papatsoris AG, Triantafyllidis A, Kollias A, Schweppe KW. Endometriosis of the urinary tract in women of reproductive age. Int J Urol. 2006;13:902–4.
98. Vercellini P, Pisacreta A, Pesole A, Vicentini S, Stellato G, Crosignani PG. Is ureteral endometriosis an asymmetric disease? BJOG. 2000;107:559–61.
99. Scioscia M, Molon A, Grosso G, Minelli L. Laparoscopic management of ureteral endometriosis. Curr Opin Obstet Gynecol. 2009;21:325–8.
100. Ghezzi F, Cromi A, Bergamini V, Serati M, Sacco A, Mueller MD. Outcome of laparoscopic ureterolysis for ureteral endometriosis. Fertil Steril. 2006;86:418–22.
101. Mereu L, Gagliardi ML, Clarizia R, Mainardi P, Landi S, Minelli L. Laparoscopic management of ureteral endometriosis in case of moderate–severe hydroureteronephrosis. Fertil Steril. 2010;93:46–51.
102. Smith IA, Cooper M. Management of ureteric endometriosis 59 associated with hydronephrosis: an Australian case series of 13 patients. BMC Res Notes. 2010;3:45.
103. Chapron C, Fauconnier A, Vieira M, et al. Anatomical distribution of deeply infiltrating endometriosis: surgical 60 implications and proposition for a classification. Hum Reprod. 2003;18:157–61.
104. Mmm Kondo W, Bourdel N, Tamburro S, et al. Complications after surgery for deeply infiltrating pelvic endometriosis. BJOG. 2011;118:292–8.
105. Azaïs H, Collinet P, Delmas V, Rubod C. Uterosacral ligament and hypogastric nerve anatomical relationship. Application to deep endometriotic nodules surgery. Gynecol Obstet Fertil. 2013;41:179–83.
106. Campagnacci R, Perretta S, Guerrieri M, et al. Laparoscopic colorectal resection for endometriosis. Surg Endosc. 2005;19:662–4.
107. Donnez J, Squifflet J. Complications, pregnancy and recurrence in a prospective series of 500 patients operated on by the shaving technique for deep rectovaginal endometriotic nodules. Hum Reprod. 2010;25:1949–58.
108. Fanfani F, Fagotti A, Gagliardi ML, et al. Discoid or segmental rectosigmoid resection for deep infiltrating endometriosis: a case–control study. Fertil Steril. 2010;94:444–9.
109. Oliveira MA, Crispi CP, Oliveira FM, Junior PS, Raymundo TS, Pereira TD. Double circular stapler technique for bowel resection in rectosigmoid endometriosis. J Minim Invasive Gynecol. 2014;21:136–41.
110. Koh CE, Juszczyk K, Cooper MJ, Solomon MJ. Management of deeply infiltrating endometriosis involving the rectum. Dis Colon Rectum. 2012;55:925–31.

111. Moawad NS, Guido R, Ramanathan R, Mansuria S, Lee T. Comparison of laparoscopic anterior discoid resection and laparoscopic low anterior resection of deep infiltrating rectosigmoid endometriosis. JSLS. 2011;15:331–8.
112. Koninckx PR, Ussia A, Adamyan L, Wattiez A, Donnez J. Deep endometriosis: definition, diagnosis, and treatment. Fertil Steril. 2012;98:564–71.
113. Wattiez A, Puga M, Albornoz J, Faller E. Surgical strategy in endometriosis. Best Pract Res Clin Obstet Gynaecol. 2013;27:381–92.
114. Kavallaris A, Banz C, Chalvatzas N, et al. Laparoscopic nerve-sparing surgery of deep infiltrating endometriosis: description of the technique and patients' outcome. Arch Gynecol Obstet. 2011;284:131–5.
115. Keckstein J, Wiesinger H. Deep endometriosis, including intestinal involvement – the interdisciplinary approach. Minim Invasive Ther Allied Technol. 2005;14:160–6.
116. Leroy J, Costantino F, Cahill RA, et al. Laparoscopic resection with transanal specimen extraction for sigmoid diverticulitis. Br J Surg. 2011;98:1327–34.
117. Moustafa MM, Elnasharty MAA. Systematic review of the outcome associated with different surgical technique of bowel and rectovaginal endometriosis. Gynaecol Surg. 2014;11:37–52.
118. Koninckx P, Craessaerts M, Timmerman D, Cornillie F, Kennedŷ S. Anti- TNF-a treatment for deep endometriosis-associated pain: a randomized placebo-controlled trial. Hum Reprod. 2008;23:2017–23.

Standardized Ultrasonographic Diagnostic Protocol to Diagnose Endometriosis Based on the International Deep Endometriosis Analysis (IDEA) Consensus Statement

3

Mathew Leonardi and George Condous

3.1 Introduction

In April of 1978, Sandler et al. published a series of ten cases entitled "The Spectrum of Ultrasonic Findings in Endometriosis" [1]. The authors made the recommendation that sonographers should consider endometriosis in the differential diagnosis when a pelvic mass was visualized on ultrasound. In the almost 40 years since this publication, the international scientific community has contributed to the literature on the utility of ultrasound in the diagnosis and management of endometriosis. The recent consensus statement on the systematic approach to sonographic evaluation of the pelvis in patients with suspected endometriosis demonstrates broad international collaboration [2]. This landmark paper was published in *Ultrasound in Obstetrics and Gynecology* in 2016 by the International Deep Endometriosis Analysis (IDEA) group, which was comprised of clinicians, gynecological sonologists, advanced laparoscopic surgeons, and radiologists. The 29 members of 15 different countries were invited to participate based on their expertise in the diagnosis and management of endometriosis. The primary goal of this consensus is to standardize terminology, including definitions of anatomy, measurements of sonographic findings, and nomenclature of endometriosis lesions, for uniform use on the international scientific stage. The downstream objective is to encourage homogeneity in terminology to enhance comparison between future studies, promote multicenter studies, and improve patient outcomes.

The purposes of ultrasound in patients with suspected endometriosis are threefold: (1) attempt to explain the patient's symptoms, (2) map the disease location, and (3) assess the severity of disease. The systematic approach to this ultrasound technique involves four basic steps (Table 3.1), which will be outlined in the section, "How We Do It." Each of the four steps will then be expanded upon in greater detail in subsequent chapters.

3.2 How We Do It

Prior to beginning the ultrasound scan, one should explain the nature of procedure to the patient and obtain consent to proceed. A transvaginal ultrasound (TVS) is the recommended imaging modality in the diagnosis of endometriosis [3]. Patients should be instructed to empty their bladder immediately prior to the TVS. They

M. Leonardi (✉) · G. Condous
Acute Gynaecology, Early Pregnancy and Advanced Endosurgery Unit, Sydney Medical School Nepean, Nepean Hospital, University of Sydney, Sydney, NSW, Australia
e-mail: mathew.leonardi@mail.utoronto.ca; george.condous@omnigynaecare.com.au

S. Guerriero et al. (eds.), *How to Perform Ultrasonography in Endometriosis*, https://doi.org/10.1007/978-3-319-71138-6_3

Table 3.1 Four basic sonographic steps, which can be adopted in this or any order as long as all four steps are performed to confirm/exclude the different forms of endometriosis

First step	Routine evaluation of the uterus and adnexa (+ sonographic signs of adenomyosis/presence or absence of endometrioma)
Second step	Evaluation of transvaginal sonographic "soft markers" (i.e., site-specific tenderness and ovarian mobility)
Third step	Assessment of status of POD using real-time ultrasound-based "sliding sign"
Fourth step	Assessment for DE nodules in anterior and posterior compartments

POD pouch of Douglas, *DE* deep endometriosis

should then be positioned and draped appropriately. A wedged cushion or medical couch, with stirrups or lowering bottom section, can be used to ensure adequate mobility with the transvaginal probe. After sanitary protocols have been followed for probe cleaning, ultrasound gel should be placed on the tip of the probe. A probe cover can then be placed overtop, followed by lubricating gel to ease insertion of the probe into the patient's vagina. The scan can then begin. It is recommended to implement a local protocol to ensure all steps are completed, though they may differ in order than that presented here. Most importantly, the operator needs to be experienced in the evaluation of patients with potential deep endometriosis (DE).

3.2.1 First Step

The first structure often identified is the uterus. The orientation (anteverted, retroverted, or axial) should be noted. Any uterine abnormalities should be noted. Specifically with endometriosis in mind, one should inspect carefully for signs of adenomyosis as there is significant correlation between the two processes [4]. These findings should be described using the terms and definitions published in the Morphological Uterus Sonographic Assessment (MUSA) consensus opinion [5]. Though not included in the MUSA group's opinion, the "question mark sign" should be noted when seen as this can represent adenomyosis and/or endometriosis [5, 6]. In the context of endometriosis, this sign generally signifies a fixed (i.e., nonmobile) anteverted/retroflexed uterus with the fundus adhered posteriorly to the rectum and/or sigmoid colon.

Next the adnexa should be evaluated. Ovarian size and characteristics should be documented. The presence or absence of endometriomas should be noted. The following three elements are critical when assessing endometriomas. *First*, the size, measured in three orthogonal planes. To achieve appropriate orthogonal plane measurements, the length is obtained in the midsagittal plane, thickness in the anteroposterior plane, and transverse diameter in the transverse plane. *Second*, the number of endometriomas should be noted. *Third* and lastly, the sonographic characteristics should be described according to terminology published by the International Ovarian Tumor Analysis (IOTA) group [7]. When an endometrioma is visualized, there is significantly higher likelihood of multiple lesions of DE [8]. Though the IDEA consensus statement recommends all four steps in all patients with suspected endometriosis, operators performing the ultrasound should be more vigilant for DE when an endometrioma is diagnosed.

The Fallopian tubes, though not usually visible on ultrasound in a normal state, may be distorted or blocked by adhesions in patients with endometriosis. If a hydrosalpinx or hematosalpinx is seen on ultrasound, endometriosis should be considered as an etiology.

3.2.2 Second Step

The next element of the scan is a dynamic assessment of "soft markers" – site-specific tenderness (SST) and ovarian mobility [2]. "Soft markers" are defined as sonographic features that indirectly suggest the presence of endometriosis, specifically superficial endometriosis and intra-abdominal adhesions, neither of which can be directly visualized [9, 10]. These "soft markers" are elicited using the transvaginal probe [10].

Firstly, before evaluating for SST, it is important to inform the patient that he or she may experience discomfort or pain. Their feedback to the operator performing the scan is essential to this step. The key anatomic locations to assess in this component of the scan include the uterus, adnexa, uterosacral ligaments (USL), and pouch of Douglas (POD). No scoring system has been validated as yet for SST. Currently, the IDEA group recommends a scoring system of 0 or 1: 0 for no pain and 1 for pain. It may be prudent to complete this aspect of the ultrasound at the very end to prevent interruption or termination of the scan secondary to pain.

Secondly, ovarian mobility should be judged by applying pressure to the ovaries using the transvaginal probe. The ovaries may be fixed laterally to the pelvic side wall, medially to the uterus, or inferiorly to the USLs. In some cases, the ovaries may be adhered to each other, known as "kissing" ovaries (Fig. 3.1). Not only does this particular ultrasound sign indirectly indicate intra-abdominal adhesions, but it may also represent underlying DE of the Fallopian tubes and/or bowel [11].

3.2.3 Third Step

The third step is another dynamic, real-time ultrasound technique involving assessment of the status of the POD called the "sliding sign." When the uterus and cervix move independently (i.e., slide) along the anterior rectum and sigmoid, the test is *positive* and the POD is *not* obliterated. When the uterus and cervix move in unison with the anterior rectum and sigmoid, the test is *negative* and the POD is thought to be obliterated [12, 13]. Depending on the orientation of the uterus, the method to test for POD obliteration is slightly different (Table 3.2).

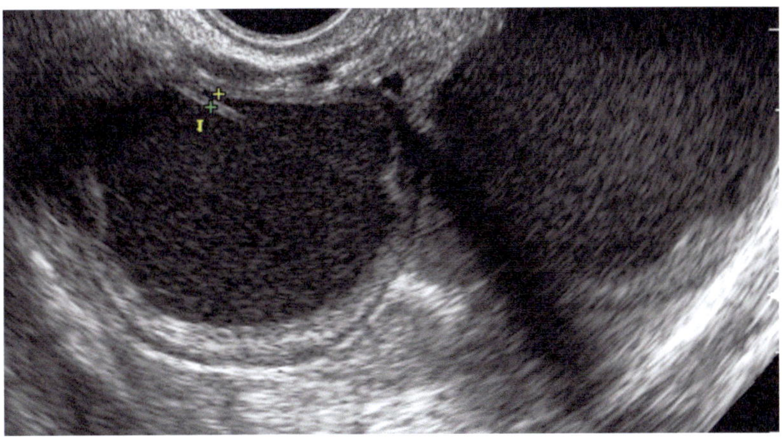

Fig. 3.1 "Kissing" ovaries sign; indirectly indicates intra-abdominal adhesions, and possibly underlying DE of posterior compartment. This ultrasound image depicts a right (Rt) ovarian endometrioma and a left (Lt) ovarian hemorrhagic cyst [2]

Table 3.2 Pouch of Douglas assessment for obliteration using "sliding sign"

	Anteverted	Retroverted
Step 1	Place gentle pressure against the retro-cervix using the transvaginal probe. Observe whether the anterior rectum glides freely across the posterior aspect of the cervix and posterior vaginal wall	Place gentle pressure against the posterior upper uterine fundus with the transvaginal probe. Observe whether the anterior rectum glides freely across the posterior upper uterine fundus
Step 2	Place one hand over lower anterior abdominal wall and ballot the uterus between the palpating hand and the transvaginal probe. Assess whether the anterior bowel glides freely over the posterior aspect of the upper uterine fundus	Place one hand over lower anterior abdominal wall and ballot the uterus between the palpating hand and transvaginal probe. Assess whether the anterior sigmoid glides freely over the anterior lower uterine segment

3.2.4 Fourth Step

The fourth and last step entails searching for DE lesions in the anterior and posterior compartments (Fig. 3.2). The anterior compartment is comprised of the urinary bladder, uterovesical region, and ureters. The posterior compartment sites include USLs, posterior vaginal fornix, rectovaginal septum (RVS), anterior rectum/anterior rectosigmoid junction and sigmoid colon [2, 14].

The IDEA group has recommended that DE lesions located in the bladder, RVS, vagina, USLs, anterior rectum, and rectosigmoid should be measured, like endometriomas, systematically in three orthogonal planes (Fig. 3.3) [2].

3.2.5 Anterior Compartment

Ideally by the time the bladder is scanned, some urine has accumulated. A small amount of urine reduces the frequency of false-negative findings [2]. The anatomical landmarks of the bladder will be discussed in greater detail in Chap. 8. To meet diagnostic criteria for a DE lesion, the muscularis of the bladder wall must be affected. Generally, this is the most common layer impacted by endometriosis. Lesions may appear as hypoechoic linear or spherical lesions, with or without regular contours [15–21]. With respect to the uterovesical region, the most important aspect to understand is whether the posterior bladder is tethered to the uterus (i.e., obliteration of the space). The concept of the "sliding sign" can be applied here as well, but one must interpret the results in the context of the patient's past surgical history, including cesarean sections [22].

The ureters can also be imaged and assessed for damage secondary to endometriosis. First, identify the urethra in the sagittal plane and move the probe toward the lateral pelvic wall. Along this path, and in order, is the intravesical segment of the ureter, the site of ureter exiting bladder, and finally, where it crosses the bifurcation of the common iliac vessels. The examiner should evaluate for ureteric dilatation, and if present, the distance between the dilatation and the distal ureteric orifice should be measured [23–25]. In the event of DE on TVS, a transabdominal scan of the kidney is necessary [2]. The purpose of the ultrasound is to rule out hydroureteronephrosis, which may exist in asymptomatic ureteral stenosis [26, 27].

3.2.6 Posterior Compartment

DE nodules in the posterior compartment should be sonographically localized based on the anatomic landmarks specified in the IDEA consensus statement. Moreover, it is critical to document the size and characteristics of these nodules. Generally, they appear as hypoechoic thickening of the bowel wall or vagina, or as hypoechoic solid nodules with variable sizes and contours [2]. Chapters 9–12 will focus on the various aspects of the posterior compartment in greater detail.

In order to satisfactorily perform a TVS of the posterior compartment with the intention of diagnosing DE, one must understand the anatomy. The IDEA group has developed a schematic to delineate the RVS and the posterior vaginal fornix (Fig. 3.4). Involvement of the RVS should be suspected when a DE nodule is seen on TVS in the rectovaginal space below the line passing along the lower border of the posterior lip of the cervix (under the peritoneum) [20]. Involvement of the posterior vaginal fornix and/or lateral vaginal fornix should be suspected when a DE nodule is seen on TVS in the rectovaginal space below the line passing along the caudal end of the peritoneum of the lower margin of the POD and above the line passing along the lower border of the posterior lip of the cervix (under the peritoneum) (Fig. 3.4). In the same vicinity, a rectovaginal nodule could be identified, extending from the posterior vaginal fornix to the anterior rectum. These appear as hourglass-shaped or "diabolo"-like nodules (Fig. 3.5) [28]. As these lesions lie beneath the peritoneum of the POD, they are not visible on laparoscopy. However, they are usually large at an average of 3 cm [29].

To evaluate for endometriotic lesions of the USLs, place the transvaginal probe in the posterior vaginal fornix in the midline in the sagittal plane and then sweep the probe inferolaterally to

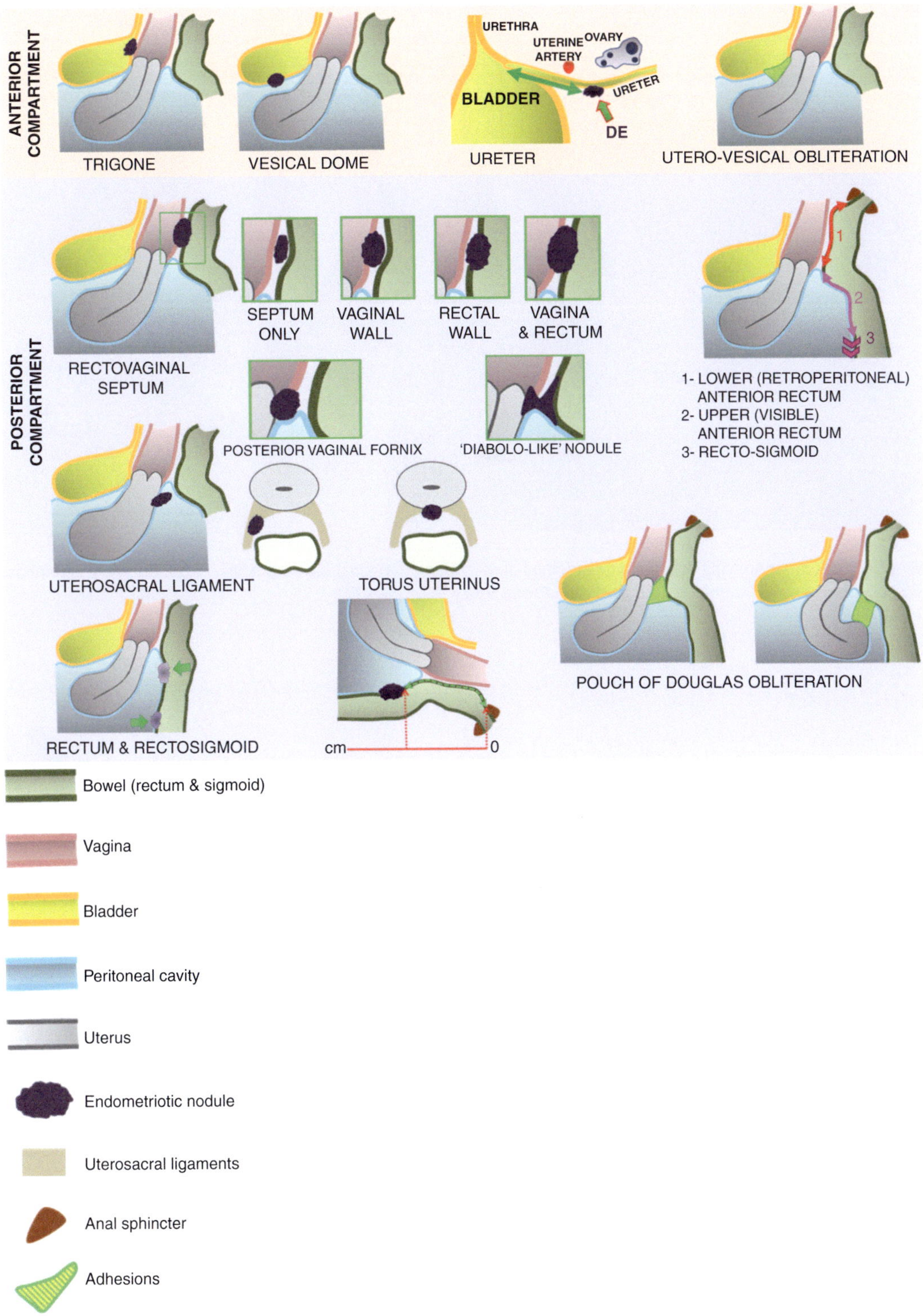

Fig. 3.2 Overview schematic demonstrating various sites of endometriotic nodules and adhesions in the anterior and posterior compartments, with associated legend. Reprinted with permission from Wiley Publishers [2]

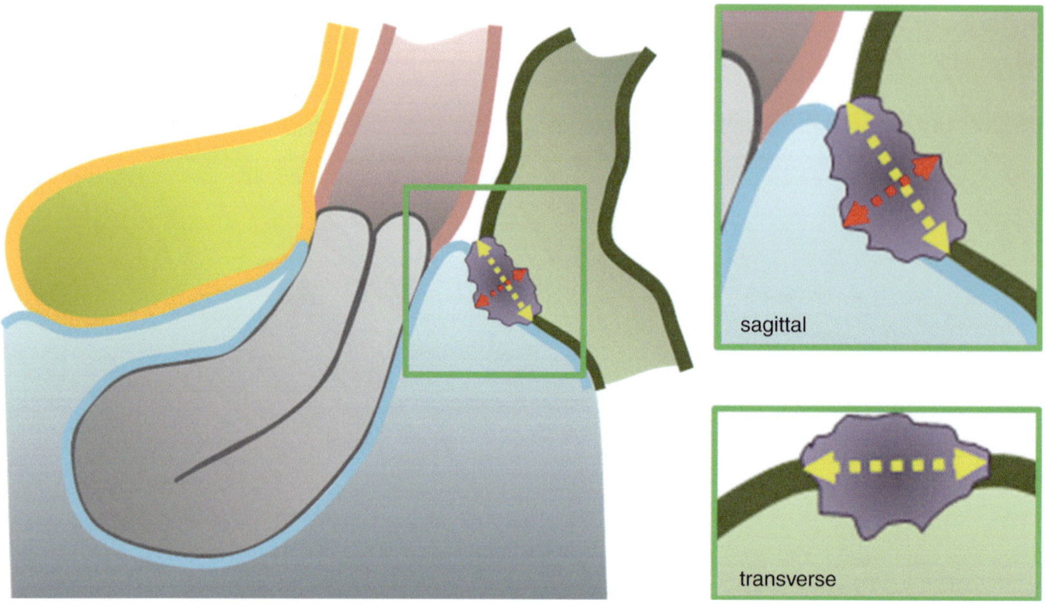

Fig. 3.3 Schematic drawing demonstrating method of obtaining orthogonal measurements, i.e., midsagittal, anteroposterior, and transverse. Reprinted with permission from Wiley Publishers [2]

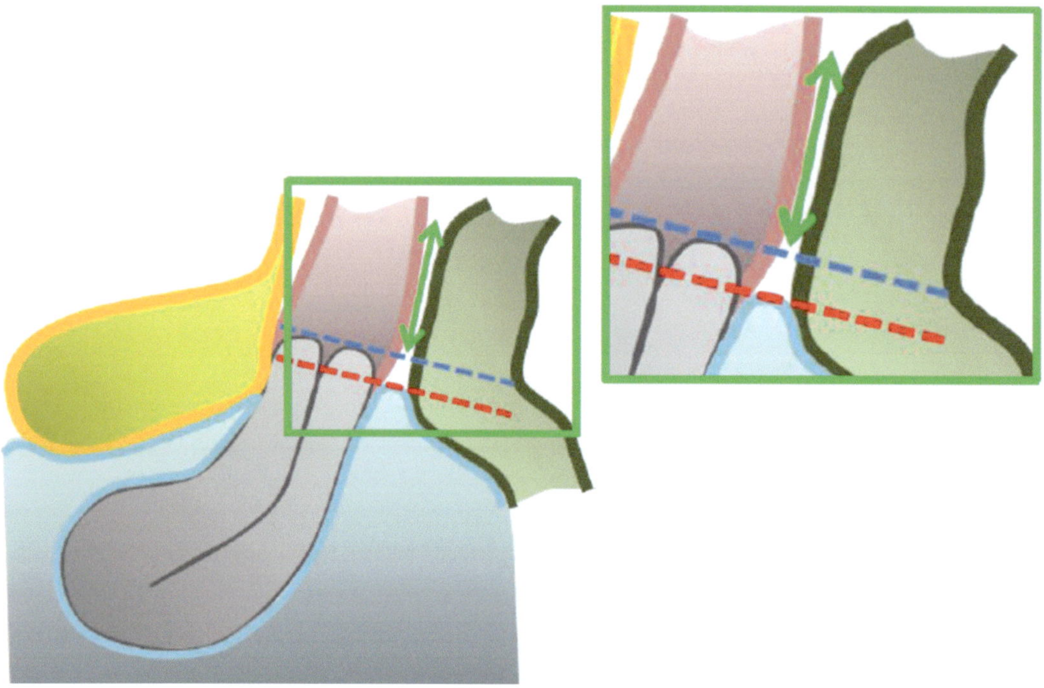

Fig. 3.4 Schematic drawing demonstrating ultrasound definition of the rectovaginal septum (RVS) (double-headed *green arrow*) and the posterior vaginal fornix (space between the *blue line* and the *red line*). Reprinted with permission from Wiley Publishers [2]

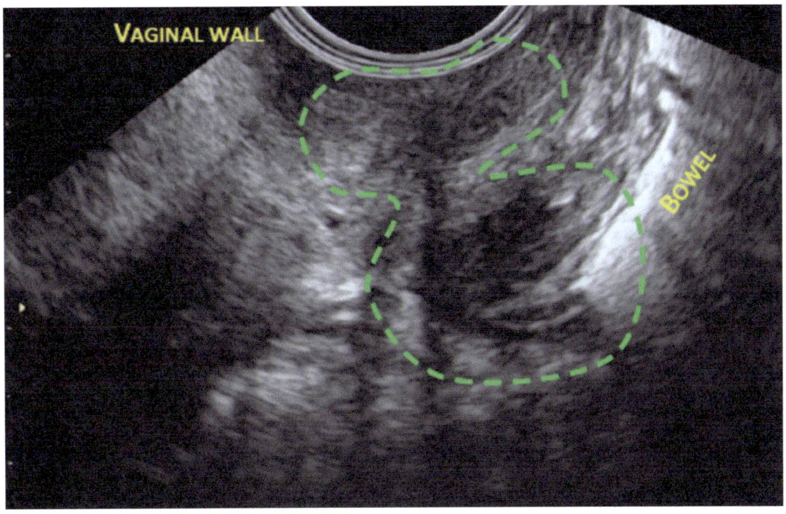

Fig. 3.5 Ultrasound image demonstrating a "diabolo-like" nodule of deep endometriosis from the posterior vaginal fornix extending into the anterior rectum. Reprinted with permission from Wiley Publishers [2]

the cervix [2]. Normal USLs are not usually visualized on TVS. If a hypoechoic thickening is seen within the peritoneal fat surrounding the USLs, it is felt that the USLs are harboring DE. An attempt should be made to identify whether the lesion is part of a larger complex, encompassing other nearby anatomic sites.

Bowel endometriosis generally involves the anterior rectum, rectosigmoid junction, and/or sigmoid colon [14]. The schematic in Fig. 3.6 delineates these areas but also dichotomizes the anterior rectum into lower (retroperitoneal) and upper (visible at laparoscopy). Bowel DE usually appears on TVS as a thickening of the hypoechoic muscularis propria or as hypoechoic nodules, with or without hyperechoic foci (Fig. 3.7). Any nodule recognized in the bowel wall should be recorded in three orthogonal planes, and the distance between the lower margin of the most caudal lesion and the anal verge should be measured using TVS. Lastly, the morphological appearance should be documented based on the types of lesions described in the IDEA consensus opinion [2].

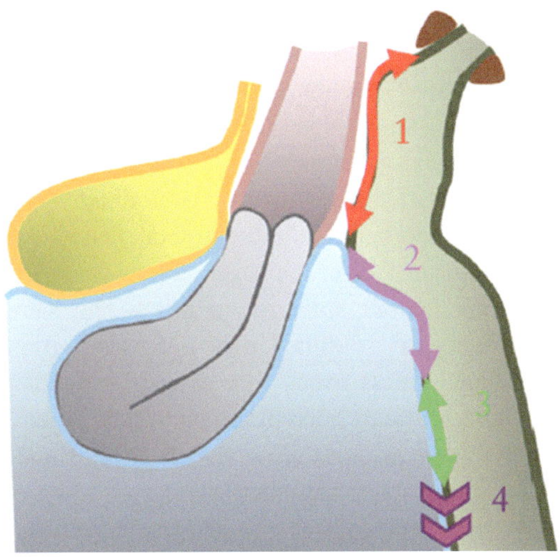

Fig. 3.6 Schematic drawing identifying distinct segments and the rectum and sigmoid colon: lower (or retroperitoneal) anterior rectum (1), upper (visible at laparoscopy) anterior rectum (2), rectosigmoid junction (3), and anterior sigmoid (4). Reprinted with permission from Wiley Publishers [2]

3.3 Important Technical Tips

- Various ultrasound techniques for the diagnosis of endometriosis have been published in the literature [30, 31] prior to the publication of the IDEA consensus statement. No single method has been externally validated. The consensus opinion approach is currently undergoing a multicenter study to externally validate its recommendations.
- The patient should understand the nature of the ultrasound, including the indication, benefits, and risks. They should provide their informed consent. They should be aware that

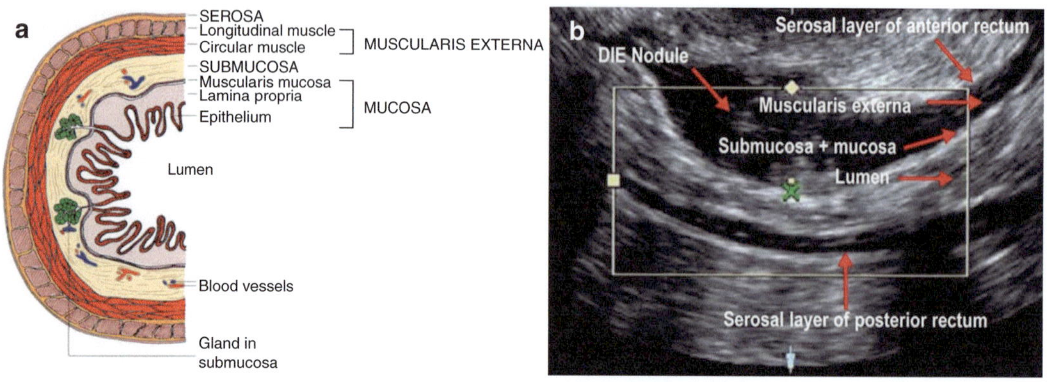

Fig. 3.7 Schematic image showing the histological layers of the rectum (**a**), which can be seen on the adjacent ultrasound image (**b**); a DE nodule can be seen as labeled. Reprinted with permission from Wiley Publishers [34]

this is a dynamic ultrasound involving testing for SST, which may cause discomfort or pain.

- The operator should understand the indications for the ultrasound and ensure appropriate patient selection.
- A strong knowledge of pelvic anatomy and the ultrasound appearance of anatomy is critical to a successful scan, regardless of findings.
- Operators should follow a protocol that encapsulates all four of the steps for all scans. The protocol *does not* have to follow the same order of steps outlined in the IDEA consensus. Thoroughness every time is key, but when more routinely identified abnormalities such as endometriomas are seen, operators should be on high alert for other lesions.
  - It may be advisable to perform aspects that are pain-evoking toward the end of the procedure.
- When DE is visualized, it should be described in detail in a standardized fashion as outlined in the IDEA consensus statement.
  - Ultrasound features
  - Location
  - Size (three orthogonal planes)
  - Proximity to important structures (e.g., anal verge, ureteric orifice)
- When DE is diagnosed on ultrasound, a transabdominal ultrasound of the kidneys should be done to ensure there is no evidence of hydroureteronephrosis.
- Importantly, the absence of DE on ultrasound scan does not mean the patient does not have endometriosis [32].

3.4 Future Perspectives

From a general perspective, there are two natural next steps. Presently, an observational noninterventional academic multicenter study is underway. This study will evaluate the use of the IDEA terminology in different groups of patients in whom pelvic ultrasound is currently routinely performed, e.g., dysmenorrhea, dyspareunia, and/or dyschezia. The IDEA group will evaluate prospectively if the ultrasound appearances of the pelvis in patients with chronic pelvic pain can predict the different phenotypes of endometriosis in patients scheduled for laparoscopic surgery.

Secondly, educational studies are necessary to understand the learning curves to reach competency in the techniques described above. Tammaa et al. have suggested that in gynecologists experienced in ultrasound for general gynecologic problems (defined as having performed approximately 2500 transvaginal scans), roughly 40 endometriosis-focused scans are required to reach competency in the prediction of POD obliteration and DE of the rectum [33]. Lesser experienced operators' learning curve is still to be determined. As an advanced ultrasound approach, operators of diverse backgrounds may require different amounts of time, number of scans, or levels of supervision before they can independently perform this scan. Implementation of this approach as standard of care requires a stronger appreciation of this concept.

We have described the IDEA group's systematic approach, using dynamic ultrasound, to examine the pelvis in patients with suspected endometriosis. The published defined anatomical terms and measurements used to describe the appearances of all endometriosis phenotypes should represent the benchmark standard for endometriosis ultrasound henceforth. This in turn will not only raise the standard of diagnostic ultrasound in this field but also ensure that experienced operators, regardless of country of origin, describe the location and extent of disease in a way which is uniform and easily interpretable.

References

1. Sandler M, Karo J. The spectrum of ultrasonic findings in endometriosis. Radiology. 1978;127(1):229–31.
2. Guerriero S, Condous G, van den Bosch T, Valentin L, Leone FPG, Van Schoubroeck D, et al. Systematic approach to sonographic evaluation of the pelvis in women with suspected endometriosis, including terms, definitions and measurements: a consensus opinion from the International Deep Endometriosis Analysis (IDEA) group. Ultrasound Obstet Gynecol. 2016;48(3):318–32.
3. Piketty M, Chopin N, Dousset B, Millischer-Bellaische AE, Roseau G, Leconte M, et al. Preoperative work-up for patients with deeply infiltrating endometriosis: transvaginal ultrasonography must definitely be the first-line imaging examination. Hum Reprod. 2009;24(3):602–7.
4. Kunz G, Beil D, Huppert P, Noe M, Kissler S, Leyendecker G. Adenomyosis in endometriosis--prevalence and impact on fertility. Evidence from magnetic resonance imaging. Hum Reprod. 2005;20(8):2309–16.
5. Van Den Bosch T, Dueholm M, Leone FPG, Valentin L, Rasmussen CK, Votino A, et al. Terms, definitions and measurements to describe sonographic features of myometrium and uterine masses: a consensus opinion from the Morphological Uterus Sonographic Assessment (MUSA) group. Ultrasound Obstet Gynecol. 2015;46(3):284–98.
6. Di Donato N, Bertoldo V, Montanari G, Zannoni L, Caprara G, Seracchioli R. Question mark form of uterus: a simple sonographic sign associated with the presence of adenomyosis. Ultrasound Obstet Gynecol. 2015;46(1):126–7.
7. Timmerman D, Valentin L, Bourne TH, Collins WP, Verrelst H, Vergote I. Terms, definitions and measurements to describe the sonographic features of adnexal tumors: a consensus opinion from the International Ovarian Tumor Analysis (IOTA) group. Ultrasound Obstet Gynecol. 2000;16(5):500–5.
8. Chapron C, Pietin-Vialle C, Borghese B, Davy C, Foulot H, Chopin N. Associated ovarian endometrioma is a marker for greater severity of deeply infiltrating endometriosis. Fertil Steril. 2009;92(2):453–7.
9. Guerriero S, Ajossa S, Lai MP, Mais V, Paoletti AM, Melis GB. Transvaginal ultrasonography in the diagnosis of pelvic adhesions. Hum Reprod. 1997;12(12):2649–53.
10. Okaro E, Condous G, Khalid A, Timmerman D, Ameye L, Huffel SV, et al. The use of ultrasound-based "soft markers" for the prediction of pelvic pathology in women with chronic pelvic pain - can we reduce the need for laparoscopy? BJOG. 2006;113(3):251–6.
11. Ghezzi F, Raio L, Cromi A, Duwe DG, Beretta P, Buttarelli M, et al. "Kissing ovaries": a sonographic sign of moderate to severe endometriosis. Fertil Steril. 2005;83(1):143–7.
12. Reid S, Lu C, Casikar I, Reid G, Abbott J, Cario G, et al. Prediction of pouch of Douglas obliteration in women with suspected endometriosis using a new real-time dynamic transvaginal ultrasound technique: the sliding sign. Ultrasound Obstet Gynecol. 2013;41(6):685–91.
13. Hudelist G, Fritzer N, Staettner S, Tammaa A, Tinelli A, Sparic R, et al. Uterine sliding sign: a simple sonographic predictor for presence of deep infiltrating endometriosis of the rectum. Ultrasound Obstet Gynecol. 2013;41(6):692–5.
14. Chapron C, Chopin N, Borghese B, Foulot H, Dousset B, Vacher-Lavenu MC, et al. Deeply infiltrating endometriosis: pathogenetic implications of the anatomical distribution. Hum Reprod. 2006;21(7):1839–45.
15. Hudelist G, Ballard K, English J, Wright J, Banerjee S, Mastoroudes H, et al. Transvaginal sonography vs. clinical examination in the preoperative diagnosis of deep infiltrating endometriosis. Ultrasound Obstet Gynecol. 2011;37(4):480–7.
16. Fedele L, Bianchi S, Raffaelli R, Portuese A. Pre-operative assessment of bladder endometriosis. Hum Reprod. 1997;12(11):2519–22.
17. Guerriero S, Ajossa S, Gerada M, Virgilio B, Angioni S, Melis GB. Diagnostic value of transvaginal "tenderness-guided" ultrasonography for the prediction of location of deep endometriosis. Hum Reprod. 2008;23(11):2452–7.
18. Guerriero S, Ajossa S, Gerada M, D'Aquila M, Piras B, Melis GB. "Tenderness-guided" transvaginal ultrasonography: a new method for the detection of deep endometriosis in patients with chronic pelvic pain. Fertil Steril. 2007;88(5):1293–7.
19. Abrao MS, Gonçalves MODC, Dias JA, Podgaec S, Chamie LP, Blasbalg R. Comparison between clinical examination, transvaginal sonography and magnetic resonance imaging for the diagnosis of deep endometriosis. Hum Reprod. 2007;22(12):3092–7.
20. Bazot M, Thomassin I, Hourani R, Cortez A, Darai E. Diagnostic accuracy of transvaginal sonography for deep pelvic endometriosis. Ultrasound Obstet Gynecol. 2004;24(2):180–5.
21. Savelli L, Manuzzi L, Pollastri P, Mabrouk M, Seracchioli R, Venturoli S. Diagnostic accuracy and potential limitations of transvaginal sonography for bladder endometriosis. Ultrasound Obstet Gynecol. 2009;34(5):595–600.
22. Moro F, Mavrelos D, Pateman K, Holland T, Hoo WL, Jurkovic D. Prevalence of pelvic adhesions on

ultrasound examination in women with a history of Cesarean section. Ultrasound Obstet Gynecol. 2015;45(2):223–8.
23. Pateman K, Holland TK, Knez J, Derdelis G, Cutner A, Saridogan E, et al. Should a detailed ultrasound examination of the complete urinary tract be routinely performed in women with suspected pelvic endometriosis? Hum Reprod. 2015;30(12):2802–7.
24. Pateman K, Mavrelos D, Hoo WL, Holland T, Naftalin J, Jurkovic D. Visualization of ureters on standard gynecological transvaginal scan: a feasibility study. Ultrasound Obstet Gynecol. 2013;41(6):696–701.
25. León M, Vaccaro H, Alcázar JL, Martinez J, Gutierrez J, Amor F, et al. Extended transvaginal sonography in deep infiltrating endometriosis: use of bowel preparation and an acoustic window with intravaginal gel: preliminary results. J Ultrasound Med. 2014;33(2):315–21.
26. Carmignani L, Vercellini P, Spinelli M, Fontana E, Frontino G, Fedele L. Pelvic endometriosis and hydroureteronephrosis. Fertil Steril. 2010;93(6):1741–4.
27. Knabben L, Imboden S, Fellmann B, Nirgianakis K, Kuhn A, Mueller MD. Urinary tract endometriosis in patients with deep infiltrating endometriosis: prevalence, symptoms, management, and proposal for a new clinical classification. Fertil Steril. 2015;103(1):147–52.
28. Squifflet J, Feger C, Donnez J. Diagnosis and imaging of adenomyotic disease of the retroperitoneal space. Gynecol Obstet Investig. 2002;54(Suppl 1):43–51.
29. Deura I, Harada T. Surgical management of endometriosis. In: Endometriosis: pathogenesis and treatment. New York: Springer; 2014. p. 385–98.
30. Holland TK, Cutner A, Saridogan E, Mavrelos D, Pateman K, Jurkovic D. Ultrasound mapping of pelvic endometriosis: does the location and number of lesions affect the diagnostic accuracy? A multicentre diagnostic accuracy study. BMC Womens Health. 2013;13(1):43.
31. Menakaya U, Reid S, Infante F, Condous G. Systematic evaluation of women with suspected endometriosis using a 5-domain sonographically based approach. J Ultrasound Med. 2015;34(6):937–47.
32. Nisenblat V, Bossuyt PMM, Farquhar C, Johnson N, Hull ML. Imaging modalities for the non-invasive diagnosis of endometriosis. Cochrane Database Syst Rev. 2016;(2):Art. No.: CD009591. https://doi.org/10.1002/14651858.CD009591.
33. Tammaa A, Fritzer N, Strunk G, Krell A, Salzer H, Hudelist G. Learning curve for the detection of pouch of Douglas obliteration and deep infiltrating endometriosis of the rectum. Hum Reprod. 2014;29(6):1199–204.
34. Reid S, Winder S, Condous G. Sonovaginography: redefining the concept of a "normal pelvis" on transvaginal ultrasound prelaparoscopic intervention for suspected endometriosis. AJUM. 2011; 14(2):21–4.

4 Uterine Evaluation Using a Diagnostic Protocol Based on MUSA

Thierry Van den Bosch

4.1 Introduction

In 2015, the MUSA group published a consensus paper on how to report the myometrium and myometrial lesion at ultrasound examination. Myometrial lesions are mostly benign including fibroids and adenomyosis, while malignant myometrial lesions or sarcomas are rare.

Fibroids are typically well-defined round lesions (Fig. 4.1) with circumferential vascularity. The echogenicity of fibroids varies from hypoechogenic to highly hyperechogenic. In the latter case, this causes strong retrolesional shadowing.

Adenomyosis gives rise to ill-defined lesions of mixed echogenicity, myometrial cysts, fan-shaped shadowing, hyperechogenic islands, and irregular junctional zone with subendometrial lines and buds. At color Doppler imaging, translesional vascularization is seen [1, 2] (Figs. 4.2 and 4.3).

Sarcomas are reportedly large, oval shaped, inhomogeneous, and highly vascularized lesions without calcifications [3–5].

T. Van den Bosch
Department of Obstetrics and Gynecology, University Hospitals KU Leuven, Leuven, Belgium

RZ Tienen, Tienen, Belgium
e-mail: thierry.vandenbosch@uzleuven.be

This chapter gives an overview of how to describe the myometrium based on the MUSA consensus [2].

4.2 How We Do It

The *total length* of the uterus includes the thickness of the fundus, the length of the cavity, and the length of the cervix.

Myometrial walls are reported as *symmetrical* or *asymmetrical*. It is important to realize that transient focal myometrial contractions may give a false impression of asymmetry. Therefore, wall asymmetry should be interpreted with caution. The presence of wall asymmetry should at least be confirmed at the end of the examination or, preferably, during a second scan later in time. Given the possible transient nature of wall asymmetry, the diagnosis of adenomyosis should never be based only on myometrial asymmetry, in the absence of other adenomyosis features.

The overall *echogenicity* of the myometrium is recorded as *homogeneous* or *heterogeneous*. It has to be taken into account that the myometrium echogenicity depends on, e.g., focal depth, uterine flection, the presence of an intrauterine device, transient uterine contractions, or extra-uterine structures such as bladder filling or overlying bowel loops. If the myometrium appears heterogeneous, the reason for this should be search for and reported.

S. Guerriero et al. (eds.), *How to Perform Ultrasonography in Endometriosis*,
https://doi.org/10.1007/978-3-319-71138-6_4

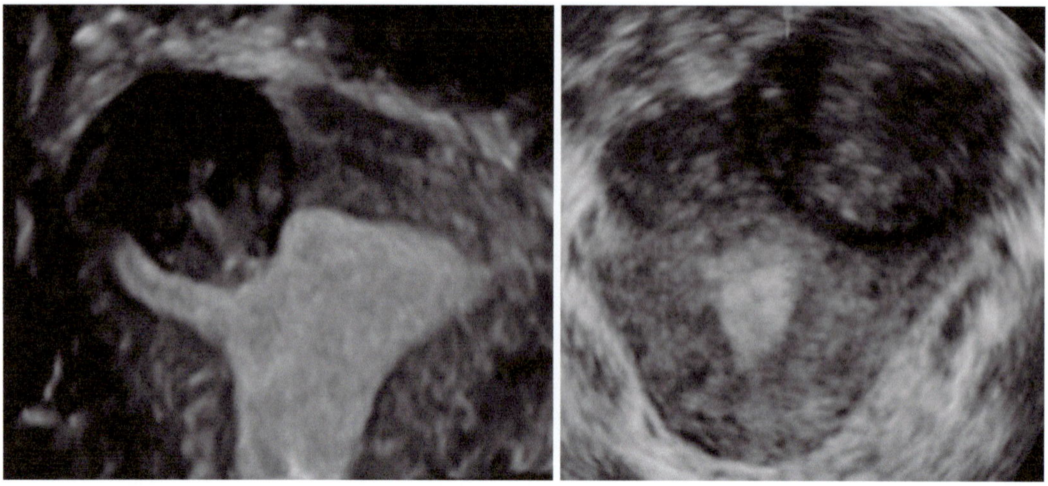

Fig. 4.1 Ultrasound images of fibroids

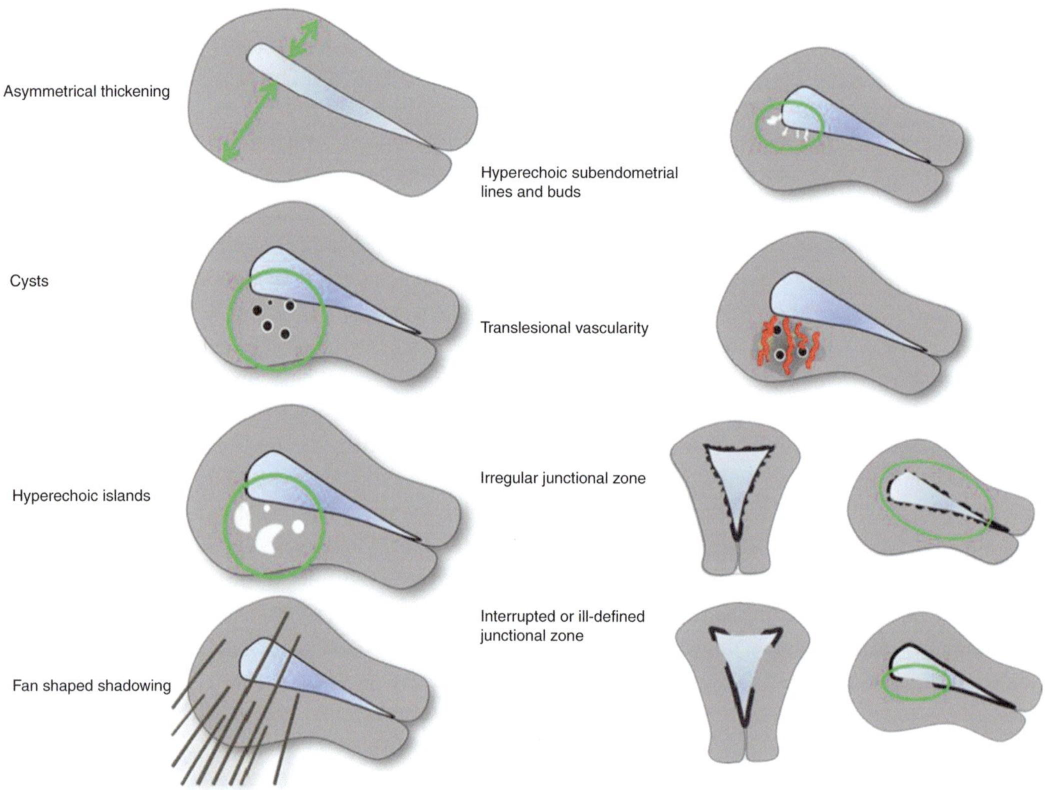

Fig. 4.2 Ultrasound features of adenomyosis (From Van den Bosch et al. [2])

Myometrial lesions may be *well-defined* or *ill-defined*. A fibroid is typically a well-defined lesion, while adenomyosis is often ill-defined.

In clinical practice, an accurate lesion mapping is particularly relevant if surgical removal is planned. The surgeon will plan his/her procedure according to the *number*, the *location*, the *site*, and the *size* of each lesion. However, in a polymyomatous uterus, in which the number, the site, and the size of the lesions preclude myomectomy, the estimation of the total volume of the uterus may be more relevant.

The lesion *location* is reported as anterior, posterior, fundal, right lateral, left lateral, or global. Although lesion location can be defined during 2D scanning, the use of 3D ultrasonography may help illustrating the findings for the surgeon. Tomographic ultrasound imaging (TUI) is especially suited in the reporting to the surgeons who are confident with the interpretation of similar tomographic images from CT scan or MRI. Uterine *fibroids* are further recorded according to the *FIGO classification* 1–7 [6] (Fig. 4.4).

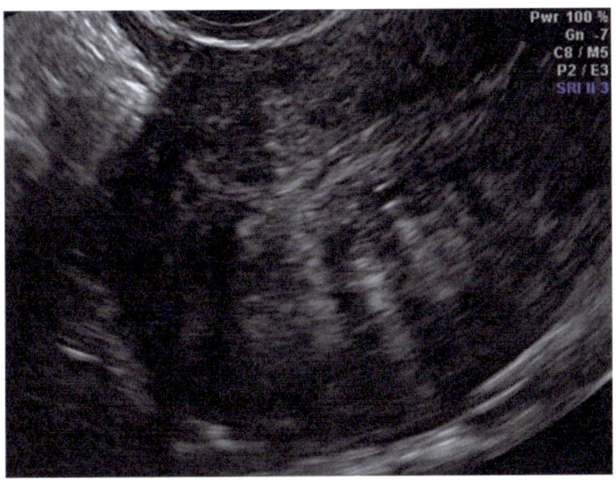

Fig. 4.3 Ultrasound image of adenomyosis (asymmetrical thickening of the posterior myometrium, multiple myometrial cysts, fan-shaped shadowing, echogenic islands, endometrial line, interrupted junctional zone)

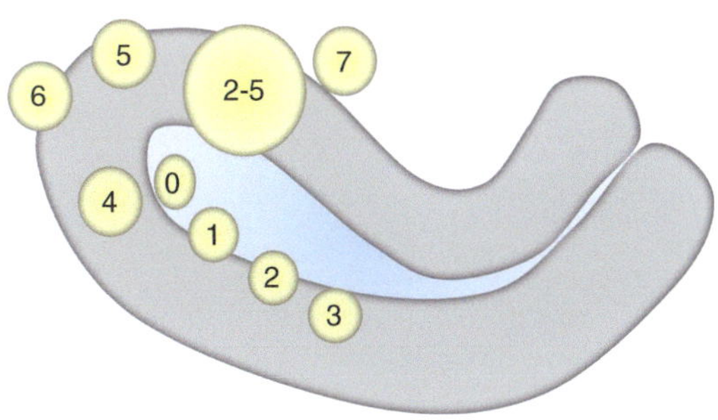

Fig. 4.4 FIGO classification of fibroids (adapted from Munro [6])

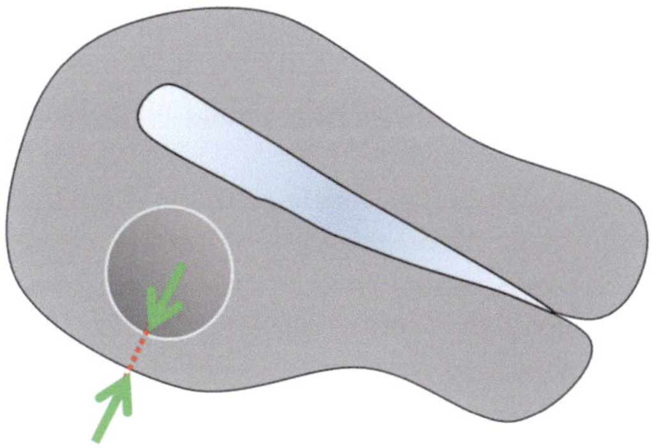

Fig. 4.5 Outer lesion-free margin (OFM) (From Van den Bosch et al. [2])

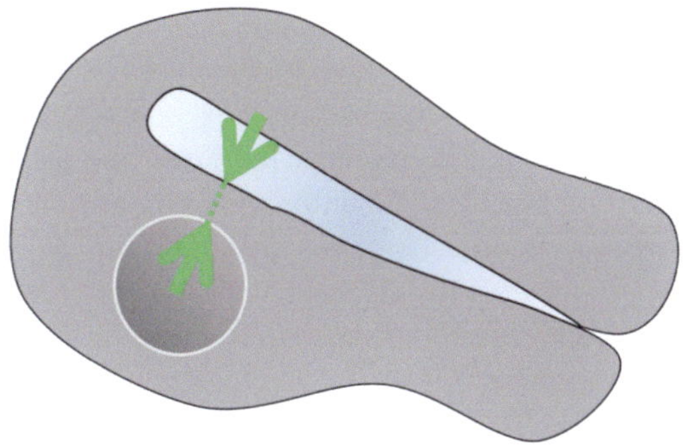

Fig. 4.6 Inner lesion-free margin (IFM) (From Van den Bosch et al. [2])

Well-defined lesions are measured in three *perpendicular diameters*. This can be measured on 2D or after acquisition of a 3D volume. In the latter case, sectional planes are selected, and the central *dot* is placed at the center of the target lesion in plane A. The lesion is measured in plane A in two perpendicular diameters, and the third diameter is measured in plane B.

In fibroids, the outer and the inner lesion-free margin is measured. The *outer lesion-free margin* (*OFM*) is the minimal distance between the serosal surface and the outermost border of the lesion (Fig. 4.5).

The *inner lesion-free margin* (*IFM*) is the minimal distance between the endometrium and the inner border of the lesion (Fig. 4.6).

In ill-defined lesions, the *penetration* is reported (Fig. 4.7). The penetration is defined as the ratio between the thickness of the lesion (measured as the maximal lesion diameter perpendicular to the endometrium) and the total uterine wall thickness (measured perpendicular to the endometrium). Both should be measured on the same image.

The *extent* of an ill-defined lesion is reported as *localized,* if less than 50% of the total uterine is involved, or as *diffuse,* if at least half of the uterine volume is involved. The extent may also be recorded as the percentage of the myometrium involved. The estimation of ill-defined lesions is a rough subjective estimation and is deemed difficult and probably not optimally reproducible.

The *echogenicity* of a myometrium lesion is reported as *uniform* or *nonuniform.* A uniform lesion may be *hypo-*, *iso-*, or *hyperechogenic* as compared with the surrounding (unaffected) myometrium. For research purposes, the relative echogenicity can be scored as very hypoechogenic (−−), hypoechogenic (−), isoechogenic, hyperechogenic (+), or very hyperechogenic (++). As stated before, the overall myometrial echogenicity may be heterogeneous, making the *reference echogenicity* less reliable. The subjectivity of the scoring system had to be taken into account in the interpretation of the report.

Shadowing originating from the myometrium may present as *edge shadows*, *internal shadows*, or *fan-shaped shadowing* (Fig. 4.8). The *degree* of shadowing is recorded as *slight*, *moderate*, or *strong* (Fig. 4.9).

Myometrial *cysts* may be present. Cyst may be caused by adenomyosis, atrophy, and necrosis or may be drug induced (e.g., tamoxifen). The cyst fluid may be *anechogenic* and have a *low level* echogenicity, a *ground-glass appearance*, or a *mixed echogenicity*. The cyst size may vary considerably. At least in the presence of larger cysts, the *number* of cysts and the *maximal*

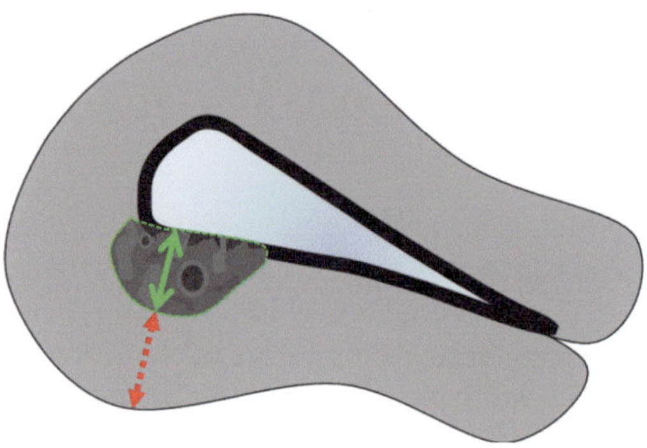

Fig. 4.7 Penetration of ill-defined lesions (From Van den Bosch et al. [2])

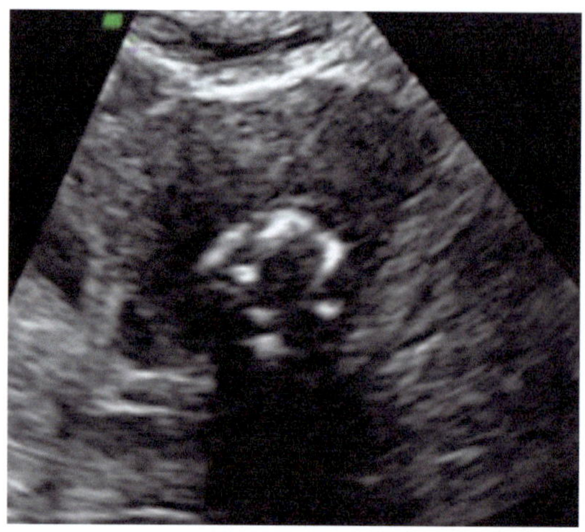

Fig. 4.9 Ultrasound image of a calcified fibroid causing intense internal shadows

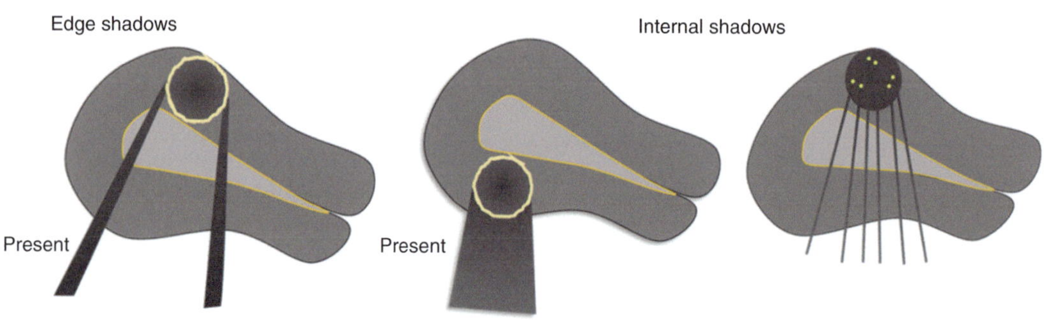

Fig. 4.8 Shadowing caused by fibroids (From Van den Bosch et al. [2])

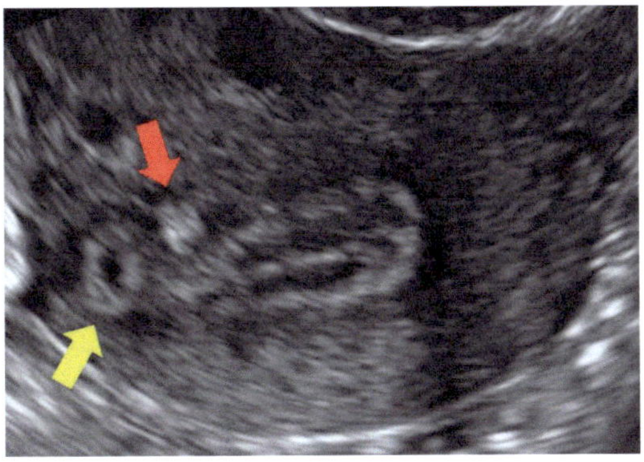

Fig. 4.10 Ultrasound image of adenomyosis: myometrial cyst surrounded by an echogenic rim (yellow arrow) and endometrial bud (red arrow)

diameter of the largest cyst are recorded. In adenomyosis numerous small cysts may be present. In this case, it is not feasible to record the exact number nor the size of the cysts. A typical adenomyosis cyst has an *echogenic rim* caused by endometrial tissue surrounding the cyst cavity (Fig. 4.10).

In adenomyosis, the presence of endometrium tissue within the myometrium may be seen as *hyperechogenic islands*. The outline of these hyperechogenic islands is often ill-defined or irregular but may also be quite regular. For research purposes, the maximum diameter and the number may be recorded.

Early myometrial invasion by endometrial tissue may be apparent at ultrasound examination as *subendometrial echogenic lines and buds*. For research purposes, their number and location may be recorded.

The *junctional zone* (JZ) or *inner myometrium* is the hypoechogenic rim surrounding the endometrium. The junctional zone may appear regular, irregular, or interrupted or may not be visible (Fig. 4.11). The clinical relevance of the measurement of the minimal and maximal JZ thickness remains to be proven and is restricted to research protocols. In case of irregular or interrupted JZ, the location of the irregularity/interruption may be specified as anterior, posterior, fundal, lateral right, lateral left, or global. The extent of the irregular JZ may also be estimated and recorded as the percentage of the JZ being irregular. In case of interruption of the JZ, the

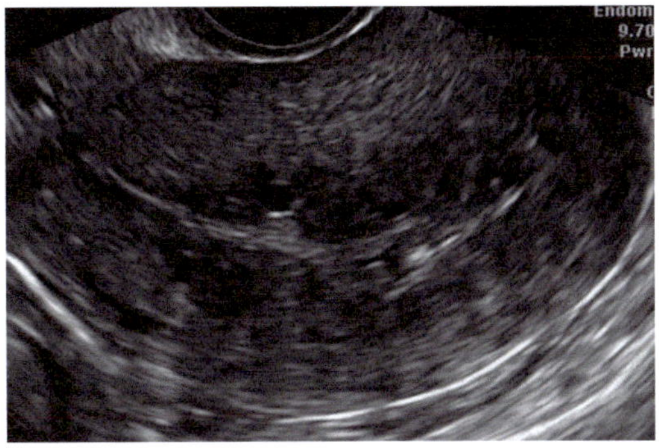

Fig. 4.11 Ultrasound image of adenomyosis: irregular junctional zone

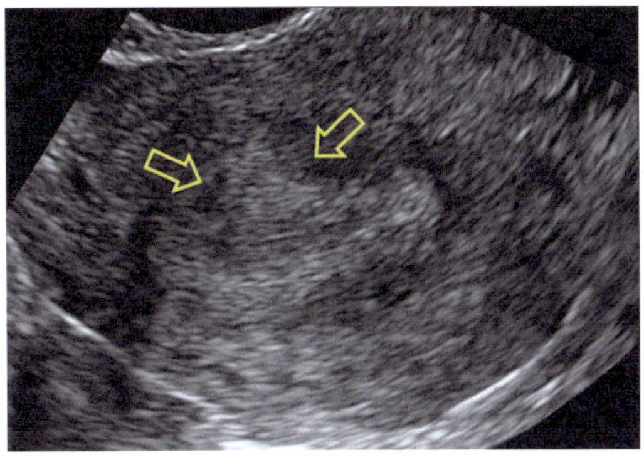

Fig. 4.12 Ultrasound image of adenomyosis: interruption of the junctional zone caused by and echogenic bud

percentage of the JZ not visualized may be recorded. If possible, the reason for the irregularity/interruption may be specified (e.g., cystic areas, hyperechogenic dots, hyperechogenic buds and lines, fibroid) (Fig. 4.12). The *vascularity* of the myometrium using color or power Doppler imaging starts with the assessment of the overall vessel pattern within the uterine walls, reported as *uniform* or *nonuniform*.

The vascularization of the myometrial lesion may be clinically relevant in the diagnosis, the management choice, and the follow-up. The amount of color in a lesion is reported as a *color score*. Both the percentage of the lesion being vascularized and the color hue are taken into account. The color score ranges from 1 to 4: *score 1* meaning no color, *score 2* minimal color, *score 3* moderate color, and *score 4* abundant flow. In case of uneven spread of vascularization, the color score of the most vascularized part may be reported using the same color score ranging from 1 to 4, and the percentage of solid tissue with color signal can be specified (0–100%). The vascularity within the lesion may be compared to the adjacent myometrium and reported as *iso-*, *hypo-*, or *hyper-vascularization.*

The l*ocation* of vessels is reported as *circumferential*, *intralesional*, or *translesional* (Fig. 4.13). Circumferential flow is typical for fibroids, whereas translesional vascularity is characteristic for adenomyosis (Fig. 4.14). The vessel spread within a lesion may be uniform or not uniform. In the latter case, there are areas with increased or decreased vascularity within the lesion.

The *vessel morphology* can further be described as to vessel *number*, *size*, *branching*, and *direction*. The number of vessels is recorded as *single* or *multiple*. The vessel size may be *large and equal*, *small and equal*, or *unequal*. Vessels may exhibit *regular* or *irregular branching*, or no branching. The direction of the vessels is recorded as *perpendicular* or *not perpendicular* to the uterine cavity.

4.3 Technical Tips

Using 2D, the uterus is scanned in sagittal and transverse plane to assess its position, shape, and volume. In transverse plane, a section high in the

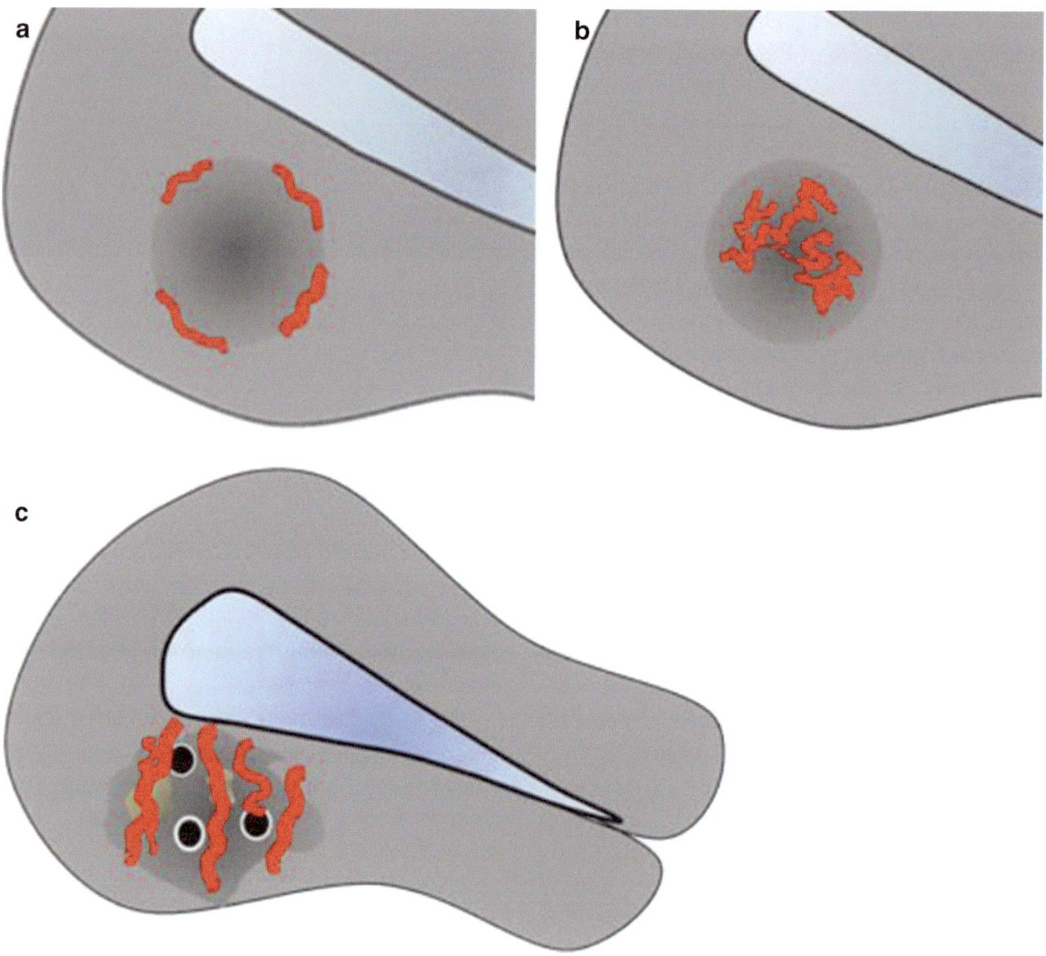

Fig. 4.13 Color imaging: circumferential (**a**), intralesional (**b**), and translesional (**c**) vascularization (adapted from Van den Bosch et al. [2])

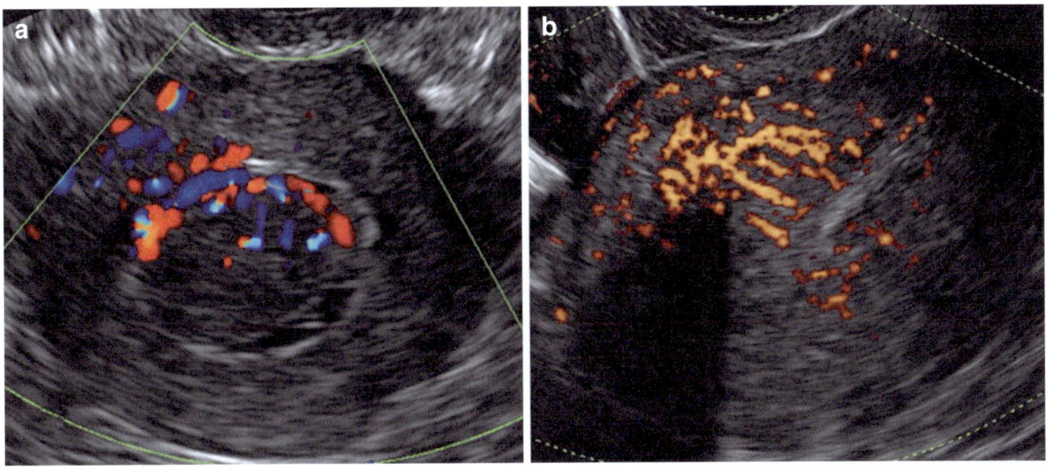

Fig. 4.14 Ultrasound image of a fibroid with circumferential flow (**a**) and adenomyosis with translesional flow (**b**)

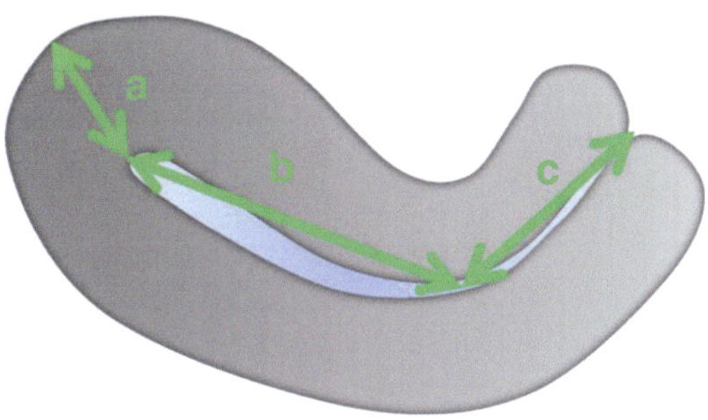

Fig. 4.15 Measurement of the length of the uterus (From Van den Bosch et al. [2])

cavity, at the level of both tubal ostia, is important to *exclude congenital uterine anomalies* (e.g., unicornuate uterus, bicornuate uterus).

Measuring the *total length of the uterus* is not always easy due to the flexion of the uterus. Unless the uterus is outstretched, the true size of the uterine length will be underestimated using a straight line. Therefore the use of a curved measure line will be more accurate. Often an approximated measurement is made using three straight measure lines: [total length] = [fundus] + [cavity] + [cervix] (Fig. 4.15).

Clinician should be aware of these limitations. In clinical follow-up, it is important to use the same methodology. For myometrial lesions, the measurement of the *uterine corpus* is the most relevant. The topographic zone between the corpus and the cervix is the *isthmus* and is often hard to distinguish. Using color Doppler and scanning the lateral border of the cervix and lower corpus, the visualization of the uterine arteries may be helpful to define the level of the isthmus.

Some uteri are rotated around the craniocaudal axis. This may render it more difficult to obtain a *midsagittal section*. Moreover, if the sagittal section is not perpendicular to the frontal plane of the uterus, the measurement of the endometrial thickness and of the anteroposterior diameter of the uterus may be significantly overestimated.

A *3D acquisition* enables to visualize all three section planes: the sagittal, transverse, and coronal planes. The frontal or coronal section is essential in the diagnosis of congenital uterine anomalies as well as in the assessment of the junctional zone [7, 8].

The *outer border* of the myometrium is the uterine serosa, the *inner border* the endometrium. The serosa is usually seen as a regular white line. It is of clinical importance to assess the mobility of the uterus against the surrounding organs (bowel, bladder). This has been referred to as the *sliding sign* [9], being a marker for the presence of adhesions caused by endometriosis, infection, or cancer. For the assessment of the *sliding sign*, the examiner applies some gentle pressure on the uterus with the vaginal probe and uses his/her freehand push on the patient's lower abdomen

(Fig. 4.16). It is important to ask the patient if she experiences some discomfort or pain during the scanning. Site-specific tenderness [10] when applying some pressure on the uterus may be caused by, e.g., adenomyosis or infection.

It is not always easy to identify the *JZ* on ultrasound examination. The use of volume contrast imaging (VCI) set at 2 mm after 3D volume acquisition has been reported to yield the best ultrasound images of the JZ [11] (Fig. 4.17). If the endometrium is not clearly visible, the junctional zone cannot be evaluated neither. In those cases, fluid instillation may be helpful.

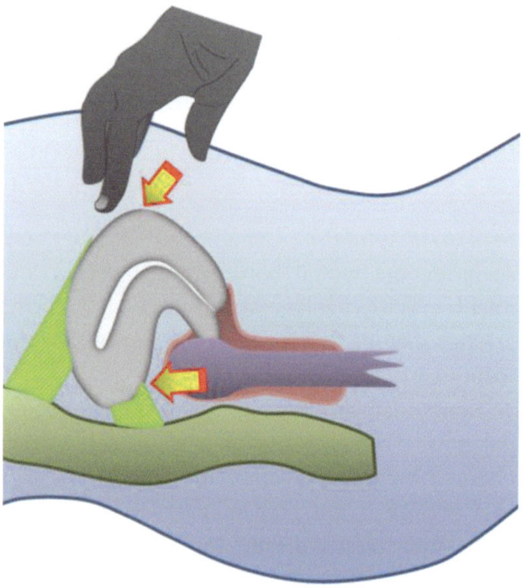

Fig. 4.16 Examining the sliding sign (From Guerriero et al. [9])

To detect *vessels* of lower velocity, the pulse rate frequency (PRF) should be set low enough (e.g., 0.3). In most cases, the *arcuate* and the *radial vessels* are visible, providing an appropriate setting (Fig. 4.18). However, the vessels in the myometrial wall nearest to the ultrasound probe are more readily detectable than in the opposite wall. An apparent asymmetrical vascularity between anterior and posterior myometrium is mostly due to a difference in focal depth and acoustic attenuation. Transient myometrial contractions may cause a temporary disappearance of the blood flow [12].

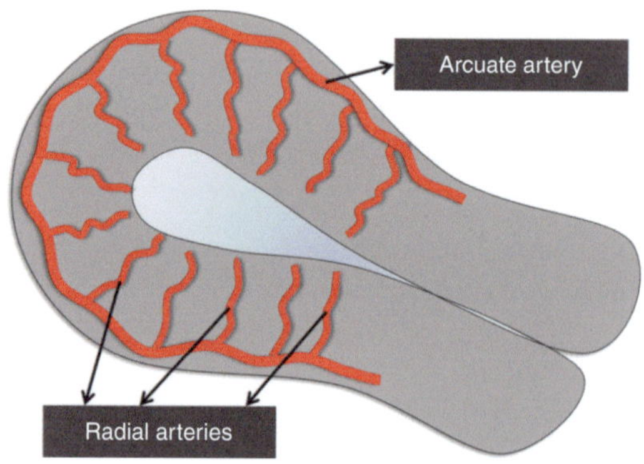

Fig. 4.18 Vascularization of the uterus

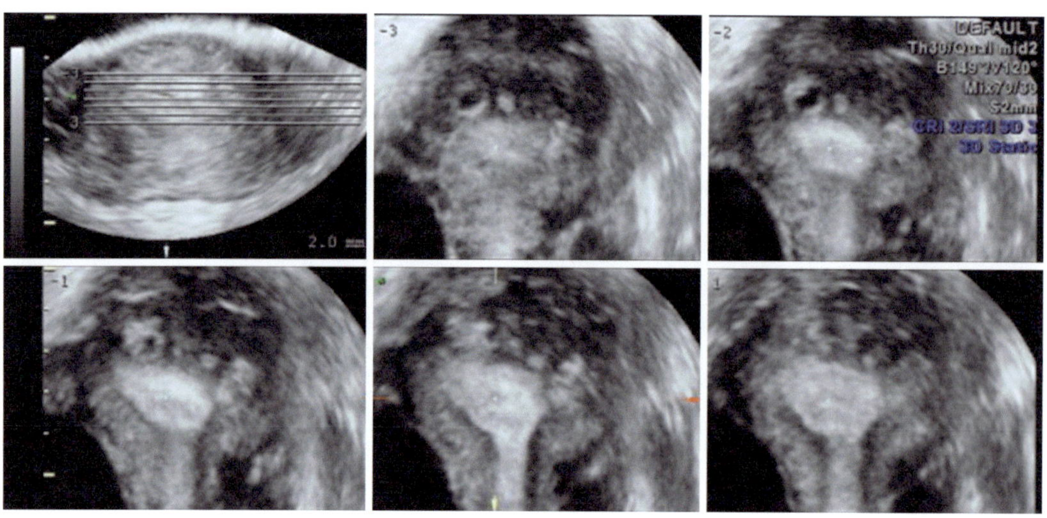

Fig. 4.17 Ultrasound image of adenomyosis using VCI and TUI: irregular junctional zone

4.4 Future Perspectives

Future studies will address the value of ultrasonography and color Doppler imaging in the prediction of fibroid growth. Ultrasonography may prove to be a key examination in the management of fibroids and in the choice between expectant management, medical therapy, ablation, and selective embolization.

A better understanding of the association between adenomyosis and pain or bleeding symptoms as well as the role of adenomyosis in infertility and adverse obstetrical outcome should be addressed in future research. The exact correlation between ultrasonographic features and histological findings [13] also deserves more attention. These issues should be solved before deciding on the place—if any—of surgery in the management of adenomyosis [14].

Finally, a better understanding of ultrasonography in the detection and—more importantly—in the exclusion of sarcomas is a crucial challenge. To date, there is no evidence whatsoever for any screening for sarcomas given their low prevalence and the absence of pathognomonic features (Van den [15]).

References

1. Exacoustos C, Manganaro L, Zupi E. Imaging for the evaluation of endometriosis and adenomyosis. Best Pract Res Clin Obstet Gynaecol. 2014;28:655–81.
2. Van den Bosch T, Dueholm M, Leone FP, Valentin L, Rasmussen CK, Votino A, Van Schoubroeck D, Landolfo C, Installé AJ, Guerriero S, Exacoustos C, Gordts S, Benacerraf B, D'Hooghe T, De Moor B, Brölmann H, Goldstein S, Epstein E, Bourne T, Timmerman D. Terms, definitions and measurements to describe sonographic features of myometrium and uterine masses: a consensus opinion from the Morphological Uterus Sonographic Assessment (MUSA) group. Ultrasound Obstet Gynecol. 2015;46:284–98.
3. Amant F, Van den Bosch T, Vergote I, Timmerman D. Morcellation of uterine leiomyomas: a plea for patient triage. Lancet Oncol. 2015;16:1454–6.
4. Brölmann H, Tanos V, Grimbizis G, Ind T, Philips K, van den Bosch T, Sawalhe S, van den Haak L, Jansen FW, Pijnenborg J, Taran FA, Brucker S, Wattiez A, Campo R, O'Donovan P, de Wilde RL, European Society of Gynaecological Endoscopy (ESGE) steering committee on fibroid morcellation. Options on fibroid morcellation: a literature review. Gynecol Surg. 2015;12:3–15.
5. Exacoustos C, Romanini ME, Amadio A, Amoroso C, Szabolcs B, Zupi E, Arduini D. Can gray-scale and color Doppler sonography differentiate between uterine leiomyosarcoma and leiomyoma? J Clin Ultrasound. 2007;35:449–57.
6. Munro MG, Critchley HO, Broder MS, Fraser IS. FIGO classification system (PALM-COEIN) for causes of abnormal uterine bleeding in nongravid women of reproductive age. Int J Gynaecol Obstet. 2011;113:3–13.
7. Naftalin J, Hoo W, Nunes N, Mavrelos D, Nicks H, Jurkovic D. Inter- and intraobserver variability in three-dimensional ultrasound assessment of the endometrial-myometrial junction and factors affecting its visualization. Ultrasound Obstet Gynecol. 2012;39:587–91.
8. Naftalin J, Jurkovic D. The endometrial-myometrial junction: a fresh look at a busy crossing. Ultrasound Obstet Gynecol. 2009;34:1–11.
9. Guerriero S, Condous G, van den Bosch T, Valentin L, Leone FP, Van Schoubroeck D, Exacoustos C, Installé AJ, Martins WP, Abrao MS, Hudelist G, Bazot M, Alcazar JL, Gonçalves MO, Pascual MA, Ajossa S, Savelli L, Dunham R, Reid S, Menakaya U, Bourne T, Ferrero S, Leon M, Bignardi T, Holland T, Jurkovic D, Benacerraf B, Osuga Y, Somigliana E, Timmerman D. Systematic approach to sonographic evaluation of the pelvis in women with suspected endometriosis, including terms, definitions and measurements: a consensus opinion from the International Deep Endometriosis Analysis (IDEA) group. Ultrasound Obstet Gynecol. 2016;48:318–32.
10. Okaro E, Condous G, Khalid A, Timmerman D, Ameye L, Van Huffel SV, Bourne T. The use of ultrasound-based 'soft markers' for the prediction of pelvic pathology in women with chronic pelvic pain--can we reduce the need for laparoscopy? BJOG. 2006;251-6(11):113.
11. Votino A, Van den Bosch T, Installé AJ, Van Schoubroeck D, Kaijser J, Kacem Y, De Moor B, Van Pachterbeke C, Timmerman D. Optimizing the ultrasound visualization of the endometrial-myometrial junction (EMJ). Facts Views Vis Obgyn. 2015;7:60–3.
12. Van den Bosch T, Van Schoubroeck D, Chuan L, De Brabanter J, Van Huffel S, Timmerman D. Color Doppler and gray-scale ultrasound evaluation of the postpartum uterus. Ultrasound Obstet Gynecol. 2002;20:586–91.
13. Vandermeulen L, Cornelis A, Kjaergaard Rasmussen C, Timmerman D, Van den Bosch T. Guiding histological assessment of uterine lesions using 3D in vitro ultrasonography and stereotaxis. Facts Views Vis Obgyn. 2017;9:77–84.
14. Grimbizis GF, Mikos T, Tarlatzis B. Uterus-sparing operative treatment for adenomyosis. Fertil Steril. 2014;101:472–87.
15. Van den Bosch T. Exabundanti cautela: from the tragedy of inadvertent sarcoma morcellation to inappropriate myoma screening. Gynecol Surg. 2016;13:73–4.

5 Ovarian Endometriosis

Juan Luis Alcázar

5.1 Introduction

Ovarian endometriosis is a common form of endometriosis. Typically, on ultrasound, it appears as a cystic lesion with "ground-glass" echogenicity with no papillary projection or solid areas. This cystic lesion is also known as an ovarian endometrioma or "chocolate cyst" due to the cyst's content.

Ovarian endometriosis occurs in about 17–44% of women affected by endometriosis [1]. In a large series of surgically removed ovarian lesions, endometrioma constituted 21–33% of all benign masses [2, 3]. The left ovary is more frequently affected than the right one but bilaterally is found in 30–50% of the cases [4].

The pathogenesis of ovarian endometrioma is a source of controversy. Three different theories have been proposed for explaining the formation of ovarian endometrioma: (1) the invagination of the ovarian cortex affected by active superficial implants on the ovarian surface, (2) the endometriotic transformation of ovarian functional cysts, and (3) the metaplastic potential of pelvic mesotelium [5].

Electronic Supplementary Material The online version of this chapter (https://doi.org/10.1007/978-3-319-71138-6_5) contains supplementary material, which is available to authorized users.

J. L. Alcázar
Department of Obstetrics and Gynecology, Clinica Universidad de Navarra, University of Navarra, Pamplona, Spain
e-mail: jlalcazar@unav.es

Ovarian endometrioma usually appears in women during the third and fourth decade of life. Many of them are asymptomatic. When symptoms occur, the most frequent are pelvic pain, dysmenorrhea, and dyspareunia. It should be noted that the finding an ovarian endometrioma is associated to deep endometriosis (DE) in up to 23% of the cases [6]. Therefore, all patients with ovarian endometrioma should be thoroughly scanned searching other lesions of DE.

The risk of malignant transformation of an ovarian endometrioma has been estimated as 0.6–0.8% of the cases [7].

Asymptomatic ovarian endometrioma may be managed expectantly with serial ultrasound scans [8]. However, symptomatic endometrioma should be treated. Laparoscopic cystectomy is considered as the first-line treatment [9]. Fine-needle aspiration and sclerotherapy may be an option [9]. More radical treatment such as oophorectomy or adnexectomy may be considered for women with completed families [9]. Medical treatment is not an effective cure for ovarian endometriosis but might be used to relief symptoms [9].

In this overview, we shall review the sonographic spectrum of ovarian endometriomas. We also shall discuss the diagnostic performance of ultrasound for the specific diagnosis of this kind of ovarian lesion, as well as the role of adjuvant ultrasound techniques such as Doppler and three-dimensional ultrasound.

S. Guerriero et al. (eds.), *How to Perform Ultrasonography in Endometriosis*,
https://doi.org/10.1007/978-3-319-71138-6_5

5.2 How We Do It

5.2.1 Technique

Transvaginal ultrasound (TVS) is the optimal approach for assessing the ovary and the endometrium. In cases where TVS cannot be performed, transrectal ultrasound is a very good alternative as it provides quite similar images to TVS. Transabdominal ultrasound may be also an option; however, the resolution of the ultrasound image is worse.

TVS does not require any specific preparation by the patient before the procedure is done. Mandatory cleaning of the transvaginal probe by an acceptable disinfectant technique prior to its use in a new patient and placement of a condom or ultrasound sheath for covering the ultrasound probe is essential.

For transrectal ultrasound, rectal cleansing is recommended before ultrasound is performed, and the same measures for probe covering than TVS are mandatory.

For transabdominal ultrasound, full bladder is required.

After inserting the endovaginal probe into the vagina, a thorough scanning of the pelvis is always advised including the uterus and ovaries (see Chap. 3), for ruling out the presence of any uterine or adnexal pathology, such as congenital uterine anomalies, fibroids, adenomyosis (see Chap. 4), or adnexal masses. For assessing ovarian endometrioma, special attention must be paid to the adnexal regions in order to identify any cystic lesion.

If a cystic lesion is found, then we must try to identify whether the lesion is derived from the ovary itself or from other areas (uterus, para-ovarian or paratubal regions, or even from another pelvic organ such as the bladder, rectum, or sigmoid).

5.2.2 Spectrum of Sonographic Findings

The typical ultrasound appearance of an ovarian endometrioma is a cystic lesion with low-level homogeneous echogenic content, representing the blood within the cystic cavity, and is commonly termed "ground-glass" echogenicity [10, 11]. The cyst is clearly demarcated from the surrounding ovarian parenchyma and usually does not exhibit any papillary projection or solid area (Fig. 5.1). Mean lesion size is about 5 cm, but it may vary from 0.5 cm up to 15 cm (Figs. 5.2 and 5.3).

Although this typical appearance has been reported in 73–82% of endometriomas, the sonographic spectrum is wide [12, 13]. Ovarian endometrioma may appear as unilocular anechoic cyst (5% of the cases) (Fig. 5.4), as a cyst with hemorrhagic content (2% of the cases) (Fig. 5.5) or as an unilocular cyst with homogeneous low-level echoes, but not "ground glass" (6% of the cases) (Fig. 5.6). Thus, the main differential diagnoses are simple or serous cyst, hemorrhagic cyst, or unilocular mucinous cyst.

Multilocularity has been reported in 18–24% of endometriomas [13, 14] (Fig. 5.7). However, very probably endometriomas are not septate lesions but single lesions one adjacent to other. A clue for this is what I call the "lambda sing" in reportedly multilocular cystic lesions; a similar finding to that observed in dichorionic-diamniotic twin pregnancies (Alcazar, personal communication) (Fig. 5.8). As a matter of fact in some women, multiple endometriomas can be observed in the same ovary (Fig. 5.9).

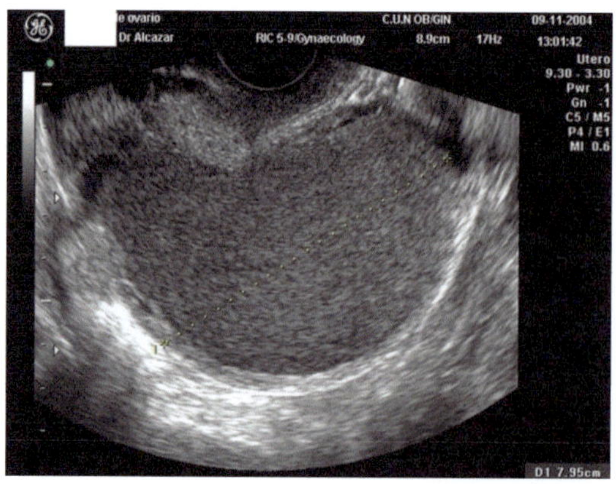

Fig. 5.1 Typical appearance of an ovarian endometrioma: unilocular cyst with ground-glass echogenicity and no papillary projections

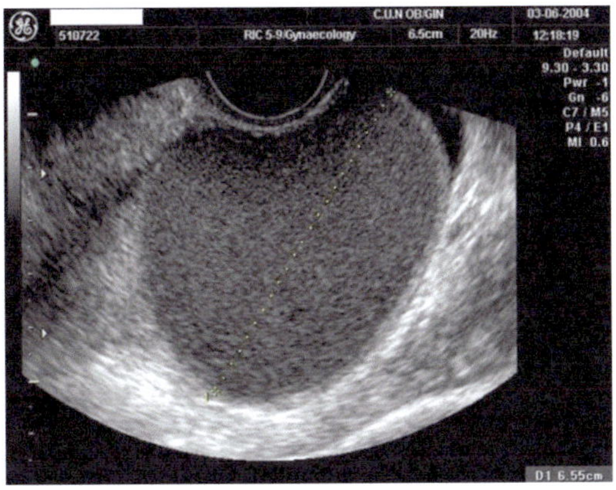

Fig. 5.2 Typical endometrioma with a clear demarcation of ovarian parenchyma (echogenic capsule surrounding the cyst)

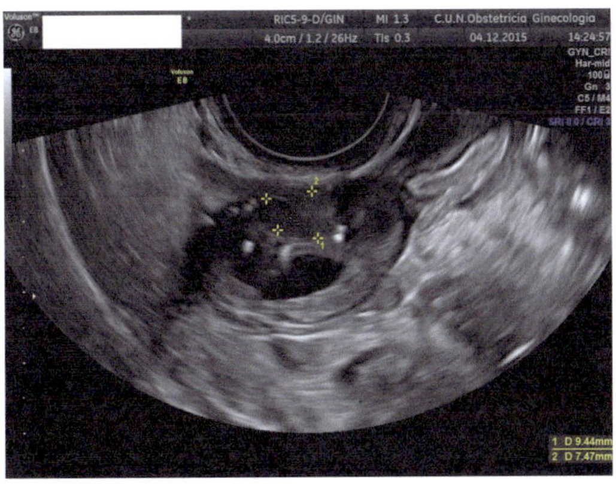

Fig. 5.3 Small ovarian endometrioma with hyperechogenic foci located close to ovarian surface

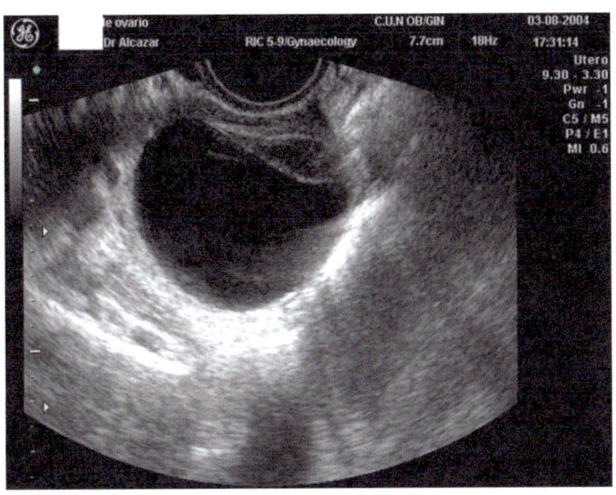

Fig. 5.4 Transvaginal ultrasound depicting an ovarian endometrioma as an anechoic cyst, some debris can be seen in the bottom of the cyst cavity

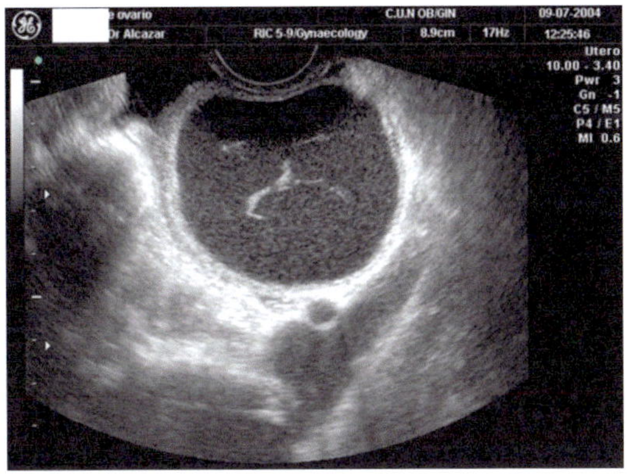

Fig. 5.5 An ovarian endometrioma showing some echogenic bands within the cyst cavity mimicking hemorrhagic echogenicity

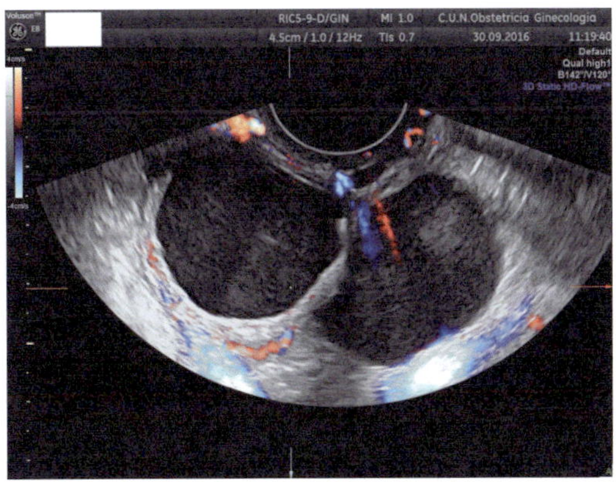

Fig. 5.6 Two ovarian endometriomas with low-level echogenicity, but not a ground-glass appearance

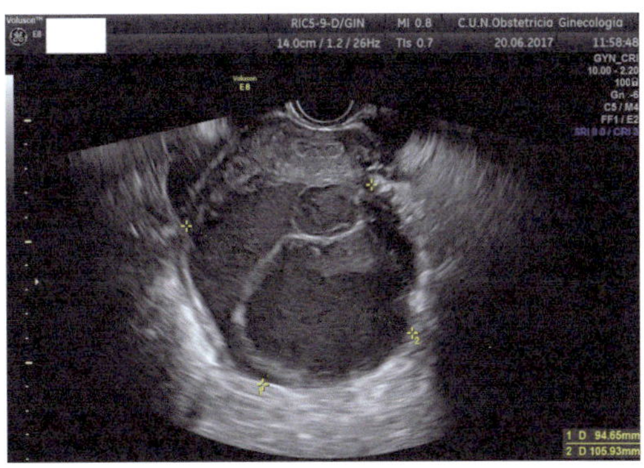

Fig. 5.7 Transvaginal ultrasound showing a "multilocular" endometrioma. Actually, this finding used to be several endometriomas one adjacent to each other

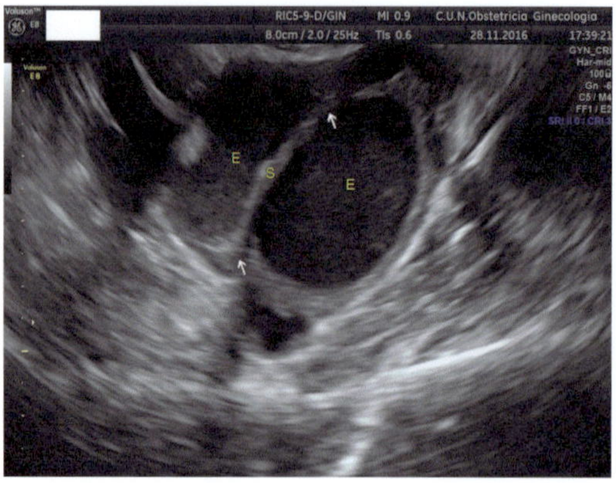

Fig. 5.8 Transvaginal ultrasound showing a "septate" endometrioma. In fact, this is two different endometriomas (E) separated by ovarian parenchyma (S). *Arrows* show the so-called "lambda sign"

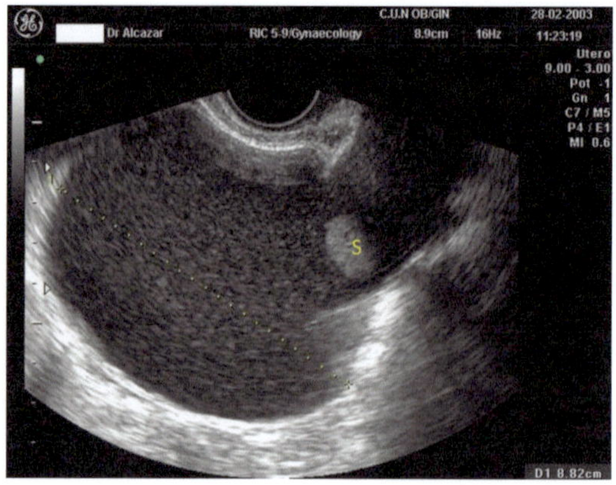

Fig. 5.10 Transvaginal ultrasound showing an atypical endometrioma containing a solid area (S) arising from internal surface of cyst's wall

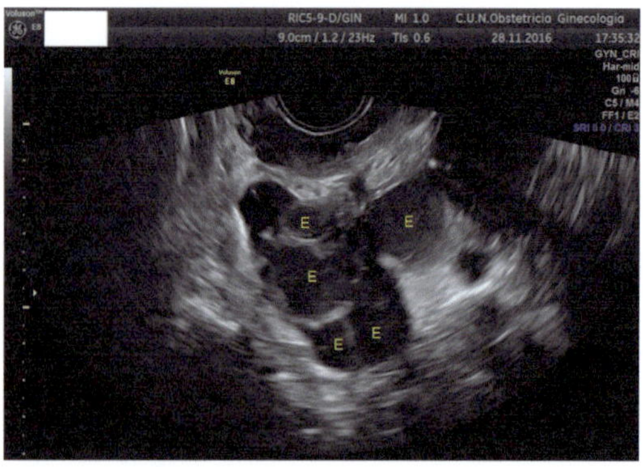

Fig. 5.9 Transvaginal ultrasound showing an ovary containing multiple small endometriomas (E)

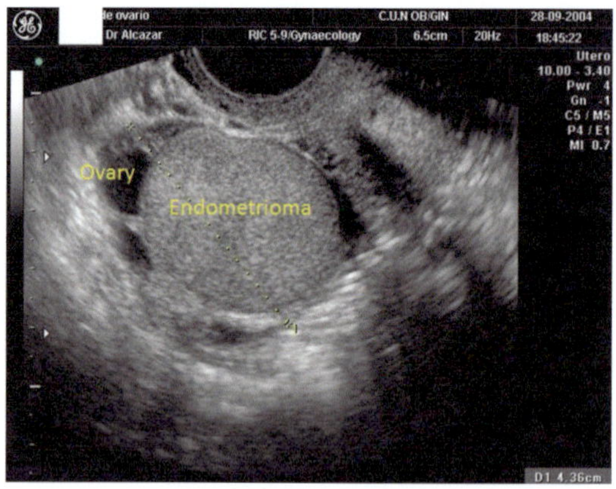

Fig. 5.11 Transvaginal ultrasound showing an ovarian endometrioma with apparent solid echogenicity

In some cases, endometriomas may show atypical features, the so-called atypical endometriomas. Usually, this term is used in endometriomas that exhibit solid areas or papillary projections [10, 11] (Fig. 5.10). In one of the largest series of sonographic findings in ovarian endometriomas, this feature has been reported in 15% of all ovarian endometriomas [13]. A purely solid appearance of ovarian endometriomas is a rare finding (<1% of the cases) (Fig. 5.11).

The presence of small hyperechoic foci in the cyst wall has been reported as a very specific sign for ovarian endometrioma (Fig. 5.12). They may appear in about one third of these lesions [15]. However, some authors have challenged this idea and consider that small hyperechoic foci are not a reliable indicator of endometrioma [16].

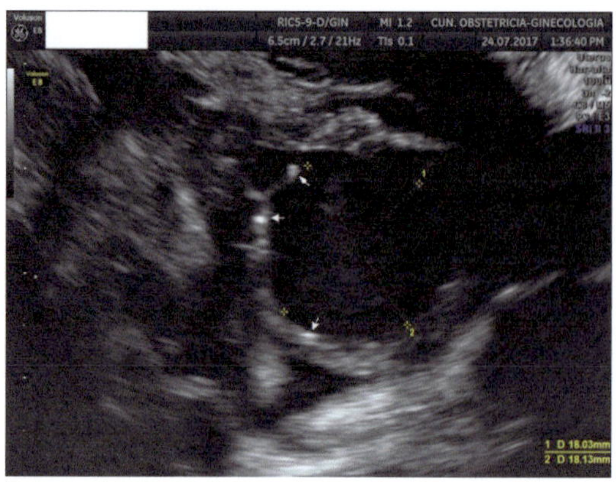

Fig. 5.12 Ovarian endometrioma showing hyperechogenic foci (*arrows*)

Another very specific feature proposed for ovarian endometrioma is the so-called acoustic streaming. Acoustic streaming is defined as the bulk movement of fluid due to the effect of a sound field caused by energy transfer from an ultrasound beam to the fluid. In other words, the energy of the ultrasound beam "pushes" the particles of the fluid away from the transducer (Video 5.1). Clarke et al. supported the concept that ovarian endometrioma never show acoustic streaming [17]. However, a subsequent study in a much large series demonstrated that acoustic streaming occurs in 9% of endometriomas, and, therefore, this feature cannot be considered as 100% specific for ovarian endometrioma [18].

The inherent dynamic nature of ultrasound evaluation allows the evaluation of two additional signs [1]. The assessment of ovarian cyst mobility is important. The lack of mobility is due to the formation of adhesions to the uterus, to the pelvic wall, or to the contralateral ovary, the so-called kissing ovaries (Fig. 5.13). The presence of ovarian adhesion to the uterus, pelvic wall, or contralateral ovary is highly predictive of ovarian endometrioma [19] (Video 5.2), but it is not always present (Video 5.3) [2]. The presence of site-specific tenderness (see Chap. 3) when moving the ultrasound probe against particular structures is also very suggestive of endometriosis [20].

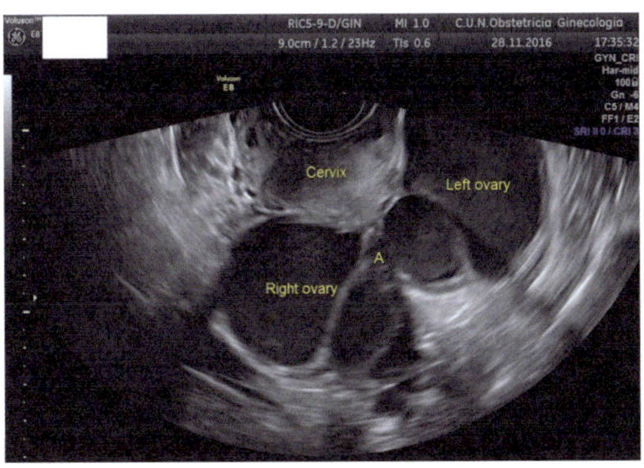

Fig. 5.13 Transvaginal ultrasound showing the two ovaries containing several ovarian endometriomas (E) and adhered one to each other (A), the so-called kissing ovaries

A recent study has shown that ultrasound features of ovarian endometriomas change with the patient's age [21]. For example, ground-glass echogenicity appears in 75% of endometriomas in premenopausal women but only in 62% of endometriomas in peri-/postmenopausal women. Anechoic cysts are uncommon in premenopausal women (3%) but may appear in up to 11% of peri-/postmenopausal women.

There are two clinical entities that deserve particular mention: decidualization of an endometrioma and ovarian cancer arising from an endometrioma. Endometrioma decidualization is a phenomenon characterized by the thickening of the ectopic endometrium due to the effect of progesterone during pregnancy. When decidualization occurs, endometriomas may mimic an ovarian cancer during ultrasound evaluation. Typical findings are the presence of one to several vascularized solid papillary projections arising from the internal surface of the cyst's wall [22, 23] (Video 5.4). The knowledge of past history of endometriosis observing the "suspicious" lesion in the same ovary where endometrioma had been diagnosed prior to pregnancy may give clues for considering decidualization. Another important tip is paying attention to the surface of the papillary projection. In decidualized endometriomas surface uses to be smooth [22], whereas in malignancy surface uses to be irregular. Serial evaluation during pregnancy can be advised in cases of suspected decidualized endometriomas [24].

Although there is a clear association between endometriosis and ovarian cancer [25], the risk of developing a malignancy from ovarian endometrioma is low [7]. Testa et al. reported a retrospective study comprising 15 malignancies arising from ovarian endometrioma [26]. They found that all malignancies were characterized by the presence of solid tissue, as compared to 16% of benign endometriomas. Blood flow within the solid component was observed in 92% of malignancies and only in 8% of benign endometriomas with solid areas. Both mean size of the lesion and mean size of the solid areas were significantly larger in malignancies. Figure 5.14 shows a case of ovarian malignancy arising from an ovarian endometrioma.

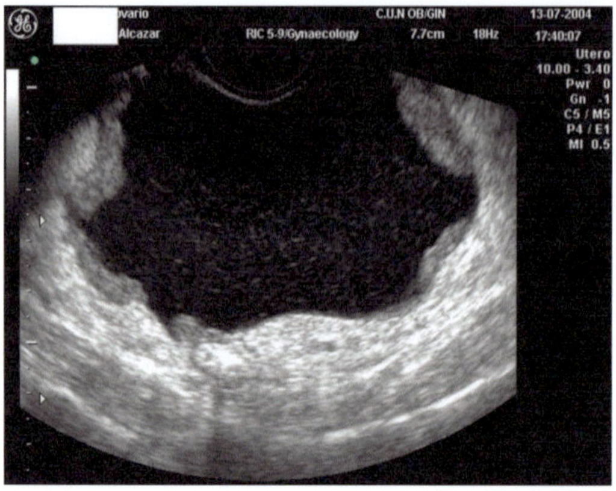

Fig. 5.14 Transvaginal sonography depicting a unilocular cyst with irregular walls. Histopathology revealed an endometrioid carcinoma arising from an endometrioma

5.2.3 Diagnostic Performance of Ultrasound for the Specific Diagnosis of Ovarian Endometriosis

Several studies have evaluated the diagnostic performance of TVS for the specific diagnosis of ovarian endometrioma. Moore et al. performed a systematic review in which sensitivity ranged from 64 to 89%, whereas specificity ranged from 89 to 100% [27]. However, most of studies included in this review were small series.

Sokalska et al. reported results of a prospective study assessing the diagnostic performance of TVS for the specific diagnosis of different types of ovarian lesions in 1066 women (199 endometriomas) [2]. They reported a sensitivity and specificity of 77% and 98%, respectively, for ovarian endometrioma.

Alcazar et al. performed a similar study comprising 2148 women (558 endometriomas) and reported a sensitivity and specificity of 88% and 97%, respectively [3]. However, these authors analyzed the diagnostic performance in premenopausal and postmenopausal women. They found that specificity was similar (96% and 99%, respectively), but sensitivity was lower in postmenopausal women as compared with premenopausal women (68% and 89%, respectively). This could be explained by the findings of Guerriero's study above cited [21].

One study has evaluated the agreement among expert examiners for the diagnosis of ovarian endometrioma [28]. This study showed that intra-observer and interobserver reproducibility were high.

5.2.4 Role of Doppler Ultrasound

The use of pulsed Doppler ultrasound was advocated in the 1990s for discriminating ovarian endometriomas from other benign ovarian lesions. However, the results of those studies were controversial [14, 29]. Guerriero and colleagues found that the addition of power Doppler mapping to conventional grayscale findings would increase the diagnostic performance of ultrasound [30]. However, these findings have not been confirmed in other studies.

Alcazar and co-workers found in a retrospective study that endometrioma vascularization was related to the presence of pain the women with ovarian endometrioma [31], supporting the concept that neoangiogenesis is related to pain symptoms in women with endometriosis. This was confirmed in a subsequent prospective study by the same group [32]. In this study, the authors found that there was a significant correlation between microvascular density in endometriomas' capsule and the amount of power Doppler signals surrounding the endometriomas. Additionally, both power Doppler and microvascular density were correlated to the severity of pain symptoms complained by the patients. However, Seckin et al. did not find a relationship of color Doppler mapping and pain symptoms [33]. These controversial results could be explained by different patient selection and because of different Doppler settings used. Because of these controversial results, the use of Doppler ultrasound should not be recommended as routine in clinical practice for assessing ovarian endometrioma.

5.2.5 The Role of Three-Dimensional (3D) Ultrasound

Few studies have assessed the role of 3D ultrasound in the evaluation of ovarian endometrioma.

Alcazar et al. evaluated the use of the so-called mean gray value (MGV) of the cyst's content for discriminating endometrioma from other benign unilocular cysts [34]. MGV represents the mean intensity of grayscale voxels contained in a given 3D region of interest and can be calculated using the virtual organ computer-aided analysis (VOCAL™) software (Fig. 5.15); the more anechoic the content, the lower MGV, and the more echogenic content, the higher MGV. They found that MGV in endometriomas was significantly higher as compared with other cysts (simple cysts, hemorrhagic cysts, and mucinous cysts).

However, Huang et al. found the opposite findings; MGV was significantly lower in ovarian endometrioma [35]. These controversial results can be explained by two facts: first, Huang's study included dermoid cysts, which tend to show highly echogenic areas. Second, MGV is highly affected by some machine settings (especially gain), so different machine settings used render different MGV values. Due to the paucity of studies and their controversial results, it could be stated that the role of 3D ultrasound still needs to be determined.

5.3 Important Technical Tips

There are several important technical tips to be considered when evaluating the ovary and ovarian endometriomas. These technical tips are basically related to the ultrasound machine settings and depth. The objective of the examination from the technical point of view is trying to get the maximum possible resolution. This is the main reason why TVS should be performed whenever possible, and the use of transrectal ultrasound is the best alternative when TVS cannot be performed.

5.3.1 Depth

The distance between the transducer and any structure under examination is a very relevant issue, especially if Doppler is used, since Doppler signal is heavily affected by attenuation. If the ovary and/or uterus are far from the transducer (>5 cm), gentle pressure with the hand over the abdomen while performing the ultrasound examination may get these structures closer to the transducer favoring image resolution.

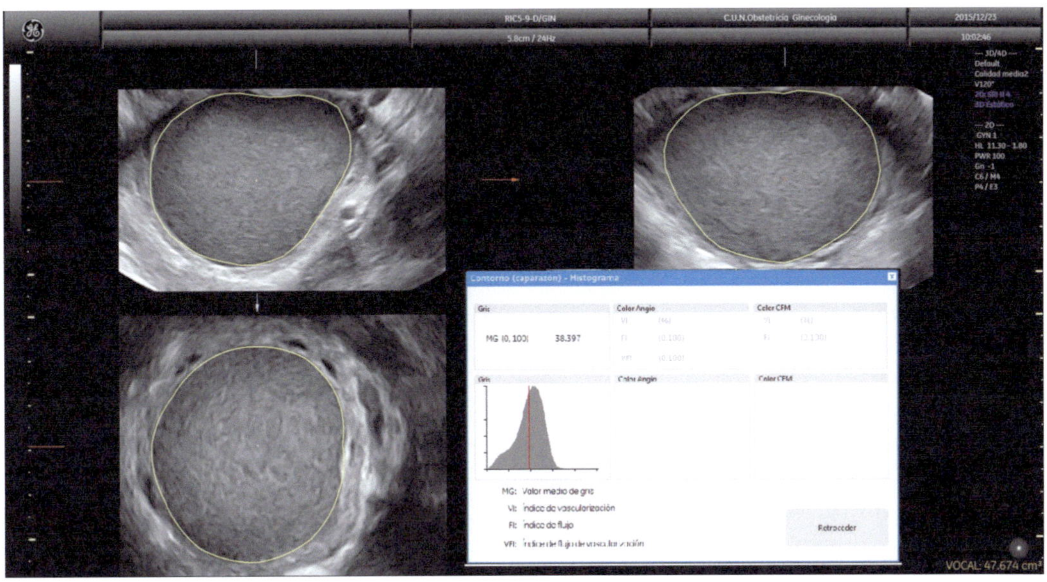

Fig. 5.15 Three-dimensional ultrasound showing mean gray value calculation from the cyst content in a case of ovarian endometrioma

5.3.2 Machine Settings

Ultrasound machine settings are also important for achieving a good resolution image. The transducer's frequency is the most important machine setting. It should not be less than 5 MHz and even higher frequency (8–9 MHz) is advisable. If Doppler is used, 5 MHz is an optimal frequency.

Gain is another important ultrasound machine setting to be considered, especially for grayscale ultrasound. Gain significantly affects the echogenicity of the structures. Thus, using adequate gain is essential for avoiding confusion between different cyst's content echogenicity. For grayscale evaluation, mid gain is initially advisable, increasing or lowering it until good quality image is obtained. Very low gain may render an endometrioma as an anechoic cyst, whereas high gain may render it as an echogenic cyst, both resulting in potential to miss ground-glass echogenicity.

For color/power Doppler assessment, it is recommended to increase gain until saturation and then reduce gain reaching sub-noise gain level.

Harmonics increases image resolution, but penetration is lower. This can also affect cyst content, and one should bear this in mind. If the ovary is very close to the transducer, the use of harmonics is advised.

Other ultrasound machine settings such as persistence, contrast, and enhancement power do not usually need to be modified for improving image quality or resolution in most circumstance.

For Doppler assessment, other important parameters are:

- Pulse repetition frequency (PRF). Since blood flow within the ovary and endometrium uses to be slow and the vessels are small, low PRF is advised (0.6–0.3 kHz).
- Wall filter should be low (50 Hz).
- Sample volume should cover the whole ovary.
- Insonation angle is not relevant for assessing ovarian vascularization since the vessels are so small that it is virtually impossible to ascertain vessel orientation.
- Pulsed Doppler sample volume size should be adjusted to vessel caliber as better as possible. If not possible, sample volume size of 0.7–1.0 mm is advisable.

5.4 Future Perspectives

Several areas in the ultrasound evaluation and follow-up of endometriomas should be evaluated in the future research studies. These include:

1. Assessment of diagnostic performance of ultrasound in hands of non-expert examiners.
2. Assessment of reproducibility on ultrasound diagnosis of ovarian endometrioma among non-expert examiners.
3. Define the role of 3D ultrasound.
4. Long-term prospective studies based on expectant management for determining the risk of developing ovarian cancer from ovarian endometrioma.
5. Prospective studies to determine if expectant management of decidualized endometriomas during pregnancy is safe and what criteria should be used for advising expectant management.

References

1. Redwine DB. Ovarian endometriosis: a marker for more extensive pelvic and intestinal disease. Fertil Steril. 1999;72:310–5.
2. Sokalska A, Timmerman D, Testa AC, Van Holsbeke C, Lissoni AA, Leone FP, Jurkovic D, Valentin L. Diagnostic accuracy of transvaginal ultrasound examination for assigning a specific diagnosis to adnexal masses. Ultrasound Obstet Gynecol. 2009;34:462–70.
3. Alcázar JL, Guerriero S, Laparte C, Ajossa S, Ruiz-Zambrana A, Melis GB. Diagnostic performance of transvaginal gray-scale ultrasound for specific diagnosis of benign ovarian cysts in relation to menopausal status. Maturitas. 2011;68:182–8.
4. Al-Fozan H, Tulandi T. Left lateral predisposition of endometriosis and endometrioma. Obstet Gynecol. 2003;101:164–6.
5. Nisolle M, Donnez J. Peritoneal endometriosis, ovarian endometriosis, and adenomyotic nodules of the rectovaginal septum are three different entities. Fertil Steril. 1997;68:585–96.
6. Chapron C, Pietin-Vialle C, Borghese B, Davy C, Foulot H, Chopin N. Associated ovarian endometrioma is a marker for greater severity of deeply infiltrating endometriosis. Fertil Steril. 2009;92:453–7.
7. Nishida M, Watanabe K, Sato N, Ichikawa Y. Malignant transformation of ovarian endometriosis. Gynecol Obstet Investig. 2000;50(Suppl 1):18–25.
8. Alcázar JL, Olartecoechea B, Guerriero S, Jurado M. Expectant management of adnexal masses in

selected premenopausal women: a prospective observational study. Ultrasound Obstet Gynecol. 2013;41:582–8.
9. Garcia-Tejedor A, Fernandez-Montoli ME, Pla Farnos MJ, Ponce Sebastia J. Management of ovarian endometrioma. In: Fernandez-Montoli ME, Gine Martinez L, Ponce Sebastia J, editors. Endometriosis. A multidisciplinary approach. New York: Nova Biomedical; 2013. p. 135–54.
10. Guerriero S, Ajossa S, Gerada M, Virgilio B, Pilloni M, Galvan R, Laparte C, Alcazar JL, Melis GB. Transvaginal ultrasonography in the diagnosis of extrauterine pelvic disease. Expert Rev Obstet Gynecol. 2008;3:731–52.
11. Sayasneh A, Ekechi C, Ferrara L, Kaijser J, Stalder C, Sur S, Timmerman D, Bourne T. The characteristic ultrasound features of specific types of ovarian pathology. Int J Oncol. 2015;46:445–58.
12. Kupfer MC, Schwimer SR, Lebovic J. Transvaginal sonographic appearance of endometriomata: spectrum of findings. J Ultrasound Med. 1992;11:129–33.
13. Van Holsbeke C, Van Calster B, Guerriero S, Savelli L, Paladini D, Lissoni AA, Czekierdowski A, Fischerova D, Zhang J, Mestdagh G, Testa AC, Bourne T, Valentin L, Timmerman D. Endometriomas: their ultrasound characteristics. Ultrasound Obstet Gynecol. 2010;35:730–40.
14. Pascual MA, Tresserra F, López-Marín L, Ubeda A, Grases PJ, Dexeus S. Role of color Doppler ultrasonography in the diagnosis of endometriotic cyst. J Ultrasound Med. 2000;19:695–9.
15. Patel MD, Feldstein VA, Chen DC, Lipson SD, Filly RA. Endometriomas: diagnostic performance of US. Radiology. 1999;210:739–45.
16. Brown DL, Frates MC, Muto MG, Welch WR. Small echogenic foci in the ovaries: correlation with histologic findings. J Ultrasound Med. 2004;23:307–13.
17. Clarke L, Edwards A, Pollard K. Acoustic streaming in ovarian cysts. J Ultrasound Med. 2005;24:617–21.
18. Van Holsbeke C, Zhang J, Van Belle V, Paladini D, Guerriero S, Czekierdowski A, Muggah H, Ombelet W, Jurkovic D, Testa AC, Valentin L, Van Huffel S, Bourne T, Timmerman D. Acoustic streaming cannot discriminate reliably between endometriomas and other types of adnexal lesion: a multicenter study of 633 adnexal masses. Ultrasound Obstet Gynecol. 2010;35:349–53.
19. Guerriero S, Ajossa S, Garau N, Alcazar JL, Mais V, Melis GB. Diagnosis of pelvic adhesions in patients with endometrioma: the role of transvaginal ultrasonography. Fertil Steril. 2010;94:742–6.
20. Guerriero S, Ajossa S, Gerada M, Virgilio B, Angioni S, Melis GB. Diagnostic value of transvaginal 'tenderness-guided' ultrasonography for the prediction of location of deep endometriosis. Hum Reprod. 2008;23:2452–7.
21. Guerriero S, Van Calster B, Somigliana E, Ajossa S, Froyman W, De Cock B, Coosemans A, Fischerová D, Van Holsbeke C, Alcazar JL, Testa AC, Valentin L, Bourne T, Timmerman D. Age-related differences in the sonographic characteristics of endometriomas. Hum Reprod. 2016;31:1723–31.
22. Mascilini F, Moruzzi C, Giansiracusa C, Guastafierro F, Savelli L, De Meis L, Epstein E, Timor-Tritsch IE, Mailath-Pokorny M, Ercoli A, Exacoustos C, Benacerraf BR, Valentin L, Testa AC. Imaging in gynecological disease. 10: Clinical and ultrasound characteristics of decidualized endometriomas surgically removed during pregnancy. Ultrasound Obstet Gynecol. 2014;44:354–60.
23. Groszmann Y, Howitt BE, Bromley B, Feltmate CM, Benacerraf BR. Decidualized endometrioma masquerading as ovarian cancer in pregnancy. J Ultrasound Med. 2014;33:1909–15.
24. Guerriero S, Ajossa S, Piras S, Parodo G, Melis GB. Serial ultrasonographic evaluation of a decidualized endometrioma in pregnancy. Ultrasound Obstet Gynecol. 2005;26:304–6.
25. Kim HS, Kim TH, Chung HH, Song YS. Risk and prognosis of ovarian cancer in women with endometriosis: a meta-analysis. Br J Cancer. 2014;110:1878–90.
26. Testa AC, Timmerman D, Van Holsbeke C, Zannoni GF, Fransis S, Moerman P, Vellone V, Mascilini F, Licameli A, Ludovisi M, Di Legge A, Scambia G, Ferrandina G. Ovarian cancer arising in endometrioid cysts: ultrasound findings. Ultrasound Obstet Gynecol. 2011;38:99–106.
27. Moore J, Copley S, Morris J, Lindsell D, Golding S, Kennedy S. A systematic review of the accuracy of ultrasound in the diagnosis of endometriosis. Ultrasound Obstet Gynecol. 2002;20:630–4.
28. Guerriero S, Alcazar JL, Pascual MA, Ajossa S, Gerada M, Bargellini R, Virgilio B, Melis GB. Diagnosis of the most frequent benign ovarian cysts: is ultrasonography accurate and reproducible? J Womens Health (Larchmt). 2009;18:519–27.
29. Alcázar JL, Laparte C, Jurado M, López-García G. The role of transvaginal ultrasonography combined with color velocity imaging and pulsed Doppler in the diagnosis of endometrioma. Fertil Steril. 1997;67:487–91.
30. Guerriero S, Ajossa S, Mais V, Risalvato A, Lai MP, Melis GB. The diagnosis of endometriomas using colour Doppler energy imaging. Hum Reprod. 1998;13:1691–5.
31. Alcázar JL. Transvaginal colour Doppler in patients with ovarian endometriomas and pelvic pain. Hum Reprod. 2001;16:2672–5.
32. Alcázar JL, García-Manero M. Ovarian endometrioma vascularization in women with pelvic pain. Fertil Steril. 2007;87(6):1271.
33. Seckin B, Oruc AS, Turkcapar F, Ugur M. The relation of pelvic pain and dense adhesions to Doppler ultrasound findings in patients with ovarian endometriomas. Arch Gynecol Obstet. 2013;287:723–8.
34. Alcázar JL, León M, Galván R, Guerriero S. Assessment of cyst content using mean gray value for discriminating endometrioma from other unilocular cysts in premenopausal women. Ultrasound Obstet Gynecol. 2010;35:228–32.
35. Huang CY, Wang HI, Wang PH, Wu YC, Yang MJ, Chen LH, Chao KC, Chen CY. Mean grey value is lower in endometriomas: differentiating a hypoechogenic adnexal cyst by 3-dimensional power Doppler ultrasound--a preliminary study. J Chin Med Assoc. 2011;74:75–80.

6 Soft Marker Evaluation

Shannon Reid

6.1 Update on Soft Markers

Transvaginal sonography (TVS) soft markers for endometriosis include ovarian immobility and site-specific tenderness (SST). In the recently published consensus statement entitled 'Systematic approach to sonographic evaluation of the pelvis in women with suspected endometriosis, including terms, definitions and measurements: a consensus opinion from the International Deep Endometriosis Analysis (IDEA)', the evaluation of soft markers is recommended as a component of the ultrasound evaluation of women with suspected pelvic deep endometriosis (DE) [1].

6.2 Ovarian Mobility

The relationship between ovarian immobility at TVS and the presence of peri-ovarian adhesions at laparoscopy has been demonstrated in women investigated for symptoms such as chronic pelvic pain (CPP), infertility, and/or endometriosis [2, 3]. The most common sites for ovarian adhesions to form are with the neighbouring uterus (Fig. 6.1) or pelvic sidewall; however, the bowel and uterosacral ligaments (USL) can also be involved. Okaro et al. found that preoperative TVS 'soft markers' (i.e. site-specific tenderness, reduced ovarian mobility) and 'hard markers' (i.e. endometrioma, hydrosalpinx) in women with a history of CPP correlated with the presence or absence of disease at laparoscopy [4]. Pre-operative TVS and transrectal ultrasound have also been used to predict endometriosis stage (including pelvic adhesions) at

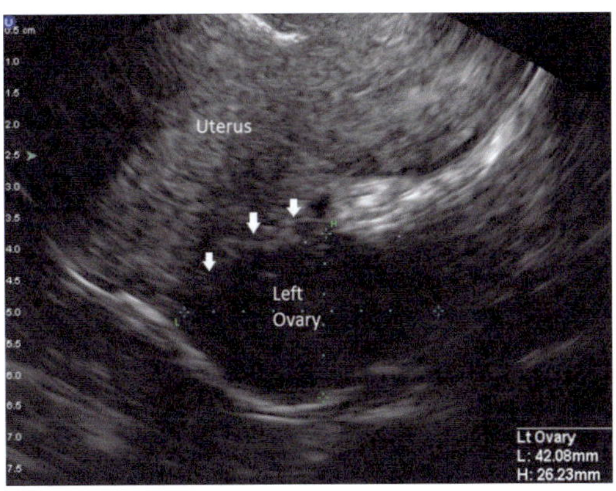

Fig. 6.1 Transvaginal sonography (TVS) image in the sagittal plane, displaying the left ovary fixed to the posterior uterine fundus; the white arrows indicate the adhesion site. The ovarian sliding sign was negative in this region during the TVS assessment, i.e. the left ovary did not glide smoothly across the posterior uterine fundus

Electronic Supplementary Material The online version of this chapter (https://doi.org/10.1007/978-3-319-71138-6_6) contains supplementary material, which is available to authorized users.

S. Reid
Department of Obstetrics and Gynaecology, Liverpool Hospital, Sydney, NSW, Australia

S. Guerriero et al. (eds.), *How to Perform Ultrasonography in Endometriosis*, https://doi.org/10.1007/978-3-319-71138-6_6

laparoscopy, with a sensitivity and specificity of 86% and 82%, respectively, for Stage III and 76% and 91%, respectively, for Stage IV disease [5].

In a recent study by Marasinghe et al., the combination of ovarian immobility and clinical findings (i.e. dyspareunia, dysmenorrhea and vaginal examination) was able to demonstrate a sensitivity/specificity of 92%/61% for the detection of endometriosis at laparoscopy [6]. More specifically, ovarian immobility at TVS is strongly associated with the presence of endometrioma [2, 7] and POD obliteration [8]. The identification of ovarian immobility at TVS may improve our ability to stage endometriosis severity preoperatively, allowing for improved surgical planning.

The diagnostic accuracy of ovarian immobility at TVS has been reported in previous studies, usually in the presence of endometriomas. In a study by Guerriero et al., women undergoing surgery for endometrioma were assessed for ovarian mobility in relation to the uterus. The sensitivity and specificity of the fixation to the uterus of at least one ovary were, respectively, 89% and 90% [2]. Holland et al. also evaluated TVS accuracy for ovarian adhesions in women with proven/suspected endometriosis by classifying adhesions as minimal, moderate or severe in accordance with the rASRM classification. For severe ovarian adhesions, the sensitivity and specificity of TVS was 83.5% and 93.5%, respectively. In another study by our group, ovarian immobility was assessed as a sonographic 'soft marker' of DE and was found to perform better in the presence of endometriomas compared with normal ovaries [7].

6.3 Site-Specific Tenderness (SST)

A relationship between SST at TVS and endometriosis at laparoscopy has also been demonstrated in previous studies. In a study that evaluated tenderness during a combination of vaginal and TVS examination, Yong et al. found that SST may be helpful in predicting abnormal laparoscopy and the presence of superficial endometriosis; however, the specificity of this study was low (22%), indicating a high false-positive rate [9]. This study did not find SST was predictive of superficial endometriosis location.

With regard to posterior compartment DE, some studies have found that tenderness-guided TVS may aid in the prediction of specific locations of posterior compartment DE [10, 11]. A recent study from our group showed that TV probe tenderness in the posterior pelvic compartment (left USL, POD and right USL) was significantly associated with both deep and superficial endometrioses in the posterior pelvic compartment ($p < 0.05$) [12]. SST appears to be a useful soft marker for the prediction of the presence/absence of endometriosis at laparoscopy [4, 9] and should be included in the sonographic evaluation of the pelvis in women with suspected endometriosis [1].

6.4 How We Do It

6.4.1 Assessment of Ovarian Mobility

In order to assess for ovarian mobility, the examiner places gentle pressure with TV probe toward the ovary of interest in order to mobilize the ovary. The examiner assesses whether the ovary glides freely along (1) the corresponding pelvic sidewall and (2) the neighbouring uterine surface. This is the same concept that is applied to the assessment of the POD for obliteration using the uterine sliding sign, where a negative sliding sign indicates adhesions are present causing limited mobility [13, 14]. Ovarian mobility is assessed in both the sagittal and transverse planes for each location (i.e. pelvic sidewall and uterine surface). If the ovary glides smoothly along the surface of the uterus and pelvic sidewall, the ovarian sliding sign is considered positive and the ovary is recorded as mobile in these regions. Video 6.1 displays a mobile right ovary (positive ovarian sliding sign) along the right pelvic sidewall, in the transverse plane. Video 6.2 displays ovarian mobility along the lateral uterus (positive ovarian sliding sign), as well as the pelvic sidewall, in the transverse plane.

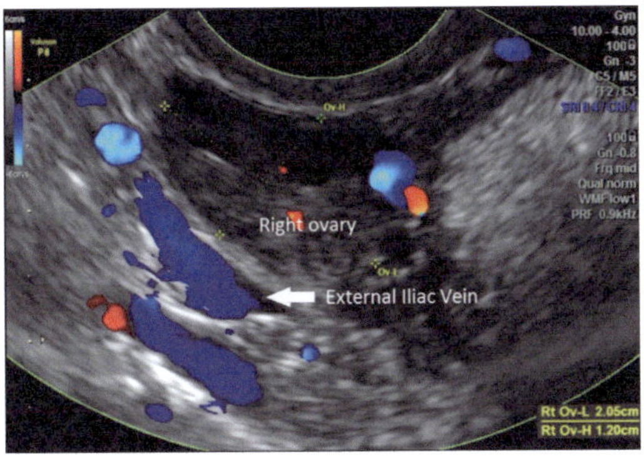

Fig. 6.2 A transvaginal sonography image in the sagittal plane demonstrating the location of the right ovary in relation to the right external iliac vein

When assessing ovarian mobility along the pelvic sidewall, colour Doppler may be used to visualize the external iliac vessels and to confirm the location of the pelvic sidewall in relation to the corresponding ovary (Fig. 6.2). By directing pressure in the region of the ovary with the TV probe, a mobile ovary will glide freely along the external iliac vessels. If the ovary is not well mobilized with the pressure from the TV probe alone, the examiner can place gentle downward pressure with the left hand (if the TV probe is being held in the right hand) over the iliac fossa region of the lower anterior abdominal wall to mobilize the ovary. If the ovary does not glide freely against the pelvic sidewall, this indicates a negative ovarian sliding sign, and the ovary is recorded as immobile or fixed in this region. Video 6.3 demonstrates ovarian fixation (negative sliding sign) at both the posterior uterus and left pelvic sidewall, in the sagittal plane. Video 6.4 demonstrates a negative ovarian sliding sign between the left ovary and the posterior uterine cervix, in the sagittal plane.

Whenever the ovarian sliding sign is negative, the examiner should then assess for the nature of the adhesion limiting ovarian mobility. In addition to adhesions between the ovary and pelvic sidewall/uterus, ovarian mobility can be limited by adhesions between the ovary and the contralateral ovary, fallopian tube, USL, POD and/or bowel.

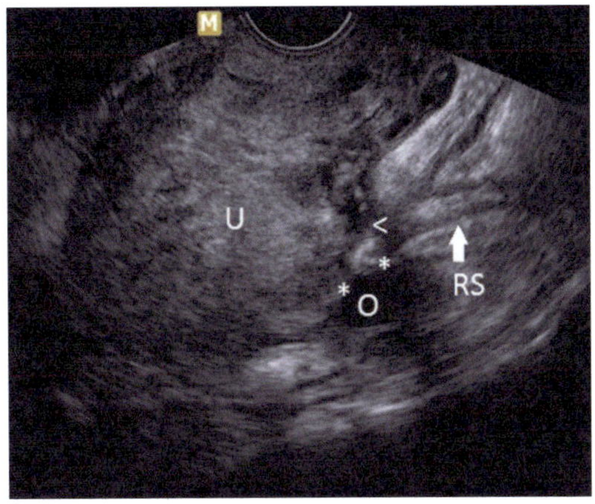

Fig. 6.3 A transvaginal sonography (TVS) image (in the sagittal plane) demonstrating an anteverted, retroflexed uterus (U). The rectosigmoid bowel (RS) is adherent posteriorly to the uterine fundus (indicated by <), causing POD obliteration. The ovary (O) is adherent posteriorly to the uterine fundus and to the rectosigmoid bowel (indicated by asterisk)

Figure 6.3 demonstrates adhesions between the ovary and posterior uterus, as well as the rectosigmoid bowel.

6.4.2 Assessment of SST

The assessment of SST during the TVS examination involves the examiner placing gentle pressure with the TV probe against each of the following six pelvic locations: anterior fornix, right adnexa, left adnexa, right USL, left USL and posterior vaginal fornix. A verbal numerical rating scale (NRS) is often used to assess for SST. Women rate their pain score on a scale from 0 (no pain) to 10 (worst pain imaginable) for each of the six locations.

6.4.3 Important Technical Tips

1. If the examiner is not able to mobilize the ovary with the TV probe alone, the left hand can be used to place downward pressure over the iliac fossa region to mobilize the ovary of interest.

2. The external iliac vessels can be used to help orientate the examiner to the pelvic sidewall when assessing ovarian mobility in this region. The colour Doppler function is used to confirm the location of the external iliac vessels.
3. The ovaries can be difficult to locate in the presence of complex endometriotic disease, as the anatomy can be severely distorted. Try to be systematic in the assessment of each ovary, carefully identifying each structure that is adherent to the ovary. These difficult scans take more time to perform as several structures may be involved, particularly in the presence of endometriomas.
4. The addition of ultrasound gel (15–20 ml) in the posterior vaginal fornix (i.e. sonovaginography) may improve the view of the structures in the posterior pelvic compartment, thereby helping the examiner to identify structures that are associated with ovarian adhesions.

6.4.4 Future Directions

The incorporation of soft markers such as ovarian mobility and SST into a standardized TVS assessment for women with pelvic pain may allow for improved surgical planning and counselling for these women. Further studies are required to evaluate the usefulness of soft markers for the prediction of endometriosis type and location. In particular, the use of soft markers to predict superficial endometriosis location could allow for improved surgical planning for women undergoing laparoscopy. This is particularly relevant for women with superficial pelvic sidewall disease overlying the ureter, as ureterolysis is an advanced laparoscopic skill that is not typically performed by general gynaecologists. If the prediction of pelvic sidewall disease at laparoscopy could be improved using preoperative TVS soft markers, then these women could be referred to an advanced laparoscopic surgeon from the outset. This may negate the need for two laparoscopies, one by a generalist who is unable to excise the disease and followed by a second laparoscopy by an advanced laparoscopic surgeon who is able to excise the disease.

In a recent study by our group, ovarian mobility and SST were included in the evaluation of an ultrasound-based endometriosis staging system (UBESS) for the prediction of level of complexity of laparoscopic surgery for endometriosis. The accuracy, sensitivity, specificity and positive and negative predictive values of UBESS I for predicting a requirement for Level 1 laparoscopic surgery were 87.5%, 83.3%, 91.7%, 90.9% and 84.6%; those of UBESS II for predicting Level 2 surgery were 87.0%, 73.7%, 90.3%, 65.1% and 93.3%; and those of UBESS III for predicting Level 3 surgery were 95.3%, 94.8%, 95.5%, 90.2% and 97.7%, respectively. This study demonstrated that UBESS has the potential to facilitate the triage of women with suspected endometriosis to the most appropriate surgical expertise required for laparoscopic endometriosis surgery [12]. External validation of UBESS is currently being performed to determine the applicability of this system for planning laparoscopic endometriosis surgery.

References

1. Guerriero S, Condous G, Van den Bosch T, Valentin L, Leone F, Van Schoubroeck D, Exacoustos C, Installé AJF, Martins WP, Abrao MS, Hudelist G, Bazot M, Alcazar J, Gonçalves MO, Pascual MA, Ajossa S, Savelli L, Dunham R, Reid S, Menakaya U, Bourne T, Ferrero S, Leon M, Bignardi T, Holland T, Jurkovic D, Benacerraf B, Osuga Y, Somigliana E, Timmerman D. Systematic approach to evaluate the pelvis in women with suspected endometriosis including terms, definitions and measurements to describe the sonographic features of deep infiltrating endometriosis: a consensus opinion from the International Deep Endometriosis Analysis (IDEA) group. Ultrasound Obstet Gynecol. 2016;48(3):318–32. Epub 2016/06/28.
2. Guerriero S, Ajossa S, Garau N, Alcazar JL, Mais V, Melis GB. Diagnosis of pelvic adhesions in patients with endometrioma: the role of transvaginal ultrasonography. Fertil Steril. 2010;94(2):742–6. Epub 2009/04/17
3. Guerriero S, Ajossa S, Lai MP, Mais V, Paoletti AM, Melis GB. Transvaginal ultrasonography in the diagnosis of pelvic adhesions. Hum Reprod. 1997;12(12):2649–53. Epub 1998/02/10
4. Okaro E, Condous G, Khalid A, Timmerman D, Ameye L, Huffel SV, et al. The use of ultrasound-based 'soft markers' for the prediction of pelvic pathology in women with chronic pelvic pain--can we reduce the need for laparoscopy? BJOG. 2006;113(3):251–6.

5. Exacoustos C, Zupi E, Carusotti C, Rinaldo D, Marconi D, Lanzi G, et al. Staging of pelvic endometriosis: role of sonographic appearance in determining extension of disease and modulating surgical approach. J Am Assoc Gynecol Laparosc. 2003;10(3):378–82. Epub 2003/10/22
6. Marasinghe JP, Senanayake H, Saravanabhava N, Arambepola C, Condous G, Greenwood P. History, pelvic examination findings and mobility of ovaries as a sonographic marker to detect pelvic adhesions with fixed ovaries. J Obstet Gynaecol Res. 2014;40(3):785–90. Epub 2014/04/17
7. Gerges BLC, Reid S, Menakaya U, Nadim B, Condous G. "Soft marker" evaluation of ovarian mobility in the normal and endometriotic ovary. Ultrasound Obstet Gynecol. 2015. https://doi.org/10.1002/uog.15990.
8. Reid S, Lu C, Condous G. Can we improve the prediction of pouch of Douglas obliteration in women with suspected endometriosis using ultrasound-based models? A multicenter prospective observational study. Acta Obstet Gynecol Scand. 2015;94(12):1297–306. Epub 2015/09/25
9. Yong PJ, Sutton C, Suen M, Williams C. Endovaginal ultrasound-assisted pain mapping in endometriosis and chronic pelvic pain. J Obstet Gynaecol. 2013;33(7):715–9. Epub 2013/10/17
10. Guerriero S, Ajossa S, Gerada M, D'Aquila M, Piras B, Melis GB. "Tenderness-guided" transvaginal ultrasonography: a new method for the detection of deep endometriosis in patients with chronic pelvic pain. Fertil Steril. 2007;88(5):1293–7.
11. Saba L, Guerriero S, Sulcis R, Pilloni M, Ajossa S, Melis G, et al. MRI and "tenderness guided" transvaginal ultrasonography in the diagnosis of rectosigmoid endometriosis. J Magn Reson Imaging. 2012;35(2):352–60. Epub 2011/10/29
12. Menakaya U, Reid S, Lu C, Gerges B, Infante F, Condous G. Performance of an Ultrasound Based Endometriosis Staging System (UBESS) for predicting the level of complexity of laparoscopic surgery for endometriosis. Ultrasound Obstet Gynecol. 2016;48(6):786–95. Epub 2016/01/15
13. Holland TK, Yazbek J, Cutner A, Saridogan E, Hoo WL, Jurkovic D. Value of transvaginal ultrasound in assessing severity of pelvic endometriosis. Ultrasound Obstet Gynecol. 2010;36(2):241–8.
14. Reid S, Winder S, Reid G, Condous G. Can we predict pouch of Douglas (POD) obliteration using a new real-time ultrasound technique: the "sliding sign". 21st World Congress on Ultrasound in Obstetrics and Gynecology. Los Angeles: Wiley-Blackwell; 2011. p. 1–55.

7 Ultrasound in the Evaluation of Pouch of Douglas Obliteration

Shannon Reid

7.1 Introduction

The pouch of Douglas (POD) is described as the region of peritoneum which occupies the deepest part of the female pelvis and is located between the lower posterior cervix and the anterior rectum. Complete POD obliteration is described when this area of peritoneum between the posterior cervix and anterior rectum is no longer visible due to adhesions or scarring in the POD. POD obliteration is most commonly associated with adhesions between the anterior rectum and posterior cervix and/or between the rectosigmoid bowel and posterior uterine fundus. Figure 7.1 displays examples of POD obliteration due to rectal/rectosigmoid deep endometriosis (DE) adhesions to the posterior cervix/uterine fundus. These adhesions in the POD are often caused by an underlying DE nodule, but may also be caused by scarring in the POD from pelvic inflammatory disease, previous surgery, or extensive ovarian/peritoneal endometriosis. Adhesions may also form unilaterally in the POD, between a structure containing a DE nodule and adjacent structure(s) (i.e., uterosacral ligament (USL) and anterior rectum). In this case, a portion of the POD may remain visible (i.e., contain normal peritoneum), and this situation is known as partial or unilateral POD obliteration.

Women with POD obliteration at laparoscopy have a threefold increased risk of rectal DE (and the need for rectal surgery) compared to women without POD obliteration at laparoscopy [1]. As with bowel DE, the surgical treatment of POD obliteration requires the skill of an advanced laparoscopic surgeon and potential colorectal input at the time of surgery. In addition to posterior compartment DE, ovarian endometrioma and ovarian immobility at TVS are also significantly associated POD obliteration at laparoscopy [2].

Studies have demonstrated that POD obliteration can be detected preoperatively with a several imaging techniques, including transvaginal sonography (TVS), computed tomography, and magnetic resonance imaging (MRI). A recent systematic review and meta-analysis assessed the accuracy of various imaging techniques for POD obliteration and found the sensitivity/specificity for TVS and MRI to be 87%/96% and 84%/93%, respectively [3]. During TVS, the POD is assessed for obliteration/utero-rectal adhesions using the uterine "sliding sign" technique [4]. TVS is recommended as the first-line imaging technique for POD obliteration due to its high accuracy, low cost, and minimal patient discomfort.

Electronic Supplementary Material The online version of this chapter (https://doi.org/10.1007/978-3-319-71138-6_7) contains supplementary material, which is available to authorized users.

S. Reid
Department of Obstetrics and Gynaecology, Liverpool Hospital, Sydney, NSW, Australia

S. Guerriero et al. (eds.), *How to Perform Ultrasonography in Endometriosis*, https://doi.org/10.1007/978-3-319-71138-6_7

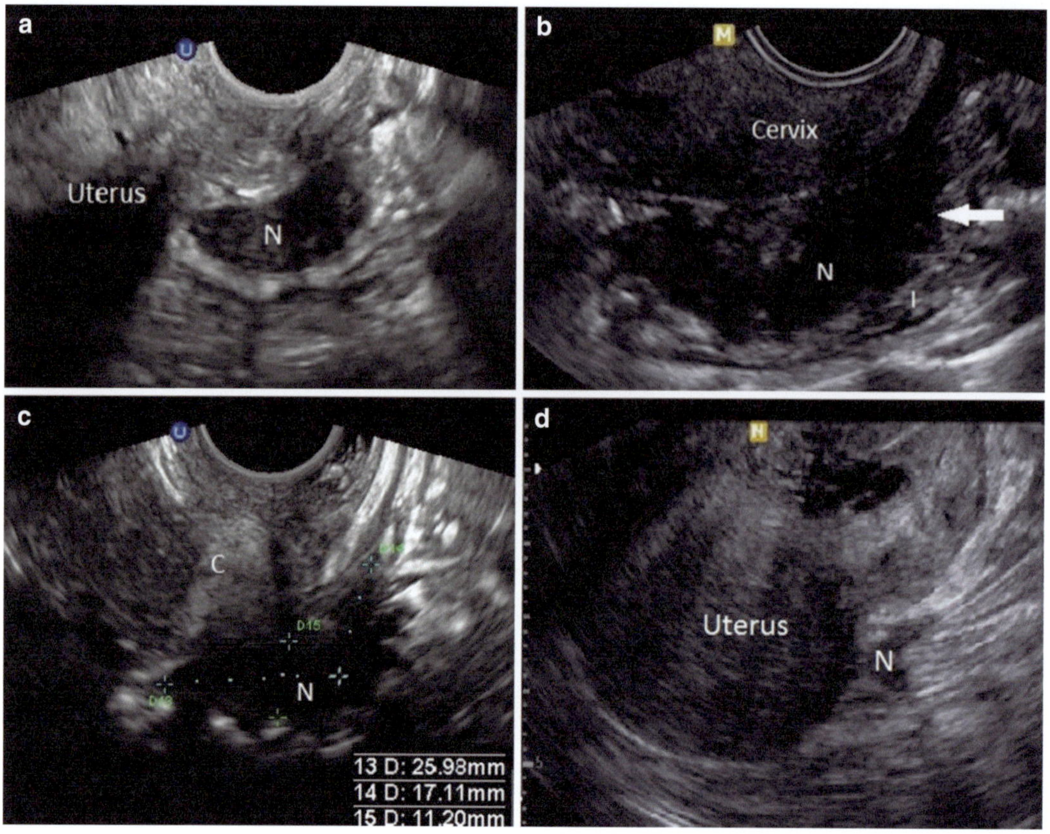

Fig. 7.1 Examples of complete POD obliteration at transvaginal ultrasound (sagittal plane). (**a**) The anterior rectum contains a DE nodule (N) and is adherent posteriorly to the uterine cervix. (**b**) The anterior rectum/rectosigmoid bowel contains a DE nodule (N) that forms an adhesion from the level of the posterior cervix to the posterior uterine fundus. (**c**) The anterior rectum contains a DE nodule (N) that infiltrates the posterior cervix (C) and rectovaginal septum posteriorly. (**d**) The rectosigmoid bowel contains a DE nodule (N) that is adherent to the posterior uterine fundus

Given the strong relationship between POD obliteration and ovarian endometrioma/posterior compartment DE, our group developed and validated two mathematical TVS models to determine whether a combination of TVS markers could improve the prediction of POD obliteration as compared with the uterine "sliding sign" alone. These models included TVS findings such as posterior compartment DE, ovarian fixation, and ovarian endometrioma, in addition to a negative uterine "sliding sign." This study found that the incorporation of additional TVS markers did not improve the prediction of POD obliteration as compared to the "sliding sign" alone [2].

The "sliding sign" has also been demonstrated to have substantial to almost perfect inter- and intra-observer agreement among sonologists/sonographers experienced in gynecological ultrasound [5] and is an easily learned technique for those with previous experience in gynecological ultrasound. Tammaa et al. determined the learning curve to be ~40 scans in order to achieve competency in predicting POD obliteration using the uterine "sliding sign" [6]. Another study found similar results, with 38 scans required to reach competency for prediction of POD obliteration using the "sliding sign" [7].

7.2 How We Do It

7.2.1 The Uterine "Sliding Sign"

In order to perform the uterine "sliding sign," the transvaginal (TV) probe (held in the right hand) is inserted into the posterior vaginal fornix, and gentle pressure is placed against the posterior cervix with the probe. In a normal pelvis (i.e., no POD obliteration), this maneuver mobilizes the posterior cervix, causing the anterior rectum to glide smoothly along the posterior vaginal wall/posterior cervix; this is termed a positive "sliding sign" (Video 7.1a). Next, the examiner places the other hand (left hand) over the lower anterior abdominal wall and gently places downward pressure to ballot the uterine fundus. If the rectosigmoid bowel glides smoothly along the posterior uterine fundus, the "sliding sign" is considered positive for this region (Video 7.1b). If the "sliding sign" is positive in both locations (i.e., posterior cervix and posterior uterine fundus), the POD is considered not obliterated. If the "sliding sign" is negative in either location (i.e., the anterior rectum does not glide smoothly against the posterior cervix or the rectosigmoid does not glide smoothly across the posterior uterine fundus), the POD is deemed obliterated. Video 7.2a demonstrates POD obliteration at the level of the cervix, and Video 7.2b demonstrates POD obliteration at the level of the posterior uterine fundus.

The anatomical relationships are somewhat different for a retroverted uterus, and as such, the "sliding sign" technique is slightly modified. The TV probe (held in the right hand) is inserted into the posterior vaginal fornix, and gentle pressure is placed against the posterior uterine fundus. If the anterior rectum glides smoothly along the posterior uterine fundus, the "sliding sign" is considered positive (Video 7.3a). The examiner then places their left hand on the lower anterior abdominal wall to ballot the uterus to determine whether the rectosigmoid bowel glides smoothly along the anterior lower uterine segment. If the rectosigmoid bowel glides smoothly over the anterior lower uterus, the "sliding sign" is considered positive in this region (Video 7.3b). If the bowel does not glide smoothly in one or both of these locations (i.e., negative "sliding sign"), the POD is deemed obliterated.

7.2.2 Important Technical Tips

1. Prior to performing the uterine "sliding sign" procedure, it is important to ascertain whether the woman has a history of painful intercourse (dyspareunia). The "sliding sign" can be painful for women with dyspareunia, and women should be informed of the possibility of pain from this procedure.
2. Before performing the "sliding sign," ensure that the anterior rectum/rectosigmoid bowel are well visualized within the frame, as you will need to assess their mobility in real time, in relation to the posterior cervix and uterine fundus.
3. Partial (or unilateral) POD obliteration may occur. This is demonstrated at TVS when the anterior rectum/rectosigmoid glides smoothly along the posterior cervix/uterus on one side of the pelvis, but not the other. This finding suggests adhesions exist between the bowel and the corresponding uterosacral ligament, pararectal space, and/or lateral posterior cervix.
4. A negative "sliding sign" carries a high risk for associated posterior compartment DE. A thorough ultrasound assessment for DE lesions, especially for DE involving the rectum/rectosigmoid, should be performed if the POD is obliterated at TVS.

7.3 Future Perspectives

POD obliteration is associated with complex surgery that requires advanced laparoscopic skills, longer operating times, and the possible need for colorectal input. Given the significant relationship between rectal DE and POD obliteration, a negative uterine "sliding sign" is an important red flag for the increased risk of bowel DE [8]. The ability to predict POD obliteration preoperatively is therefore essential for appropriate specialist referral, surgical planning, and counseling for these high-risk women.

As recommended in the recent consensus statement by the International Deep Endometriosis Analysis group [9], women with pelvic pain/suspected endometriosis, should ideally undergo a standardized TVS examination for pelvic DE, including assessment for POD obliteration with the uterine "sliding sign." Although the "sliding sign" has a high accuracy for the prediction of POD obliteration and is an easily learned technique, very few ultrasound centers currently perform an assessment for POD obliteration. Future gynecological ultrasound training programs will benefit from the integration of this important technique into their curriculum for the ultrasound assessment of women with suspected endometriosis.

References

1. Khong SY, Bignardi T, Luscombe G, Lam A. Is pouch of Douglas obliteration a marker of bowel endometriosis? J Minim Invasive Gynecol. 2011;18(3):333–7.
2. Reid S, Lu C, Condous G. Can we improve the prediction of pouch of Douglas obliteration in women with suspected endometriosis using ultrasound based models? A multicenter prospective observational study. Acta Obstet Gynecol Scand. 2015;94(12):1297–306.
3. Shakeri B, Nadim B, Reid S, Martins WP Condous G OP34.04: Accuracy of different imaging techniques to assess POD obliteration: a systematic review and meta-analysis. In: Gynecol UO, editor. 26th World Congress on Ultrasound in Obstetrics and Gynaecology; September 2016; Rome. 2016. p. 165.
4. Reid S, Lu C, Casikar I, Reid G, Abbott J, Cario G, et al. Prediction of pouch of Douglas obliteration in women with suspected endometriosis using a new real-time dynamic transvaginal ultrasound technique: the sliding sign. Ultrasound Obstet Gynecol. 2013;41(6):685–91. Epub 2012/09/25
5. Reid S, Lu C, Casikar I, Mein B, Magotti R, Ludlow J, et al. The prediction of pouch of Douglas obliteration using offline analysis of the transvaginal ultrasound 'sliding sign' technique: inter- and intra-observer reproducibility. Hum Reprod. 2013.; Epub 2013/03/14
6. Tammaa A, Fritzer N, Strunk G, Krell A, Salzer H, Hudelist G. Learning curve for the detection of pouch of Douglas obliteration and deep infiltrating endometriosis of the rectum. Hum Reprod. 2014;29(6):1199–204. Epub 2014/04/30
7. Piessens S, Healey M, Maher P, Tsaltas J, Rombauts L. Can anyone screen for deep infiltrating endometriosis with transvaginal ultrasound? Aust N Z J Obstet Gynaecol. 2014;54(5):462–8. Epub 2014/10/08
8. Hudelist G, Fritzer N, Staettner S, Tammaa A, Tinelli A, Sparic R, et al. Uterine sliding sign: a simple sonographic predictor for presence of deep infiltrating endometriosis of the rectum. Ultrasound Obstet Gynecol. 2013;41(6):692–5. Epub 2013/02/13
9. Guerriero SCG, Van den Bosch T, Valentin L, Leone F, Van Schoubroeck D, Exacoustos C, AJF I, Martins WP, Abrao MS, Hudelist G, Bazot M, Alcazar J, Gonçalves MO, Pascual MA, Ajossa S, Savelli L, Dunham R, Reid S, Menakaya U, Bourne T, Ferrero S, Leon M, Bignardi T, Holland T, Jurkovic D, Benacerraf B, Osuga Y, Somigliana E, Timmerman D. Systematic approach to evaluate the pelvis in women with suspected endometriosis including terms, definitions and measurements to describe the sonographic features of deep infiltrating endometriosis: a consensus opinion from the International Deep Endometriosis Analysis (IDEA) group. Ultrasound Obstet Gynecol. 2016;48(3):318–32.

8 Anterior Compartment Including Ureter

Luca Savelli and Maria Cristina Scifo

8.1 Introduction

Endometriosis is usually classified into three main forms: ovarian, superficial, and deep endometriosis (DE). The latter is the most severe type of endometriosis and is defined as the presence of endometrial glands and stroma infiltrating a depth of >5 mm beneath the peritoneum [1, 2]. Implants of endometriosis may be supplied by the nerves and lymphatic and blood vessels and are surrounded by a variable amount of collagen fibers and elastin. Infiltration of the urinary tract occurs in approximately 1–2% of patients with endometriosis [3], but its prevalence increases to 19–53% among patients with severe endometriosis, as for those with DE [4–6].

DE can involve the anterior pelvic compartment (anatomical region anterior to the uterine corpus) including bladder and ureters or the posterior pelvic compartment (uterosacral ligaments, torus uterinus, rectum, pouch of Douglas, sigmoid colon) or both [7]. The expression of urinary tract endometriosis (UTE) is used to indicate anterior compartment endometriosis, but it comprises even the presence of endometriosis of the retrouterine portion of the ureter and the subsequent involvement of the kidneys, organs which lie posterior (dorsal) to the level of the uterine corpus. Notably, true bladder endometriosis is defined as the infiltration of the bladder muscularis propria [8] by endometrial glands and stroma, which can reach even the bladder mucosa, thus excluding the superficial endometriosis of the peritoneal layer covering the bladder dome. Overall, bladder involvement occurs in 70–85% of cases of UTE, while ureteral involvement is found in 25–30% of UTE cases [9].

The pathogenesis of UTE has not been clearly explained; several proposed hypotheses include migration, transplantation of endometrial glands and stroma, and the iatrogenic theory. It has been even proposed that UTE can develop from the presence of remnants of the Mullerian ducts, located in the vesicouterine space and vesicovaginal septum.

Once considered a rare pathological condition, bladder endometriosis is actually underdiagnosed due to nonspecific symptoms, often mimicking recurrent cystitis such as dysuria, urgency, frequency, suprapubic pain, vesical tenesmus, incontinence, and hematuria [2, 7]. These symptoms may worsen during menstruation, or may have a noncyclical presentation.

Electronic supplementary material The online version of this chapter (https://doi.org/10.1007/978-3-319-71138-6_8) contains supplementary material, which is available to authorized users.

L. Savelli (✉) · M. C. Scifo
Gynecology and Early Pregnancy Ultrasound Unit, Department of Obstetrics and Gynecology, S.Orsola-Malpighi Hospital, University of Bologna, Bologna, Italy
e-mail: luca.savelli@aosp.bo.it

S. Guerriero et al. (eds.), *How to Perform Ultrasonography in Endometriosis*, https://doi.org/10.1007/978-3-319-71138-6_8

Moreover, a variable percentage of patients with UTE are asymptomatic until a severe grade of anatomical distortion of affected organs is reached.

In particular ureteral endometriosis is more often asymptomatic and can lead to loss of renal function due top urinary flow obstruction [10]. In most of the cases, the disease affects the pelvic portion of the ureter [9], at the level of the cross with the uterine artery. Commonly, two different types of ureteral involvement are distinguished: extrinsic and intrinsic. The first is by far the most common (80% of the patients) and is due to the extension of a fibrotic reaction around a pelvic DE nodule which narrows the ureter causing a variable degree of stricture, thus limiting the passage of urine and eventually causing a dilated distal ureteric segment. The intrinsic form represents 20% of the cases and is defined as the presence of glands and endometrial stroma directly infiltrating the wall of the ureter: adventitia, muscularis propria, and intima may be infiltrated with subsequent anatomical and functional impairment.

As stated, a common feature in anterior compartment endometriosis is the nonspecific symptoms often leading to an insidious onset and progressive anatomical distortion of the affected structures which can lead to severe hydronephrosis (Fig. 8.1).

The percentage of patients with endometriosis and a hydronephrosis is actually not known, but its silent progression up to severe cases renders a

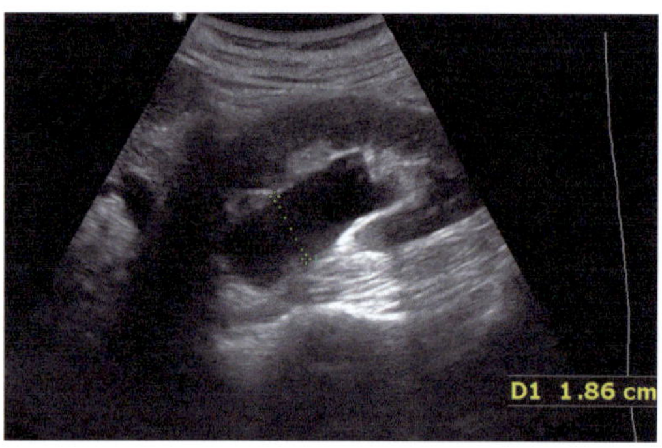

Fig. 8.1 Transabdominal scan of the right kidney stage II hydronephrosis. Both renal pelvis and calices appear anechoic. Sagittal scan shows obvious expansion of the renal pelvis (calipers) with no thinning of the renal cortex

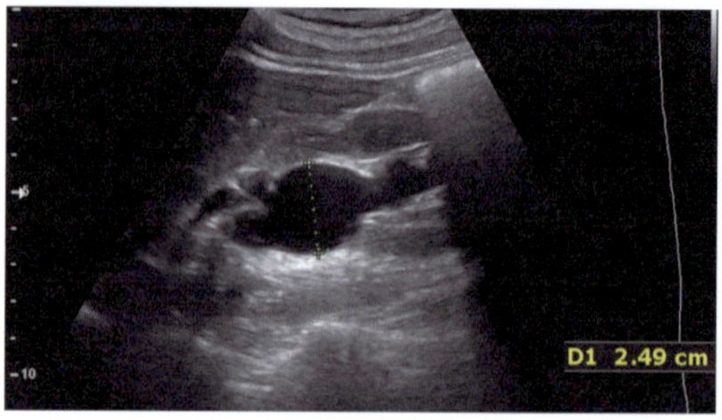

Fig. 8.2 Transabdominal scan of the cranial portion of the right ureter (same patient as in Fig. 8.1). Note the enlarged ureter (calipers) arising from the renal pelvis

thorough evaluation of the kidneys anatomy in patients with DE mandatory (Fig. 8.2). A high index of suspicion and an accurate assessment of the urinary tract are thus needed in patients with known or suspected pelvic endometriosis in order to avoid the progression of the disease, planning proper treatment, and eventually a complete surgical excision [11]; delayed or incomplete diagnosis can lead to increased morbidity and incorrect and inefficient treatment [7].

8.2 How We Do It

8.2.1 Urinary Bladder Endometriosis

Endometrial lesions may involve every part of the bladder; the most commonly affected portions are the bladder base and the dome, while the extra-abdominal bladder is rarely involved [12]. It has been proposed to divide the bladder into four zones: (a) the trigone, a smooth triangular region lying within 3 cm of the urethral opening and laterally delimited by the two ureteral orifices; (b) the bladder base, adjacent to the vagina and the supravaginal cervix; (c) the bladder dome, lying superior to the base; and (d) the extra-abdominal bladder (Fig. 8.3).

Symptoms of bladder endometriosis depend on the size and location of the nodule, the endocrine condition of the patient, and the effect of drugs assumed (such as contraceptive pills, progestins). As stated, one-third of patients remain asymptomatic or complain only minor complaints

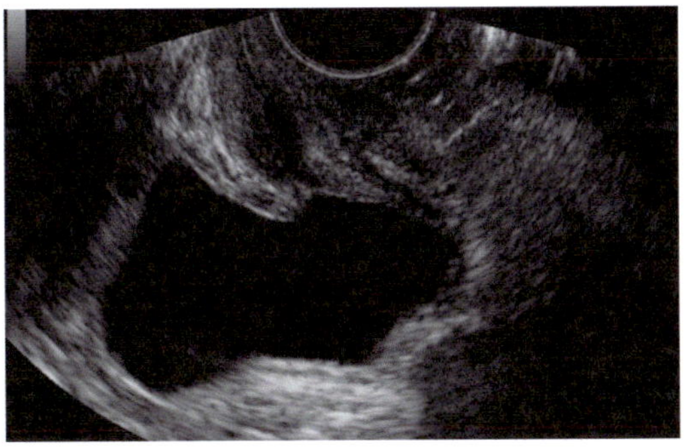

Fig. 8.3 Transvaginal longitudinal sonogram. By positioning the probe at the level of the anterior fornix, it is possible to visualize the entire bladder, moderately filled by urine. The urethra is easily identified, as a tubular sagittal structure directed downward. The trigonal zone starts at the level of the urethra up to 3 cm upward and is laterally delimited by the ureteral orifices. The bladder base faces backward and downward lies adjacent the supravaginal cervix. The bladder dome lies superior to the base and is intra-abdominal. The remaining portion is named "extra-abdominal bladder"

[13]. Symptomatic women refer a variable amount of symptoms including chronic pelvic pain, dysuria, urinary urgency and/or frequency, painful micturition, and discomfort in the retropubic area. Usually symptoms are recurrent and worsen in the peri-menstruation days. Hematuria is rare (20% of patients) because in a minor proportion of patients, the bladder mucosa is involved and penetrated by endometrial glands. Differential diagnoses should include overactive bladder, acute/chronic cystitis, and bladder cancer.

Diagnosis can be made incidentally at a pelvic examination performed due to infertility or pain symptoms or at a diagnostic imaging modality, but usually only large foci of DE are seen with any imaging technique but transvaginal ultrasound (TVS).

The accuracy of TVS performed by expert hands is high, but the sensitivity of the method is related to the size of the nodule, besides the experience of the operator [14]. Cystoscopy has been advocated as mandatory by some Authors [13] but may reveal only lesions protruding toward the lumen and infiltrating the bladder mucosa (which are a minority) or those producing hyperemia and distortion of the mucosa. Magnetic resonance imaging (MRI) has been proposed [11, 15, 16], but its diagnostic accuracy does not outperform that of TVS [17].

With any imaging modality, it is crucial to determine the size of the nodule involving the balder wall, the location, and the exact distance between the nodule and the internal ureteral orifices. In fact, the need for preoperative ureteral stent positioning, the surgical skills, and the technique needed (e.g., ureteral reimplantation requirement) depend on the sum of such information, together with the degree of symptoms.

Bladder endometriotic nodules can be seen at TVS as discrete solid hypoechoic lesions embedded in the bladder wall, altering the profile of the muscle layer. The most frequent sites involved are the posterior wall of the bladder, close to the vesicouterine pouch (Fig. 8.4), or the dome of the bladder (Fig. 8.5). This space is easily investigated if the bladder is distended by a small amount of urine; we therefore recommend asking patients not to empty their bladder before the sonographic examination. In fact, a *moderate* amount of urine, creating an anechoic acoustic window, facilitates the detection of nodules along the bladder wall.

The morphology of bladder endometriotic nodules is rather constant, either spherical or comma-shaped [14]; their borders are regular and can show a bright rim due to the presence of congested adipose tissue. At color/power Doppler, few blood vessels are seen within or around the nodule [14].

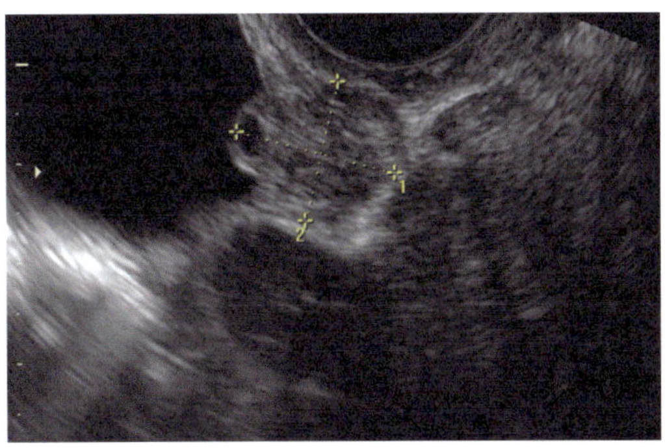

Fig. 8.4 Transvaginal scan of the bladder base (sagittal section) showing the presence of an endometriotic nodule at the level of the bladder base close to the trigonus (calipers). The nodule has blurred margins and continues with the muscle layer of the bladder (detrusor). Note the presence of a small anechoic area inside the nodule

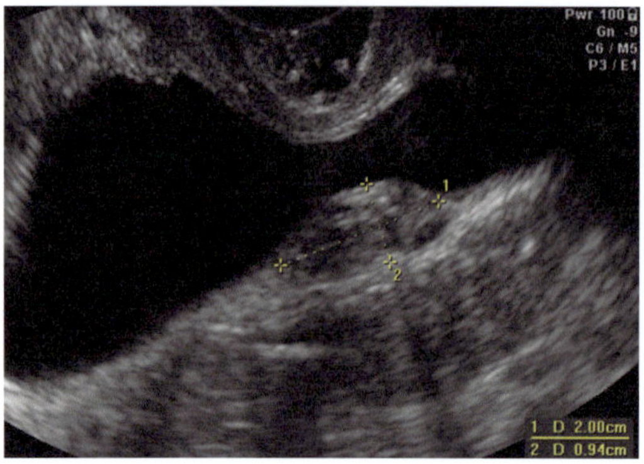

Fig. 8.5 Transvaginal scan of the bladder dome (sagittal section) showing the presence of an endometriotic nodule at this level (calipers). The nodule has a comma shape and is covered by a normal layer of bladder mucosa

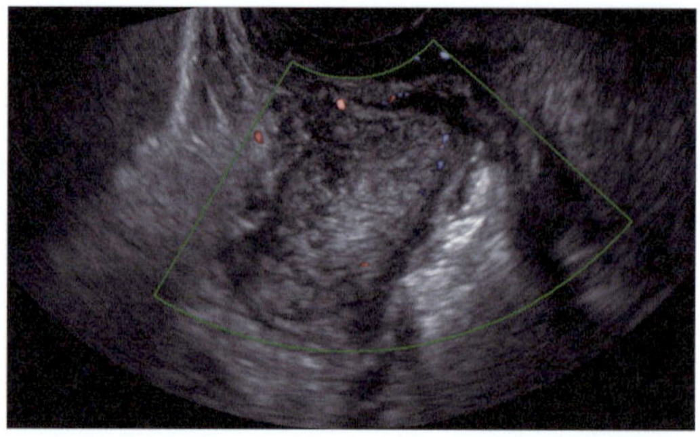

Fig. 8.6 Transvaginal scan of a patient with a bladder cancer. The neoplasm has filled the lumen of the bladder and appears as a bulky inhomogeneous mass with indistinct borders

The mean lesion diameter at TVS is usually lower than the diameter of the nodule measured at histologic examination [14] because the surgeon when removing the nodule must reach healthy margins of the bladder incised in order to obtain a good reconstruction (suture) of the bladder. In a series we recently reported, TVS showed a high overall accuracy of 95% in diagnosing bladder endometriosis, but the sensitivity is low for small nodules (<2 cm mean diameter). This is in agreement with a previous study by Bazot et al. [18] on a smaller number of cases. It is reasonable to think that the bigger the nodule, the easier the diagnosis; thus, both the physician performing the preoperative ultrasound and the surgeon managing the patient should be aware that small endometriotic nodules can be missed at TVS. We have the strong impression that implants forming a bulky nodule (either comma-shaped or spherical) are clearly detectable at TVS, while those forming a fibrous plaque along the bladder wall can be missed if the sliding of the cervix along the bladder is not systematically sought. In fact, as most nodules obliterate the vesicouterine space, and extend toward the anterior wall of the uterus, we suggest evaluating the sliding of the cervix along the bladder by gently pushing the vaginal probe while looking for the eventual presence of an endometriotic implant. The pain produced by pressing with the probe, due to the fibrosis and obliteration of the vesicouterine space, as well as the fixity of bladder and uterus, can be considered as a "soft markers" for bladder endometriosis.

Differential diagnosis with bladder cancer is mandatory: at TVS a neoplasm appears as a diffuse lesion invading the wall of the bladder and eventually leading to complete distortion of its anatomy (Fig. 8.6, AVI bladder cancer). Its outer border is ill-defined, and power Doppler may reveal an enhanced vascularization of the tumor compared to that of DE.

8.3 Ureteral Endometriosis

Endometriosis may affect one (80% of the cases) or both (20%) the ureters, being either intrinsic or extrinsic. The first type is the rarest (20% of the cases) and is due to the presence of glands and stroma directly infiltrating the ureteral wall. Extrinsic ureteral endometriosis is more common and is due to the distortion, narrowing of the ureteral lumen by the fibrotic retraction caused by a distant nodule, which may originate from the posterior pelvic compartment and extend laterally toward the parametrium, thus reaching the ureter (most frequently at the level of the uterine artery). These two pathological forms may coexist; moreover it is often impossible preoperatively to state which form of ureteral damage is present.

TVS coupled with transabdominal ultrasound (TAS) is accurate in diagnosing urinary tract involvement, and examination of the complete urinary tract should be considered an integral part of US assessment of women with suspected endometriosis. Unfortunately, ultrasound and every other imaging modality (Uro-CT, MRI, urography) have limited value in providing accurate information about the exact degree of ureteral wall infiltration [13] which might be evaluated only at surgery or at histopathologic examination. The ureters are tubular hypoechoic structures (Fig. 8.7) measuring 22–30 cm in length approximately divided in a pelvic and abdominal parts. The lumen is virtual and surrounded by transitional epithelium (mucosa), longitudinal and circular muscle layers, and outer fibrous tissue. Their course starts from the kidneys, dorsal to the renal artery, and continues caudally on the anterior edge of the psoas muscle until crossing the iliac vessels anteriorly. They are covered by the peritoneum of the pelvic side wall, behind the lateral attachment of the broad ligaments [19]. At this level they curve medially and forwards, crossing caudally the uterine arteries approximately 2 cm lateral and above the lateral fornices of the vagina. Then they reach the bladder base at the level of the upper angles of the trigone passing medially in front of the upper vagina with an oblique course. At ultrasound their function can be evaluated by visualizing the "ureteric jets," indicating normal patency (Fig. 8.8): color/power Doppler can help in visualizing the small amount of urine injected in the bladder lumen for a 1–4 s interval (AVI ureteral jet).

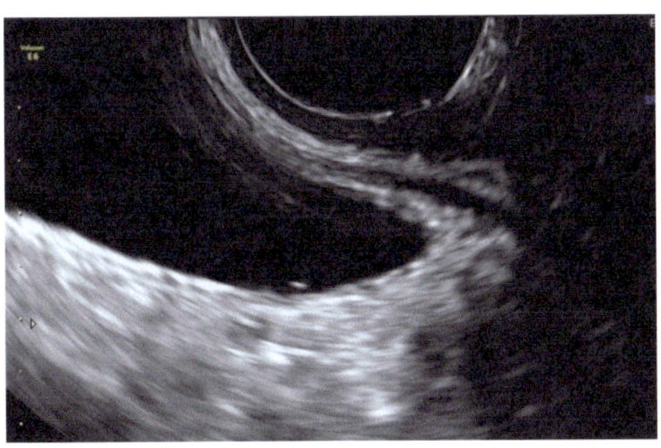

Fig. 8.7 Transvaginal scan of a left ureter (normal size) appearing as a tubular structure located besides the bladder wall. After waiting a sufficient length of time, it is possible to visualize normal peristaltic movements of the ureter

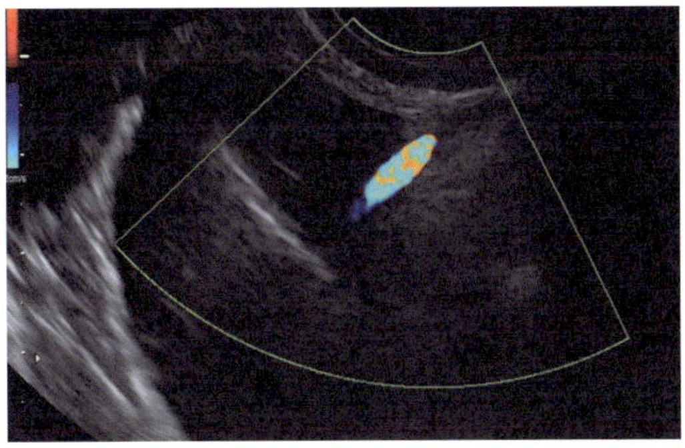

Fig. 8.8 Transvaginal scan of a filled bladder showing a ureteral jet. This appears as a colored flame pointing toward the ureteral orifice and lasting 1–3 s

The pelvic segment of normal ureters can be visualized, and their size can be measured at TVS. Starting from a longitudinal section of the urethra, the probe should be moved toward the pelvic side walls without tilting in order to visualize the distal portion of the ureter adjacent to the trigone (Fig. 8.7). Ureters can be visualized as hypoechoic tubular structures surrounded by a hyperechoic mantle running from the bladder wall toward the common iliac vessels [19]. Visualization of the ureters is possible in 96% of the patients after a handful of seconds and seems more difficult only in obese women and those with absent uteri most probably due to anatomical changes in their position. The mean diameter of the ureter is 1.7 mm at rest and 2.9 mm during peristalsis. A dilated ureter appears as a tubular structure with anechoic content and thick walls measuring >6 mm in diameter (Fig. 8.9). At TVS it is possible to visualize even the presence of a catheter, which is correctly positioned in the lumen of the ureter, as often is done before extensive laparoscopic ureterolysis (Fig. 8.10). One of the most common sites where the ureters are narrowed by DE is at the level of the cross with the uterine artery, lateral to the cervix. In fact a bulky endometriotic nodule, often originating from the pouch of Douglas, involving the uterosacral ligaments and the anterior wall of the rectum can extend laterally toward the parame-

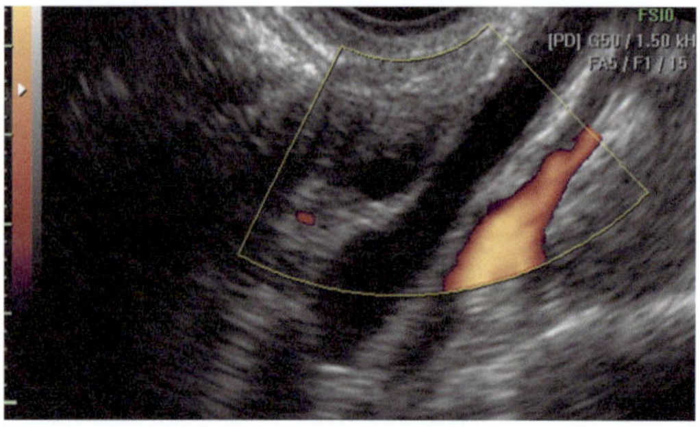

Fig. 8.9 Transvaginal scan of left pelvic sidewall showing a dilated ureter as a straight tubular structure with anechoic content. The ureter is delimited by a thick muscular wall, and this helps in differentiating with an iliac vessel. It is generally possible to visualize the peristalsis in the ureter by waiting for a few seconds. Moreover, Doppler helps in the differential diagnosis as the dilated ureter shows no blood flow inside

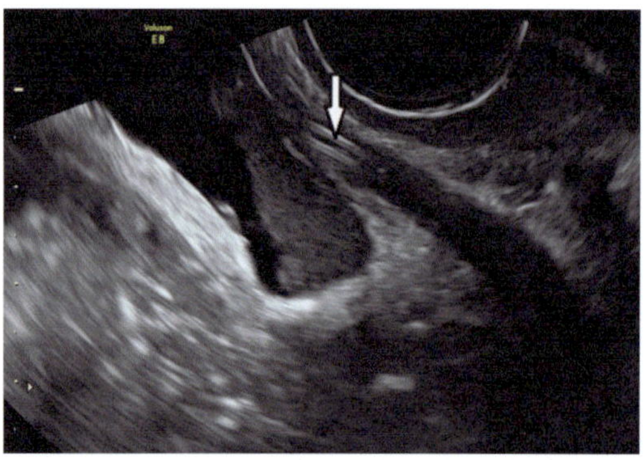

Fig. 8.10 Transvaginal scan of the bladder (parasagittal section) showing the first part of the ureter containing a catheter (arrow)

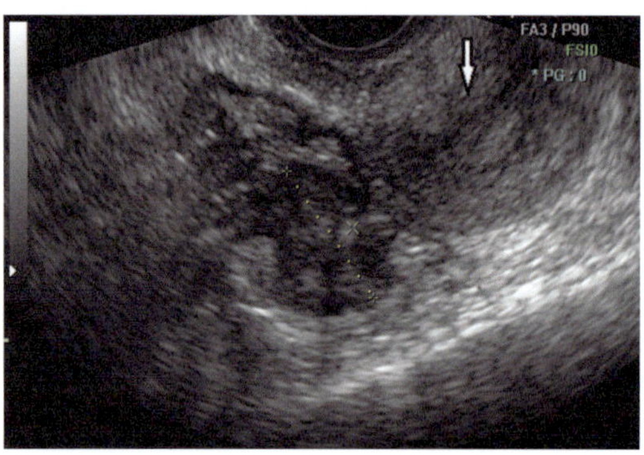

Fig. 8.11 Transvaginal scan (transverse section) of the cervix (arrow). Besides the cervix a bulky endometriotic nodule is seen at the level of the right parametrium

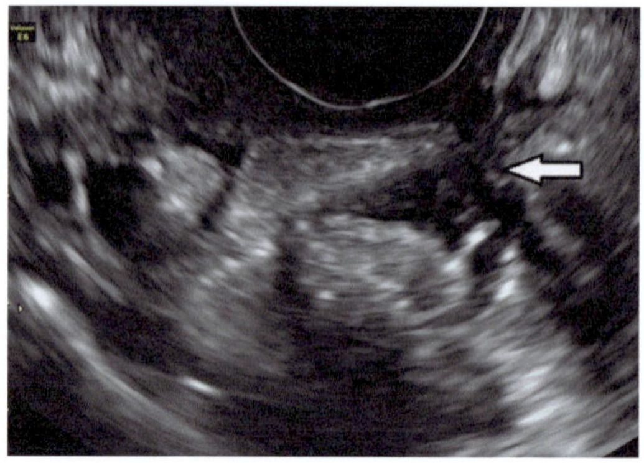

Fig. 8.12 Transvaginal scan (transverse section) of the left parametrium showing the presence of a diffuse DE involving the retroperitoneal space and narrowing the colon (arrow). The left ureter is included in the vast fibrotic retraction caused by the nodule

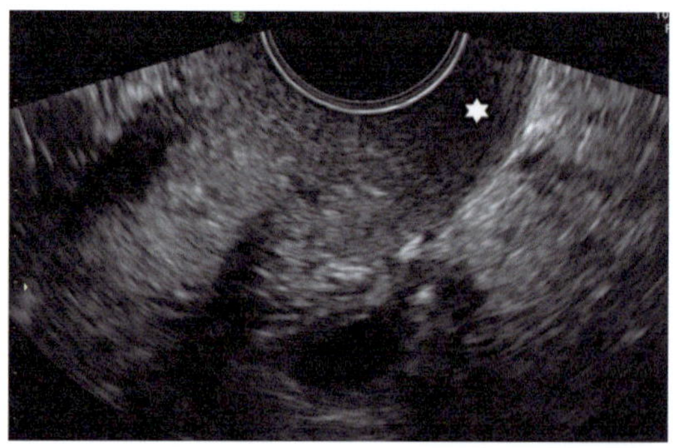

Fig. 8.13 Transvaginal scan (longitudinal section) of the posterior fornix showing an endometriotic nodule involving a uterosacral ligament, the vaginal wall, and the parametrium (star)

tria (Figs. 8.11 and 8.12). The ureter can disappear embedded in the nodule; a dilated ureter is seen cranial to the stricture as a straight tubular structure located beneath the peritoneum, devoid of blood flow, not movable by the pressure exerted with the probe, and surrounded by a thick wall (Fig. 8.9). Peristalsis is often seen even in dilated ureters after waiting a sufficient amount of seconds. Involvement of the ureter should be suspected even in case of bulky nodules extending laterally from the uterosacral ligaments to the parametrium because of the close proximity of the ureter to this anatomic structure (Fig. 8.13).

8.4 Important Technical Tips

All scans should be performed both via transabdominal (TAS) and transvaginal ultrasound (TVS). The investigator must be aware of the patients' clinical and surgical history, symptoms (dysmenorrhea, dyspareunia, chronic pelvic pain, dysuria, urgency, frequency, suprapubic pain, vesical tenesmus, infertility), and the results of a physical bimanual examination of the patient. The optimal situation would be the case in which the same physician performing TAS and TVS is expert in bimanual exploration of the female pelvis (gynecologic examination) in order to obtain the best from both exams. The ultrasound examinations must be performed in a standardized manner using ultrasound machine equipped with broadband abdominal and vaginal probes.

At first, an accurate examination of the pelvis should be undertaken to evaluate the anatomy of the uterus and the ovaries. The transvaginal transducer should then be positioned in the anterior vaginal fornix and tilted upward to visualize the vesicouterine space and the bladder, on a longitudinal and on a transverse section. In these planes, the bladder wall can easily be visualized if a moderate amount of urine is present. The sliding of the normal bladder wall toward the anterior wall of the uterus should be evaluated by gently pushing with the transvaginal probe (Video 8.1). The physician must be familiar with the normal anatomy of the bladder, in order to recognize the peritoneum covering the intra-abdominal portion (dome) of the bladder, the muscle layer, and the mucosa.

Diagnostic criteria indicative of a bladder endometriotic nodule are the following [14, 18]:

1. The presence of a hypo- or isoechogenic nodule in the bladder wall
2. The presence of a nodule with a heterogeneous echostructure containing numerous anechoic ("bubble-like") areas (Fig. 8.14).

Whenever a bladder endometriotic nodule is seen at TVS, its location, shape, mean diameter (or the three orthogonal diameters), mobility with regard to the anterior uterine wall, and pain at pressure with the probe should be recorded. Moreover, the relationship of the DE with the trigonus and the internal ureteral orifices should be evaluated, eventually waiting for the ureteral jet to appear (Video 8.3). Assessment of vascularization of the nodule by means of color/power Doppler does not seem to be crucial, but it might be of help in the differential diagnosis with a bladder neoplasm (which is usually more vascularized than DE).

Pelvic sections of the ureter should be routinely evaluated at TVS [19] both at rest and during peristalsing to identify any evidence of ureteric dilatation, abnormal bending, or differences in peristalsis frequency between the ureters [19]. In women with evidence of ureteric obstruction, the distance between the nodule and the ureteric orifice should be measured. As already discussed, the operator must be aware of the fact that nodules involving the ureter are most often large nodules of the posterior pelvic compartment extending laterally toward the parametrium (Figs. 8.11 and 8.12), at the level of the uterine cervix, thus reaching the ureter either directly or as an involvement caused by the fibrotic reaction (collagen fibers, smooth muscle cells) surrounding the DE. Thus, it is mandatory to perform a complete evaluation of the posterior pelvic compartment. As previously recommended, TVS should be performed in a dynamic and interactive manner, while asking the patient about possible complaints and looking for painful site (*pain mapping*). A normal pelvis will show the sliding of the rectum toward the posterior uterine wall (Video 8.2).

The examination is completed only after a TAS is done (which can be even done before TVS) by means of a 3.5–5.0 MHz curvilinear probe. Kidneys are easy to be evaluated by positioning the woman on a lateral decubitus position with the probe in the lower intercostal space at the level of the midaxillary line. Kidneys are scanned on a longitudinal (long axis) and transverse (short axis) views.

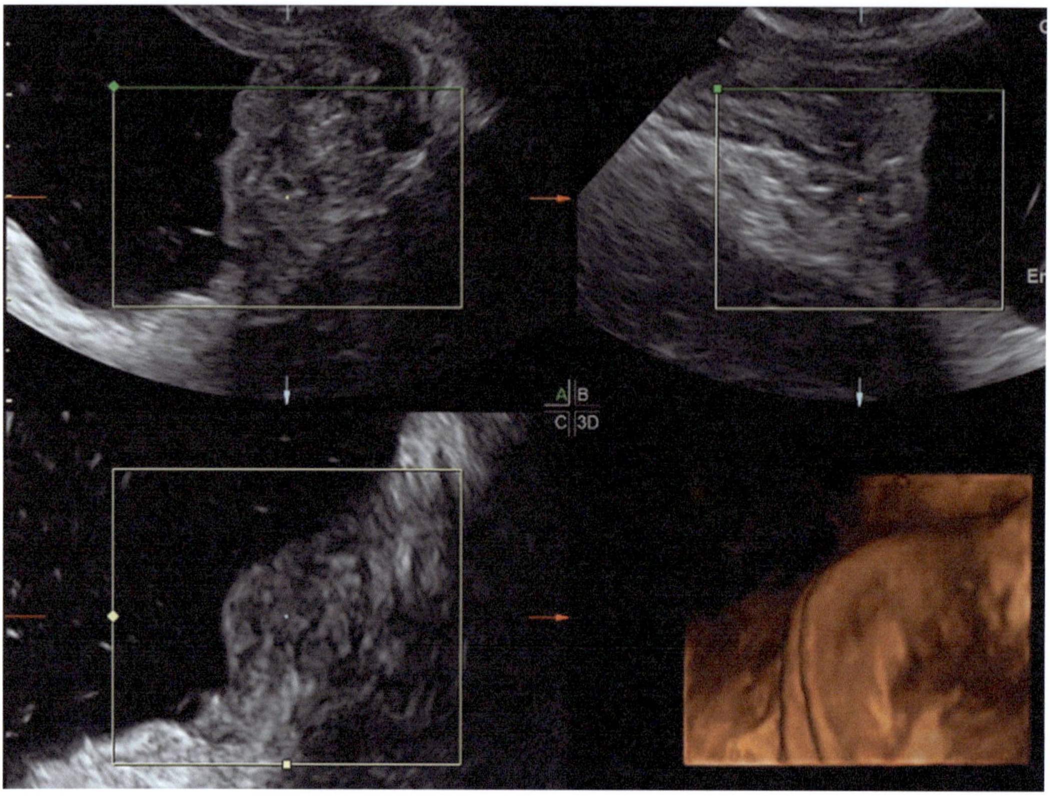

Fig. 8.14 Transvaginal scan of a bladder endometriotic nodule (multiplanar image plus 3D reconstruction). The nodule appears as hypoechoic mass containing small cystic spaces (bubble-like). Three-dimensional image (bottom right) shows the distortion of bladder anatomy and indenting of the bladder lumen. The nodule does not infiltrate the mucosal layer which is smooth and has a normal appearance

Hydronephrosis is diagnosed and graded using commonly accepted ultrasound criteria [20]. When the cranial portion of the ureter appears dilated (Figs. 8.1 and 8.2), it should be followed on its abdominal and pelvic portions to the level of obstruction if not already seen vaginally [19].

The course of the ureter at TVS can be easily followed starting from the trigonus up to the pelvic brim and to the crossing of the common iliac vessels. Color Doppler may help in differentiating the ureter from a blood vessel. Another feature which can help is the presence of peristalsis, which can be seen in the ureter keeping the probe still for up to 180 s. The diameter of the ureter can be measured both at rest and during peak of dilatation during peristalsis by placing the calipers on the outer edge of muscularis layer at the junction with the hyperechoic fibrous layer surrounding the ureter [19].

References

1. Koninckx PR, Martin D. Treatment of deeply infiltrating endometriosis. Curr Opin Obstet Gynecol. 1994;6:231–41.
2. Chapron C, Fauconnier A, Dubuisson JB, Barakat H, Viera M, Breart C. Deep infiltrating endometriosis: relation between severity of dysmenorrhoea and extent of disease. Hum Reprod. 2003;18:760–6.
3. Berlanda N, Vercellini P, Carmignani L, Aimi G, Amicarelli F, Fedele L. Ureteral and vesical endometriosis. Two different clinical entities sarin the same pathogenesis. Obstet Gynecol Surv. 2009;64:830–42.
4. Gabriel B, Nassif J, Trompoukis P, Barata S, Wattiez A. Prevalence and management of urinary tract endometriosis: a clinical case series. Urology. 2011;78:1269–74.

5. Knabben L, Imboden S, Fellmann B, Nirgianakis K, Kuhn A, Mueller MD. Urinary tract endometriosis in patients with deep infiltrating endometriosis: prevalence, symptoms, management and proposal for a new classification. Fertil Steril. 2015;103:147–52.
6. Chapron C, Fauconnier A, Vierira M, et al. Anatomical distribution of deeply infiltrating endometriosis: surgical implications and pro position for a classification. Hum Reprod. 2003;18:157–61.
7. Vercellini P, Frontino G, Pietropaolo G, Gattei U, Daguati R, Crosignani PG. Deep endometriosis: definition, pathogenesis, and clinical management. J Am Assoc Gynecol Laparosc. 2004;11:153–61.
8. Chapron C, Dubuisson JB. Laparoscopic management of bladder endometriosis. Acta Obstet Gynecol Scand. 1999;78:887–90.
9. Maccagnano C, Pellucchi F, Rocchini L, et al. Ureteral endometriosis: proposal for a diagnostic and therapeutic algorithm with a review of the literature. Urol Int. 2013;91:1–9.
10. Carfagna P, De Cicco Nardone C, Testa AC, Scambia G, Marana F, De Cicco Nardone F. The role of transvaginal ultrasound in the evaluation of ureteral involvement in deep endometriosis. Ultrasound Obstet Gynecol. 2018;51(4):550–5.
11. Del Frate C, Girometti R, Pittino M, Del Frate G, Bazzocchi M, Zuiani C. Deep retroperitoneal pelvic endometriosis: MR imaging appearance with laparoscopic correlation. Radiographics. 2006;26:1705–18.
12. Guerriero S, Condous G, Van den Bossch T, Valentin L, et al. Systematic approach to sonographic evaluation of the pelvis in women with suspected endometriosis, including terms, definitions and measurements: a consensus opinion from the International Deep Endometriosis Analysis (IDEA) group. Ultrasound Obstet Gynecol. 2016;48:318–32.
13. Kolodziej A, Krajewski W, Dolowy L, Hirnle L. Urinary tract endometriosis. Urol J. 2015;12:2213–7.
14. Savelli L, Manuzzi L, Pollastri P, Mabrouk M, Seracchioli R, Venturoli S. Diagnostic accuracy and potential limitations of transvaginal sonography for bladder endometriosis. Ultrasound Obstet Gynecol. 2009;34:595–600.
15. Chamié LP, Blasbalg R, Pereira RM, Warmbrand G, Serafini PC. Findings of pelvic endometriosis at transvaginal US, MR imaging, and laparoscopy. Radiographics. 2011;31(4):E77–100.
16. Manganaro L, Fierro F, Tomei A, Irimia D, Lodise P, Sergi ME, Vinci V, Sollazzo P, Porpora MG, Delfini R, Vittori G, Marini M. Feasibility of 3.0T pelvic MR imaging in the evaluation of endometriosis. Eur J Radiol. 2012;81(6):1381–7.
17. Thonnon C, Philip CA, Fassi-Fehri H, Bisch C, Coulon A, de Saint-Hilaire P, Dubernard G. Three-dimensional ultrasound in the management of bladder endometriosis. J Minim Invasive Gynecol. 2015;22:403–9.
18. Bazot M, Thomassin I, Hourani R, Cortez A, Darai E. Diagnostic accuracy of transvaginal sonography for deep pelvic endometriosis. Ultrasound Obstet Gynecol. 2004;24:180–5.
19. Pateman K, Mavrelos D, Hoo WL, Holland T, Naftalin J, Jurkovic D. Visualization of ureters on standard gynecological transvaginal scan: a feasibility study. Ultrasound Obstet Gynecol. 2013;41:696–701.
20. Tuma J, Trinkler F, Zát'ura F, Novakova B. Genitourinary ultrasound. In: Dietrich C, editor. EFSUMB (European Federation of Societies for Ultrasound in Medicine and Biology) course book. London: European Federation of Societies for Ultrasound in Medicine and Biology; 2017. p. 275–340. ISBN 978-0-9571581-0-8.

Uterosacral Ligament Endometriosis

9

Francesco Paolo Giuseppe Leone

9.1 Introduction

Endometriosis occurs in 15–30% of patients with endometriosis and may involve, in descending order of frequency, the uterosacral ligaments (USLs), the pouch of Douglas, the rectosigmoid colon, the rectovaginal septum, the vagina, and the bladder [1, 2]. Considerable diagnostic delay of up to 8 years from presenting symptoms often confers a heavy economic and social price [3–5].

Preoperative diagnosis of USL endometriosis is extremely relevant for the surgeon, as removal of these lesions is associated with a high risk of bladder dysfunction. Nerve-sparing surgery of the inferior hypogastric plexus is recommended to avoid this complication; it is especially feasible in women with isolated USL endometriosis, whereas more extensive endometriotic lesions are not always compatible with this conservative surgery [6].

This overview will focus on the sonographic diagnosis of USL endometriosis, by transvaginal sonography (TVS) with color and power Doppler (CD and PD) assessment, combined with sonovaginography (SVG) (using either saline contrast or gel infusion) or with three-dimensional transvaginal sonography (3D-TVS).

F. P. G. Leone
Department of Obstetrics and Gynaecology, Clinical Sciences Institute L. Sacco, University of Milan, Milan, Italy

9.2 How We Do It

9.2.1 Clinical History

A detailed clinical history is always a mandatory preliminary step. USL deep endometriosis (DE) can be associated with dysmenorrhea, deep dyspareunia (or even apareunia), and dyschezia [7].

9.2.2 Clinical Pelvic Examination

The physical pelvic examination is based on digital vaginal and/or rectal examinations, which is considered suggestive of USL DE when an area of thickening or a nodule in the uterosacral ligaments, often painful, is found [8].

9.2.3 2D-Transvaginal Sonography

TVS can be performed throughout the menstrual cycle, without bowel preparation (i.e., without use of laxatives or enema).

Conventional 2D-TVS is performed, using a wide-band 3–9-MHz vaginal high-resolution microconvex probe, to obtain an overview of the whole pelvis by a tenderness-guided and dynamic methodology according to IDEA consensus' sonographic steps (see Chap. 3). The tenderness-guided exam is performed with or without an

S. Guerriero et al. (eds.), *How to Perform Ultrasonography in Endometriosis*,
https://doi.org/10.1007/978-3-319-71138-6_9

acoustic window between the transvaginal probe and the surrounding vaginal structures, combined with an active role of the patient, who indicates the site of any tenderness experienced during the pelvic scan [9, 10]. Then, the image is magnified to contain only the upper vagina, cervix, and lower uterus, to be assessed in the sagittal plane of the cervix from uterine artery to uterine artery and in the transverse plane from the external to the internal cervical os. The magnification should be as large as possible, focusing on the area of interest. Furthermore, in order to obtain a high-quality image, a proper setting of the following is of paramount importance:

(a) Depth (the complete cervix on the screen after whole pelvic assessment)
(b) Gain (setting also overall time gain compensation)
(c) Dynamic range (less relevant for cervical assessment)
(d) Focus (single enough, below the cervix)
(e) Zoom (better high definition (HD) zoom)

However, difficulties may arise from variations in uterine position (particularly when axial) or with uterine rotation (endometriosis or previous surgery-related adhesions). This problem may be overcome in some cases by pressing on the abdomen with the non-scanning hand. The probe can be positioned either in the anterior or in the posterior vaginal fornix.

The color and power Doppler box should include the nodule with the surrounding fat and structures. Magnification and settings should be adjusted to ensure maximal sensitivity for blood flow:

(a) Ultrasound frequency "normal" (at least 5.0 MHz)
(b) Pulse repetition frequency 0.6 kHz (0.3–0.9 kHz)
(c) Wall filter "low" 40 Hz (30–50 Hz)
(d) Color and power Doppler gain (reduced until all color artifacts disappear)

The color content in the DE nodule may be scored using the standardized color score (CS), a subjective semiquantitative assessment of the amount of blood flow present: CS 1, no color flow; CS 2, only minimal color; CS 3, moderate color; and CS 4, abundant color.

Normal USLs are usually not visible on ultrasound. USL DE lesions appear as hypoechoic thickening with regular, smooth outline, or irregular, stellate margins, within the hyperechoic peritoneal fat surrounding the USLs, with homogeneous or heterogeneous echogenicity (Fig. 9.1) [2]. USL DE nodule can be seen in the parasagittal view of the cervix (Fig. 9.2):

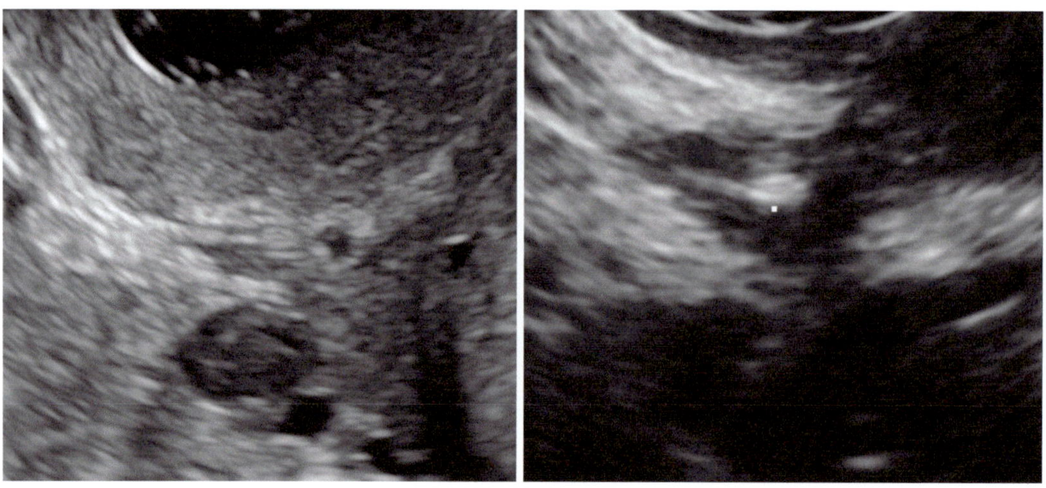

Fig. 9.1 USL DE lesion may appear as an hypoechoic, homogeneous thickened nodule with regular, smooth outline (left) or as an hypoechoic, heterogeneous thickened nodule with irregular, stellate margins (right)

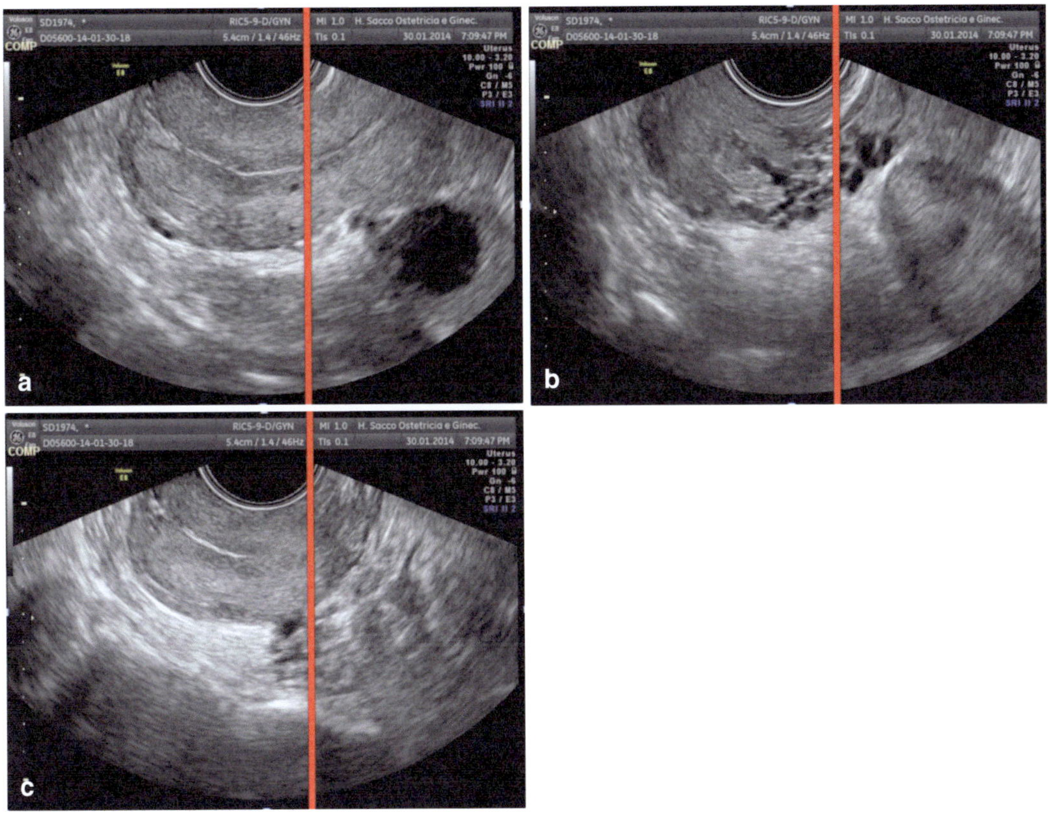

Fig. 9.2 (**a**) Sagittal image of the cervix with an imaginary line passing through the cervical internal os. (**b**) Lateral sagittal image of the cervix with an imaginary line passing at the level of uterine artery. (**c**) Sagittal image of the cervix, medial to the uterine artery, with an imaginary line passing at the level of the hypoechoic USL DE nodule

(a) Place the transvaginal probe in the anterior or in the posterior vaginal fornix.
(b) Obtain the sagittal plane of the cervix and select the midline (passing through the cervical canal).
(c) Trace an imaginary line passing through the internal cervical os.
(d) Sweep the probe laterally up to the uterine artery.
(e) Sweeping back medially to the uterine artery, the USL DE nodule appears as a hypoechoic lesion.

Similarly, USL DE nodule can be seen in the transverse view of the cervix (Fig. 9.3):

(a) Place the transvaginal probe in the anterior or in the posterior vaginal fornix.
(b) Obtain the transverse plane of the cervix.
(c) Sweep the probe cranially up to the internal cervical os, and the USL DE nodule appears as a hypoechoic lesion.

The USL lesion may be isolated or may be part of a larger nodule extending into the vagina or into other surrounding structures (rectosigmoid, ovary) (Fig. 9.4). If the nodule is seen as a central block of hypoechoic tissue of the retrocervical area (arciform abnormality), it should be considered a DE lesion of the torus uterinus [2]. In the presence of an extended nodule, a posterior negative "sliding sign" (i.e., pouch of Douglas obliteration) is usually observed [11, 12].

The thickness of the USL nodule should be measured systematically in three orthogonal planes by sagittal and transverse scans, to obtain

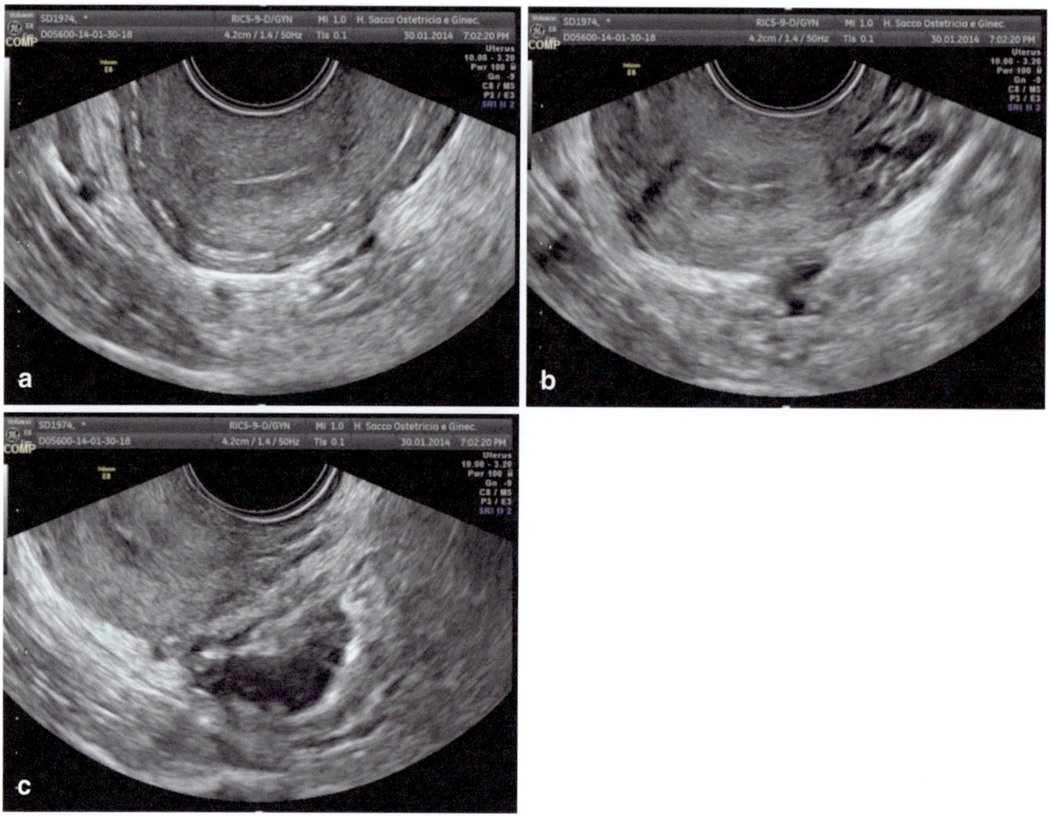

Fig. 9.3 (**a**) Transverse image of the cervix with the vaginal bright edge. (**b**) Cranial transverse image of the upper cervix with the hypoechoic left USL DE nodule. (**c**) Cranial transverse image of the uterine isthmus with the hypoechoic left USL DE nodule adherent to a rectosigmoid bowel DE nodule

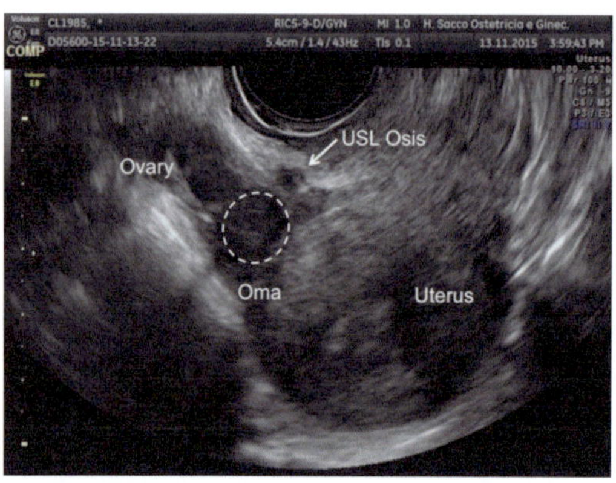

Fig. 9.4 Extended USL DE lesion, hypoechoic with irregular outline, adherent to an ovarian endometrioma and to a retrocervical DE nodule

the length (midsagittal measurement), thickness (anteroposterior measurement), and transverse diameter in millimeters.

The whole procedure should be digitally recorded for second opinion (videoclips) and the selected diagnostic images stored and/or printed. The former option is particularly relevant when discussing with surgeons the surgical strategy.

9.2.4 Sonovaginography with Saline or Gel

Sonovaginography combines TVS with injection of saline or gel into the vagina. Up to 50 mL of these contrast agents, injected into the vagina using a plastic syringe and a Foley catheter or a condom, create an acoustic window between the transvaginal probe and the structures surrounding the vagina, thus permitting more complete visualization of the vaginal walls and anterior/posterior vaginal fornices [13, 14]. The great advantage of the condom fulfilled with gel is that it lasts longer, with no backflow and no need of a specific set (catheter, syringe). SVG should be always performed when the clinical interview and the preliminary pelvic exam suggest the presence of posterior DE nodules, permitting to identify isolated (Fig. 9.5) or extended lesions (Fig. 9.6). As well as above, the whole procedure should be digitally recorded for second opinion (videoclips) and the selected diagnostic images stored and/or printed.

9.2.5 Transrectal Sonography

Transrectal sonography using transvaginal probe should be used if necessary to support TVS in selected cases or if TVS is impossible or inappropriate (virgo intacta) [15].

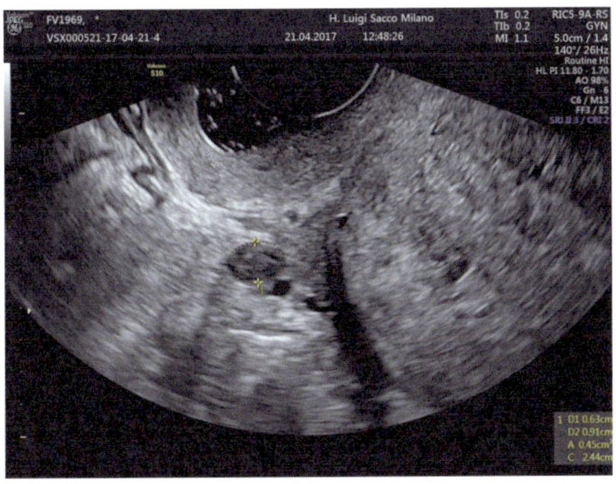

Fig. 9.5 Isolated USL DE lesion, hypoechoic with smooth outline, at gel sonovaginography

9.2.6 3D-Transvaginal Sonography

In the last decades, a large number of papers referred the usefulness of 3D-TVS in gynecological investigations, mainly focused on uterine congenital anomalies and adenomyosis but poorly on DE [16].

3D-TVS should always be performed after a detailed tenderness-guided and dynamic transvaginal exam, useful to adequately report the USL DE lesion on the three orthogonal planes and its relationship with surrounding structures, thus easily permitting to distinguish isolated and extended lesions (Fig. 9.7).

In order to obtain a high-quality 3D image, it is of paramount importance to acquire an excellent volume by a high-quality 2D image. Therefore:

(a) Obtain a good 2D image of the upper cervix and of the USL DE lesion.
(b) Select 3D/4D static mode.
(c) Select quality option (slower the speed of acquisition, longer the duration of the sweep, thus higher the quality).
(d) Select sweep angle (range of volume sweep 85°–120°; the smaller the range, the higher the quality; thus select the smallest angle fitting the target).

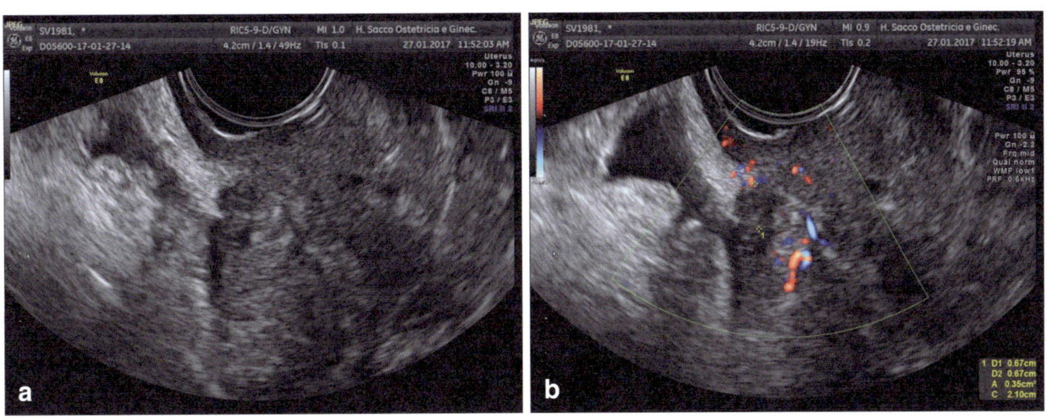

Fig. 9.6 Extended USL DE lesion, hypoechoic with smooth outline (**a**) and CS1 (**b**), at gel sonovaginography, strictly adherent to a retrocervical DE hypoechoic lesion

(e) Choose the sagittal and/or transverse plane, being sure to include the whole nodule and surrounding structures.
(f) Hold still, avoid pressure with the probe, ask the patient to remain still during the acquisition, acquire the volume, and store it electronically for later analysis.
(g) Magnification over 70% of the screen and virtual navigation on the multiplanar display, referring to the fulcrum (dot of interest) and by rotating the three orthogonal planes on the rotational axis *X*, *Y*, and *Z*.
(h) Assessment and measurements of the USL DE findings, by adding post-processing tools (volume contrast imaging (VCI), rendering mode, tomographic ultrasound imaging (TUI)).

Volume contrast imaging (VCI) is a technology based on a volume acquisition technique that leads to contrast enhancement and speckle suppression in the two-dimensional ultrasound image, by offering to increase resolution and to reduce noise and artifacts. Hence, the result of VCI is a thin surface-rendered image of the DE nodule, which thickness usually set at 2 mm by the sonographer (Fig. 9.7).

Volume rendering analysis is based on the selection of the region of interest (ROI) and of the observation plane of the acquired volume of the nodule, thus obtaining a thick slice of the lesion (Fig. 9.8).

Tomographic ultrasound imaging (TUI) is a technology which leads to multiple planes displayed at the same time, with the option of concomitant use of VCI. Similarly, the number of images and the thickness might be selected by the sonographer, with differences depending on the plane used for analysis. I would suggest the option with three or nine images with distances of 0.5–3.5 mm depending on USL lesion (isolated or extended) and involved surrounding structures (Fig. 9.9).

In particular, the following steps after volume acquisition of the USL DE lesion at 3D-TVS should be performed:

(a) Identify and magnify the selected image of the USL DE lesion, in the multiplanar display mode and add VCI.
(b) Shift the selected plane forward and backward to identify the plane containing the largest diameter of the DE lesion and evaluate involvement of surrounding structures.
(c) Rotate the DE lesion on its ideal center ("fulcrum") on the *Z*-axis until the line passes through the center of the nodule and assess extension to surrounding structures (Fig. 9.10).
(d) Report images adding TUI or rendering mode if potentially useful to discuss in a clinical multidisciplinary setting.

3D volumes can be stored and analyzed later as many times as needed, permitting a second opinion by sending volumes by internet, offering the possibility of studying an infinite number of sections through the lesions. This latter feature is particularly relevant when discussing with surgeons the surgical strategy (Figs. 9.11 and 9.12).

9.3 Future Perspectives

TVS should remain the first-line method in the evaluation of patients with suspicion of DE. The future uptake of the recent IDEA consensus on terms, definitions, and measurements of DE lesions may improve standardization of scanning and reporting and in turn potentially reduce the operator dependency. This may optimize the preoperative triage and potentially improve surgical outcomes. Furthermore, it may lead to large multicentric studies and proper meta-analyses on ultrasound diagnosis of endometriosis.

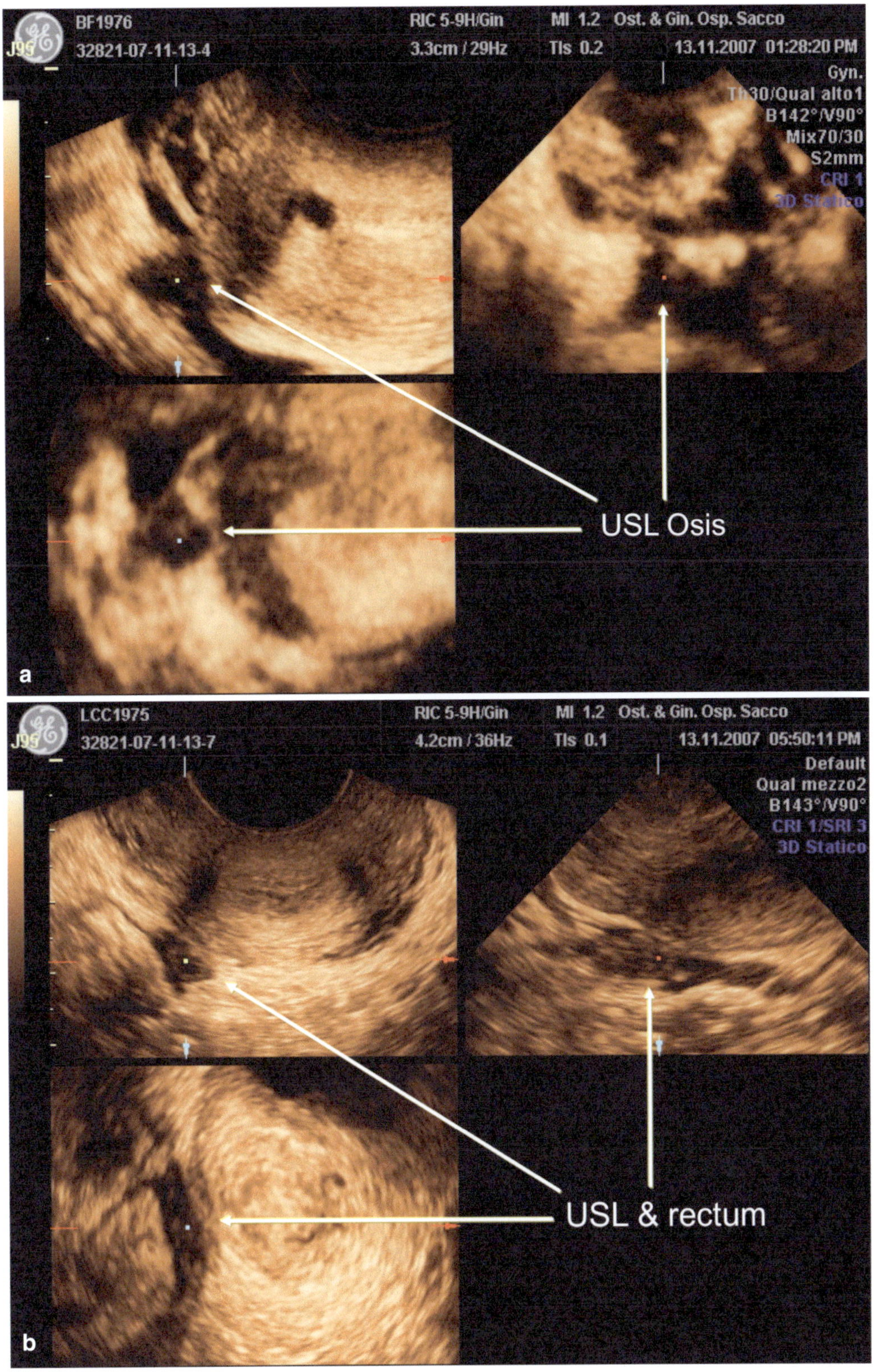

Fig. 9.7 Multiplanar images with VCI analysis (2 mm) of an isolated (**a**) and an extended nodule (**b**) infiltrating the rectosigmoid

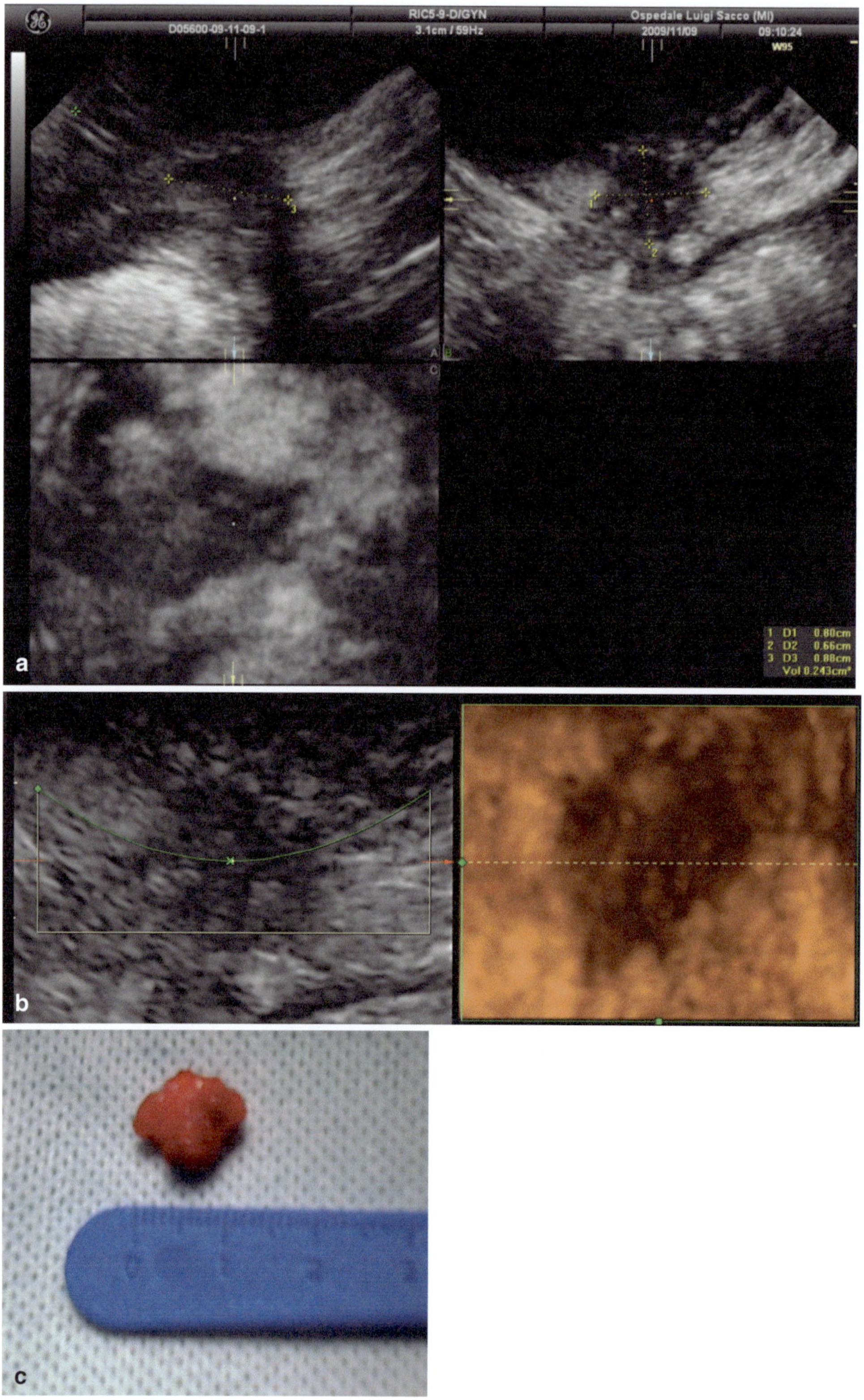

Fig. 9.8 Multiplanar images with VCI (**a**) and Volume Rendering Analysis (**b**), with the selection of the curved render ROI, of an isolated hypoechoic smooth homogeneous USL DE nodule, compared to the macroscopic surgical specimen (**c**)

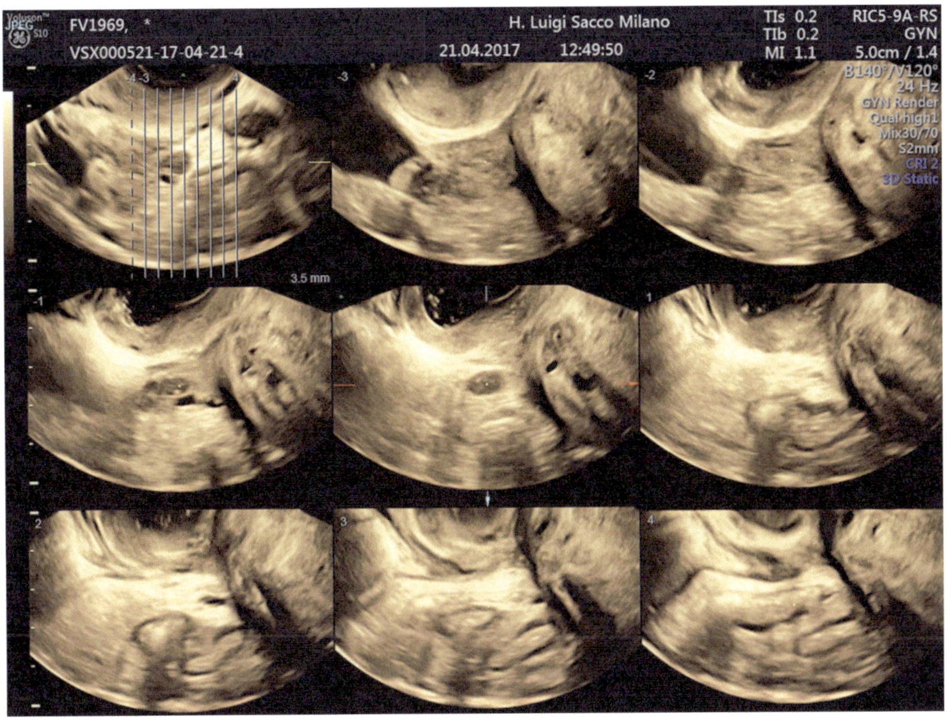

Fig. 9.9 TUI images (nine images with distance of 3.5 mm) with VCI analysis (2 mm) of an isolated hypoechoic smooth homogeneous isolated USL DE nodule

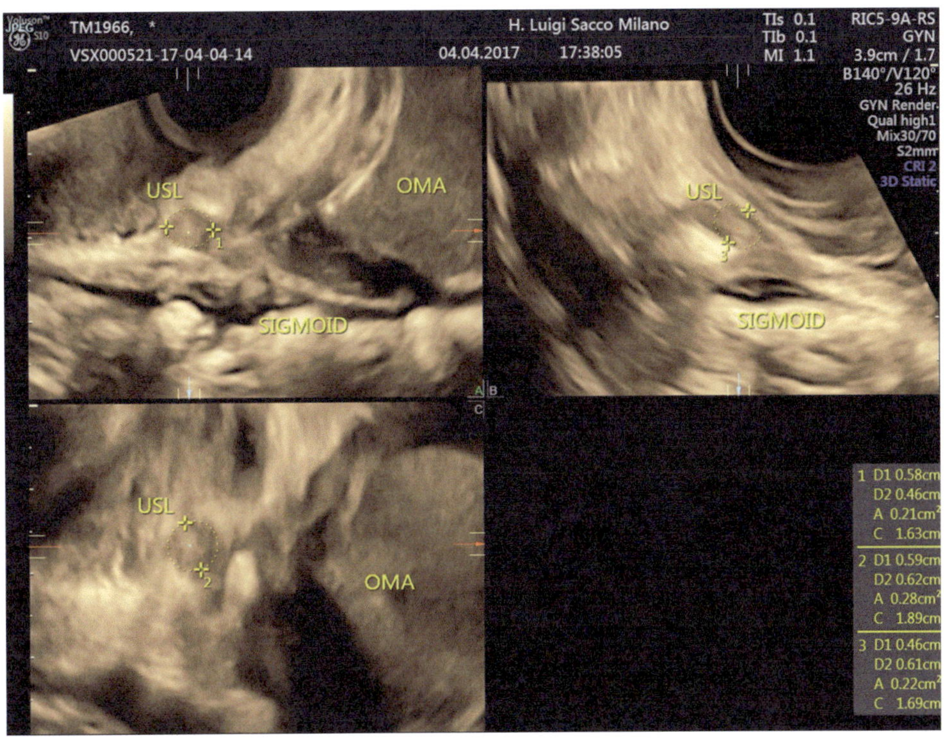

Fig. 9.10 Multiplanar images with VCI analysis (2 mm) of an extended irregular hypoechoic homogeneous USL DE nodule adherent to an ovarian endometrioma and to the sigmoid serosa

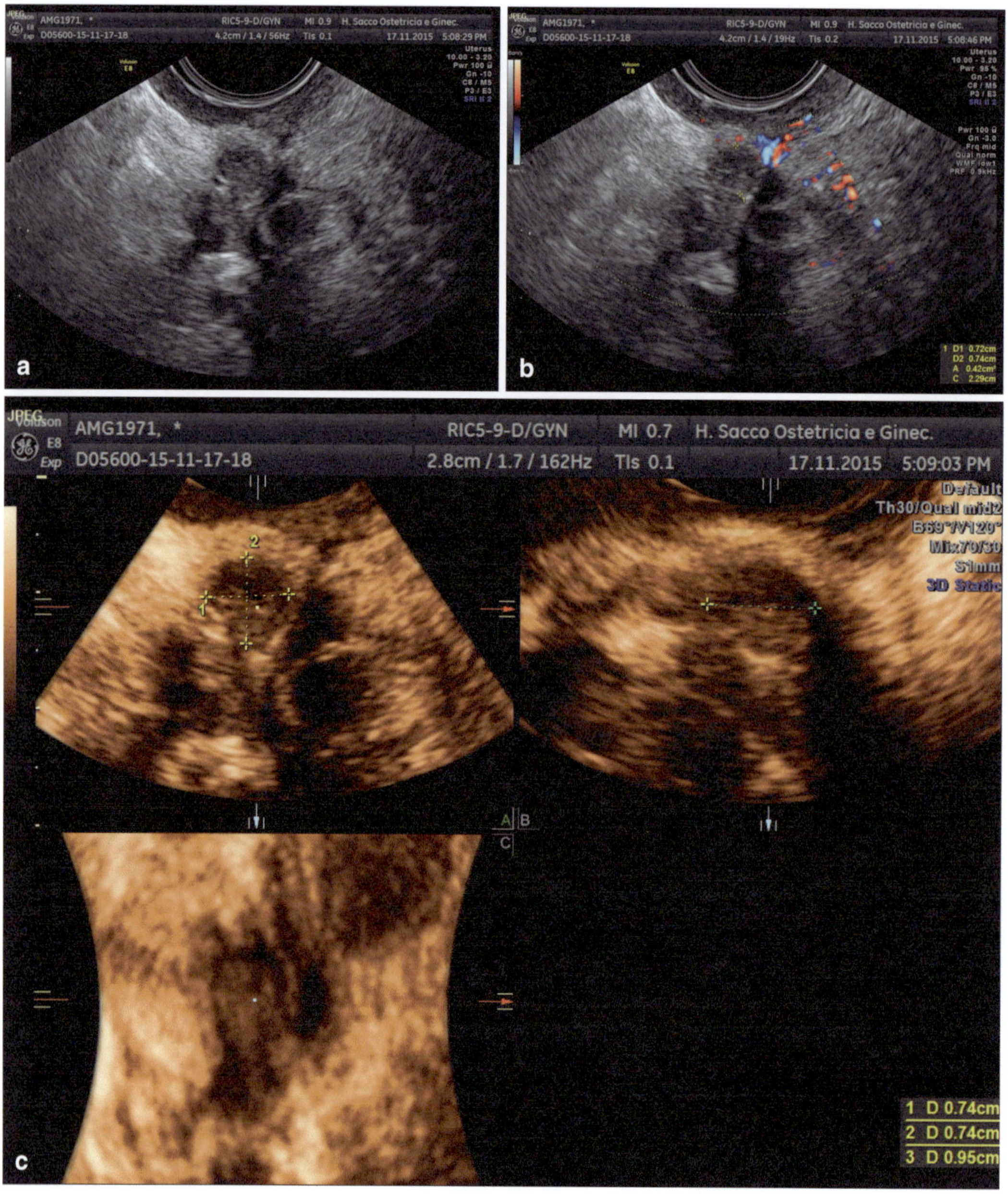

Fig. 9.11 Extended hypoechoic homogeneous USL DE lesion with irregular outline, strictly adherent to a retro-cervical DE hypoechoic lesion and to an infiltrating recto-sigmoid nodule at 2D-TVS (**a**), with CS1 (**b**), and at 3D-TVS with multiplanar images and VCI analysis (2 mm) (**c**)

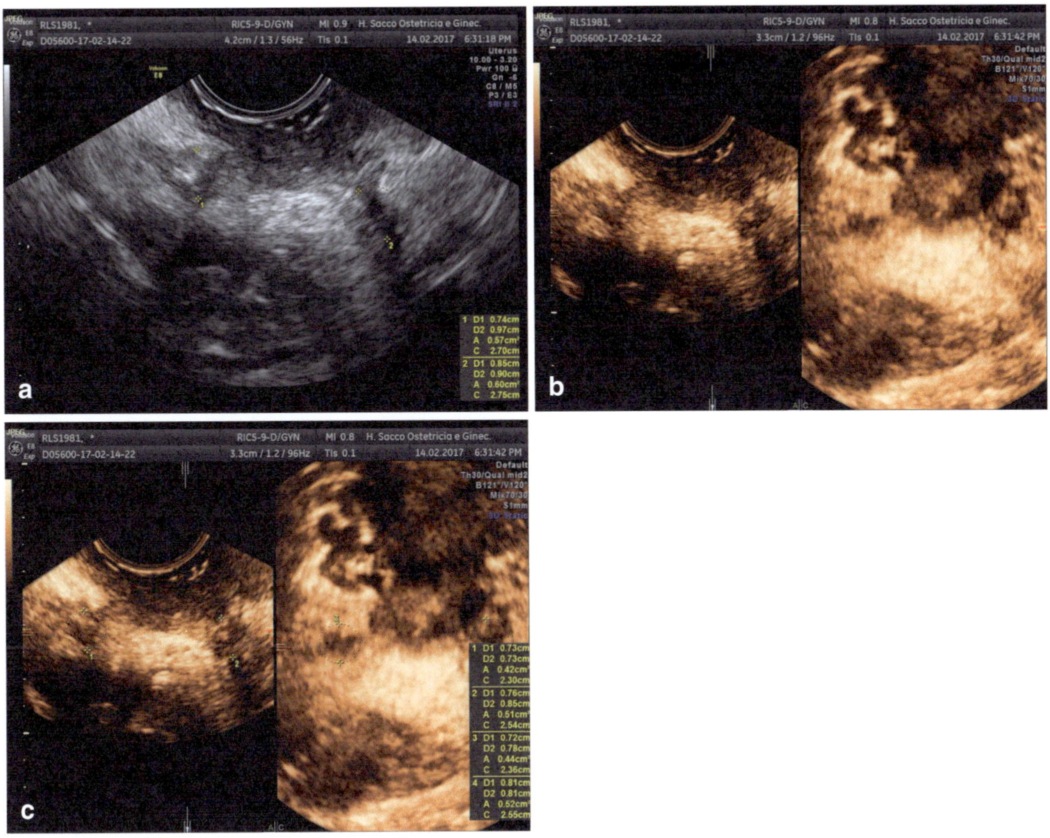

Fig. 9.12 Bilateral extended hypoechoic heterogeneous USL DE lesions with irregular outline, strictly adherent to an arciform retrocervical DE hypoechoic lesion at 2D-TVS on a transverse plane (**a**) and at 3D-TVS with multiplanar images and VCI analysis (2 mm) (**b**, **c**)

References

1. Exacoustos C, Zupi E, Piccione E. Ultrasound imaging for ovarian and deep infiltrating endometriosis. Semin Reprod Med. 2017;35(1):5–24.
2. Bazot M, Thomassin I, Hourani R, Cortez A, Darai E. Diagnostic accuracy of transvaginal sonography for deep pelvic endometriosis. Ultrasound Obstet Gynecol. 2004;24(2):180–5.
3. Dunselman GA, Vermeulen N, Becker C, Calhaz-Jorge C, D'Hooghe T, De Bie B, Heikinheimo O, Horne AW, Kiesel L, Nap A, Prentice A, Saridogan E, Soriano D, Nelen W, European Society of Human Reproduction and Embryology. ESHRE guideline: management of women with endometriosis. Hum Reprod. 2014;29(3):400–12.
4. Nisenblat V, Bossuyt PM, Farquhar C, Johnson N, Hull ML. Imaging modalities for the non-invasive diagnosis of endometriosis. Cochrane Database Syst Rev. 2016;(2):CD009591.
5. Nisenblat V, Prentice L, Bossuyt PM, Farquhar C, Hull ML, Johnson N. Combination of the non-invasive tests for the diagnosis of endometriosis. Cochrane Database Syst Rev. 2016;(7):CD012281.
6. Volpi E, Ferrero A, Sismondi P. Laparoscopic identification of pelvic nerves in patients with deep infiltrating endometriosis. Surg Endosc. 2004;18(7):1109–12.
7. Chapron C, Barakat H, Fritel X, Dubuisson JB, Bréart G, Fauconnier A. Presurgical diagnosis of posterior deep infiltrating endometriosis based on a standardized questionnaire. Hum Reprod. 2005;20(2):507–13.
8. Hudelist G, Oberwinkler KH, Singer CF, Tuttlies F, Rauter G, Ritter O, Keckstein J. Combination of transvaginal sonography and clinical examination for preoperative diagnosis of pelvic endometriosis. Hum Reprod. 2009;24(5):1018–24.
9. Guerriero S, Ajossa S, Gerada M, D'Aquila M, Piras B, Melis GB. "Tenderness-guided" transvaginal ultrasonography: a new method for the detection of deep endometriosis in patients with chronic pelvic pain. Fertil Steril. 2007;88(5):1293–7.
10. Guerriero S, Ajossa S, Gerada M, Virgilio B, Angioni S, Melis GB. Diagnostic value of transvaginal

'tenderness-guided' ultrasonography for the prediction of location of deep endometriosis. Hum Reprod. 2008;23(11):2452–7.

11. Reid S, Lu C, Casikar I, Reid G, Abbott J, Cario G, Chou D, Kowalski D, Cooper M, Condous G. Prediction of pouch of Douglas obliteration in women with suspected endometriosis using a new real-time dynamic transvaginal ultrasound technique: the sliding sign. Ultrasound Obstet Gynecol. 2013;41(6):685–91.
12. Reid S, Lu C, Casikar I, Mein B, Magotti R, Ludlow J, Benzie R, Condous G. The prediction of pouch of Douglas obliteration using offline analysis of the transvaginal ultrasound 'sliding sign' technique: inter- and intra-observer reproducibility. Hum Reprod. 2013;28(5):1237–46.
13. Saccardi C, Cosmi E, Borghero A, Tregnaghi A, Dessole S, Litta P. Comparison between transvaginal sonography, saline contrast sonovaginography and magnetic resonance imaging in the diagnosis of posterior deep infiltrating endometriosis. Ultrasound Obstet Gynecol. 2012;40:464–9.
14. Reid S, Lu C, Hardy N, Casikar I, Reid G, Cario G, Chou D, Almashat D, Condous G. Office gel sonovaginography for the prediction of posterior deep infiltrating endometriosis: a multicenter prospective observational study. Ultrasound Obstet Gynecol. 2014;44:710–8.
15. Koga K, Osuga Y, Yano T, Momoeda M, Yoshino O, Hirota Y, Kugu K, Nishii O, Tsutsumi O, Taketani Y. Characteristic images of deeply infiltrating rectosigmoid endometriosis on transvaginal and transrectal ultrasonography. Hum Reprod. 2003;18:1328–33.
16. Pascual MA, Guerriero S, Hereter L, Barri-Soldevila P, Ajossa S, Graupera B, Rodriguez I. Three-dimensional sonography for diagnosis of rectovaginal septum endometriosis: interobserver agreement. J Ultrasound Med. 2013;32(6):931–5.

10 Forniceal-Vaginal Deep Endometriosis

Stefano Guerriero, Gil Cohen, Silvia Ajossa, Ornella Comparetto, Camilla Ronchetti, Bruno Piras, Alba Piras, and Valerio Mais

10.1 Introduction

The forniceal-vaginal anatomical area is located in the recess at the vault of the vagina. Forniceal deep endometriosis (DE) is mainly located in the posterior part of the vaginal fornix but might involve also the lateral parts of the fornix [1]. The mean prevalence of vaginal DE is 17% [2], ranging from 4 to 39% [3, 4]. This wide range is probably due to the different classification systems used before the International Deep Endometriosis Analysis (IDEA) consensus [5].

The histologic findings of infiltrative lesions of deep pelvic endometriosis are mainly characterized by fibromuscular hyperplasia that surrounds foci of endometriosis, and the foci sometimes contain small cavities. The endometrial glands and stroma infiltrate the adjacent fibromuscular tissue and elicit smooth muscle proliferation and fibrous reaction, resulting in solid nodule formation [6–8]. Endometriotic glands are found to be very near to the vaginal mucosal epithelium [9].

Donnez et al. [10] proposed a classification to forniceal-vaginal endometriotic lesions, previously called "retroperitoneal" or "retrocervical" lesion. This classification is based on their theory of disease pathogenesis which states that adenomyosis originates in the retrocervical area and involves the retroperitoneal space. These authors proposed a classification that takes into account the location of the retroperitoneal lesion (Fig. 10.1) [11]. This classification has been described also by Del Frate et al. [12]:

Type I: rectovaginal septum DE nodules (10% of cases). These lesions are situated within the rectovaginal septum between the posterior wall of the vaginal mucosa and the anterior wall of the rectal muscularis [10].

Type II: posterior vaginal fornix DE nodules (65% of cases). These lesions develop from the posterior fornix toward the rectovaginal septum. The posterior fornix is retrocervical and corresponds, in the attachment of the vaginal mucosa, to the posterior face of the posterior lip of the cervix [10].

Electronic Supplementary Material The online version of this chapter (https://doi.org/10.1007/978-3-319-71138-6_10) contains supplementary material, which is available to authorized users.

S. Guerriero (✉) · S. Ajossa · O. Comparetto
C. Ronchetti · B. Piras · A. Piras · V. Mais
Department of Obstetrics and Gynecology, University of Cagliari, Policlinico Universitario Duilio Casula, Cagliari, Italy
e-mail: gineca.sguerriero@tiscali.it; gineca.sajossa@tiscali.it; camilla.ronchetti@fastwebnet.it; valerio.mais@alice.it

G. Cohen
Department of Obstetrics and Gynecology, Ultrasound Unit, Bnai-Zion Medical Center, Haifa, Israel

S. Guerriero et al. (eds.), *How to Perform Ultrasonography in Endometriosis*, https://doi.org/10.1007/978-3-319-71138-6_10

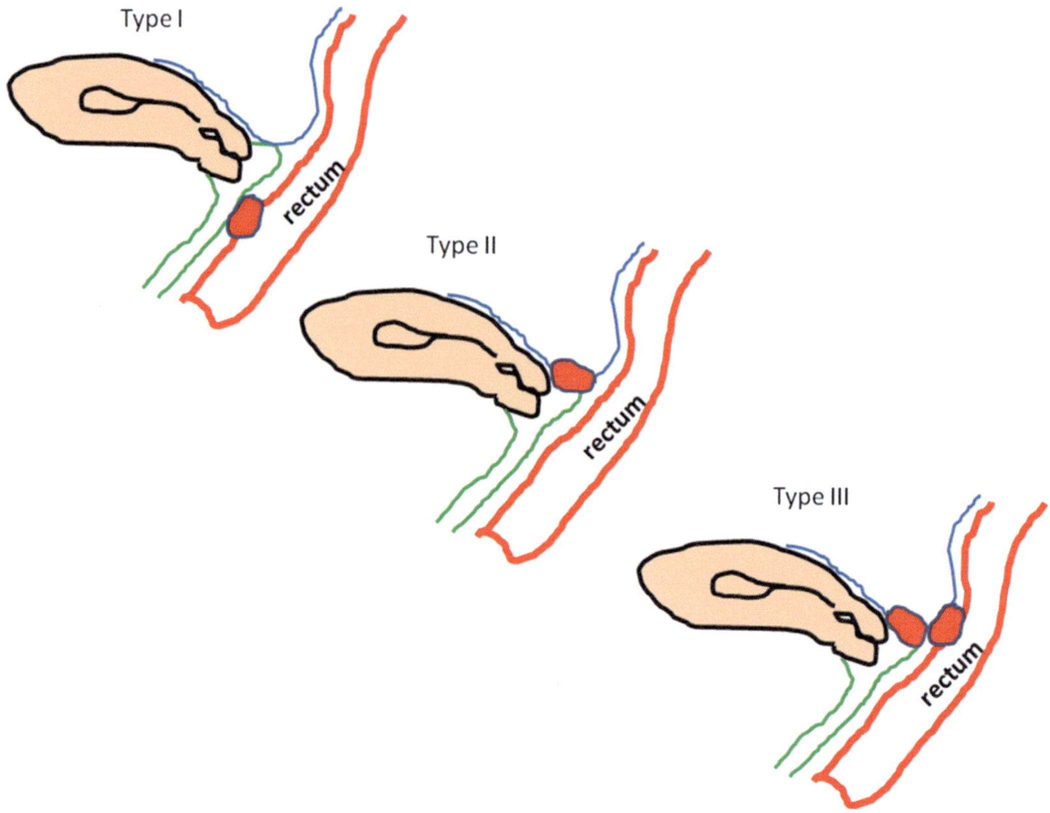

Fig. 10.1 A drawing of the three different localizations of forniceal-vaginal endometriotic lesions, previously called "retroperitoneal or retrocervical lesion" proposed by Donnez et al. [10]

Type III: hourglass-shaped or diabolo-like DE nodules (25% of cases). These lesions occur when posterior fornix lesions extend cranially to the anterior rectal wall. The part of the adenomyotic lesion situated in the anterior rectal wall is in the same size as the part situated near the posterior fornix. A small but well-observed continuum exists between these two parts of the lesion. These lesions always occur under the peritoneal fold of the recto-uterine pouch or pouch of Douglas and were found to be large (their average size estimated to be 3 cm by clinical examination) [10].

The present chapter is focused on types II and III. Type I or rectovaginal septum DE is described in Chap. 11.

Fauconnier et al. [13] found an association between the presence of vaginal DE and painful defecation during menstruation and other gastrointestinal symptoms. Chapron et al. [14] found that the presence of vaginal infiltration by the posterior DE was related to the severity of dysmenorrhea, while this correlation was not observed by Vercellini et al. study [15].

Several studies evaluated the sensitivity and specificity of transvaginal ultrasound (TVS) for vaginal DE lesions. Guerriero et al. [2] in their meta-analysis found a sensitivity of 58% and a specificity of 96%. Nisenblat et al. [16] in a Cochrane review found a mean sensitivity of 57% and a mean specificity of 99%. Noventa et al. [17] in their meta-analysis found a sensitivity of 50% with a specificity of 88.7%.

10.2 How We Do It

As suggested by IDEA consensus [5], an optimal sonographic evaluation starts with a detailed clinical history evaluation [5, 18–20]. It is mandatory to do a vaginal examination in women with a

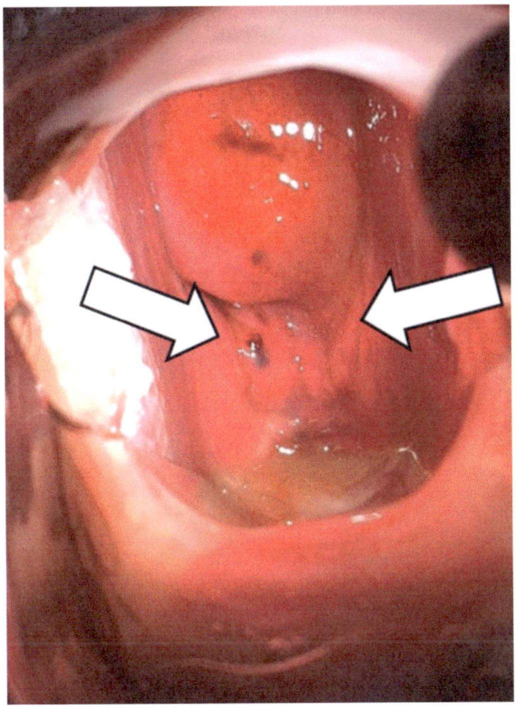

Fig. 10.2 A forniceal nodule as visualized using speculum

vaginal DE nodule. Indeed, some forniceal DE lesions can be visualized directly by a speculum examination (Fig. 10.2).

On TVS, the posterior fornix refers to the sonographic area between the lower border of the posterior lip of the cervix and the caudal end of the peritoneum of the lower margin of the recto-uterine peritoneal pouch (pouch of Douglas) (see Chap. 11). At TVS a forniceal DE lesion appears as a thickened posterior vaginal fornix or as a discrete nodule in the hypoechoic layer of the vaginal wall. The hypoechoic nodule may be homogeneous or inhomogeneous with or without large cystic areas with or without cystic areas surrounding the nodule [5] (Figs. 10.3, 10.4, 10.5, 10.6, 10.7, 10.8 and 10.9).

The sonographic assessment of the posterior fornix should aim to identify not only the presence of DE but also the size (in three orthogonal planes), the anatomical relationship with contiguous structures, and eventually the possible mobility or fixation of the surrounding organs with or without tenderness. We suggest to use the color Doppler modality for every lesion in order

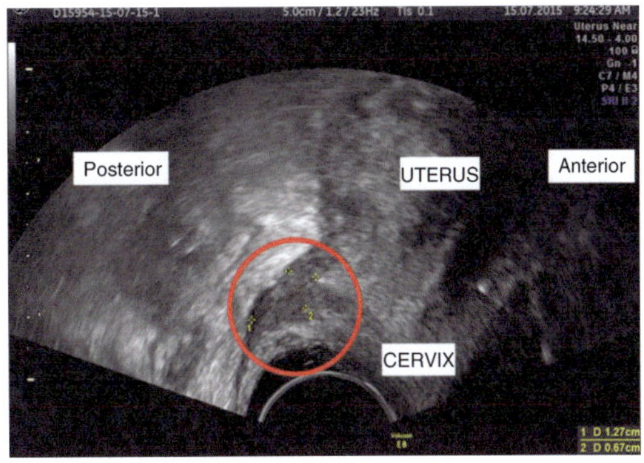

Fig. 10.3 A solid forniceal nodule as visualized using transvaginal ultrasonography

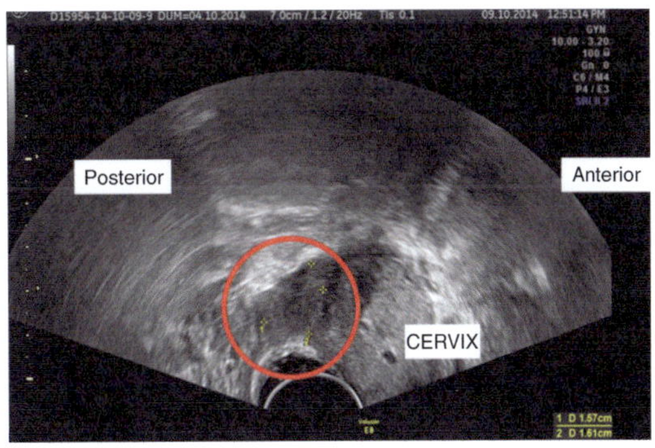

Fig. 10.4 A solid forniceal nodule as visualized using transvaginal ultrasonography

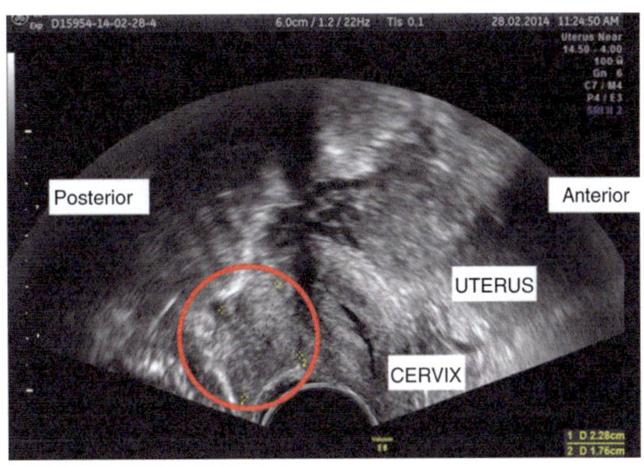

Fig. 10.5 A solid forniceal nodule as visualized using transvaginal ultrasonography

to rule out other possible diagnoses (Figs. 10.10, 10.11 and 10.12). After a careful ultrasound evaluation of the posterior vaginal fornix, the observer has to proceed with exploring the relationship with the rectal wall by sliding the transvaginal

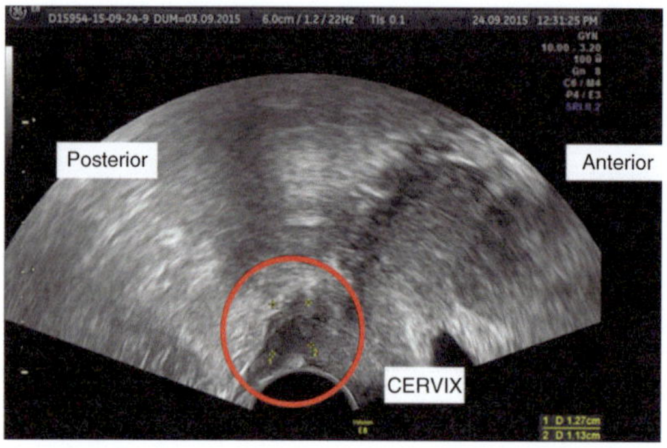

Fig. 10.6 A solid forniceal nodule as visualized using transvaginal ultrasonography

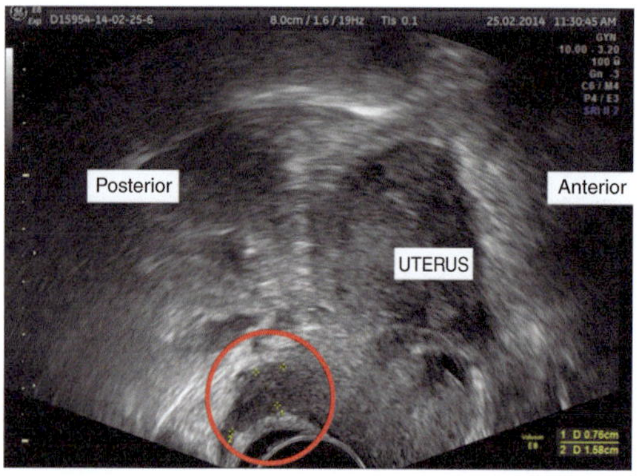

Fig. 10.7 A solid forniceal nodule as visualized using transvaginal ultrasonography

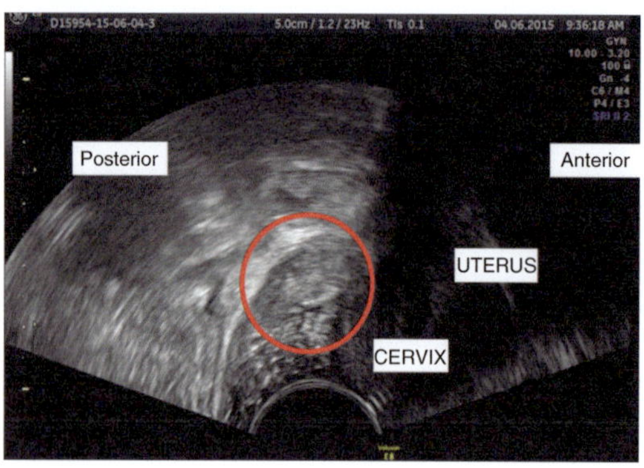

Fig. 10.8 A solid forniceal nodule as visualized using transvaginal ultrasonography

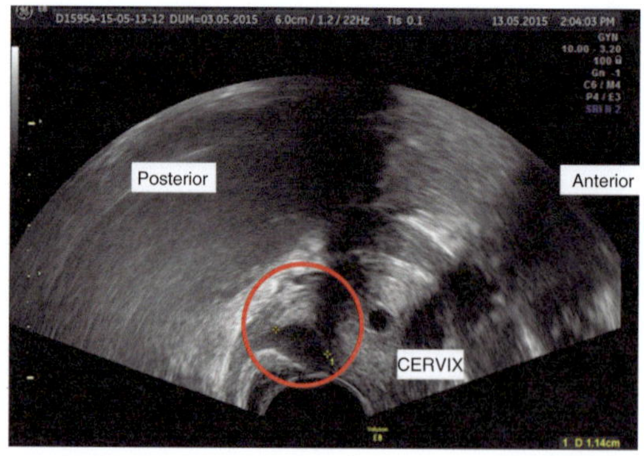

Fig. 10.9 A cystic forniceal nodule as visualized using transvaginal ultrasonography

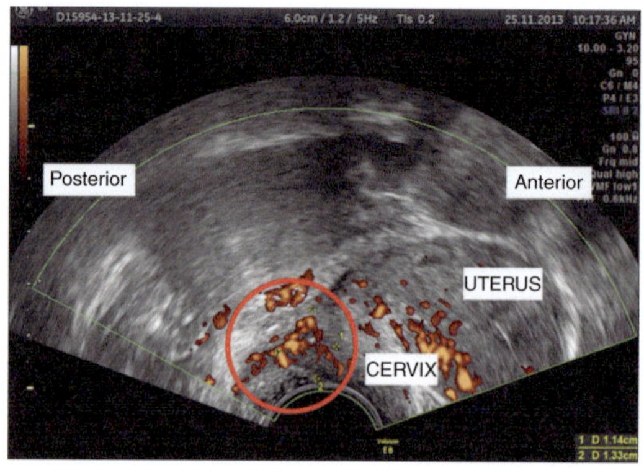

Fig. 10.10 A solid forniceal nodule as visualized using transvaginal ultrasonography and power Doppler

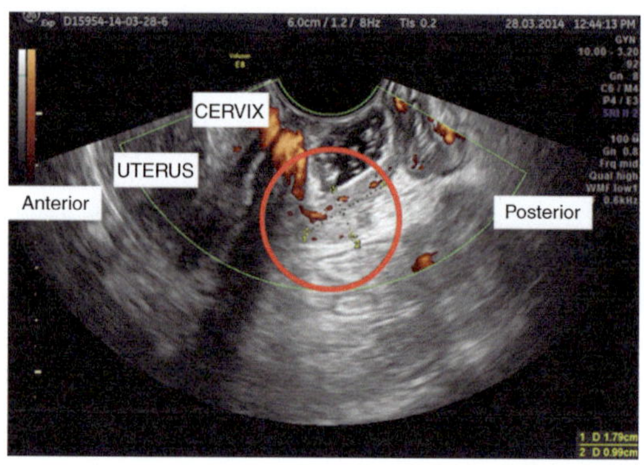

Fig. 10.11 A solid forniceal nodule as visualized using transvaginal ultrasonography and power Doppler

probe back and forth from the vaginal introitus along the rectovaginal septum.

In vaginal DE cases which are hourglass-shaped or diabolo-like in appearance, the lesions extend cranially to the anterior rectal wall where a nodule is present at the level of muscularis mucosa (further details in Chap. 12) (Figs. 10.13 and 10.14). In such cases, both DE nodules should be measured in the three planes.

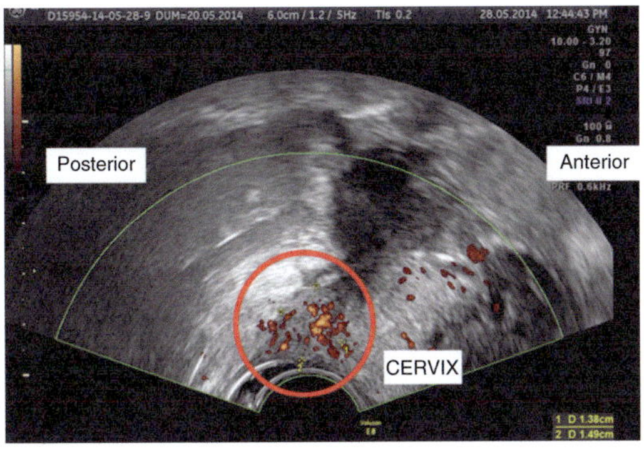

Fig. 10.12 A solid forniceal nodule as visualized using transvaginal ultrasonography and power Doppler

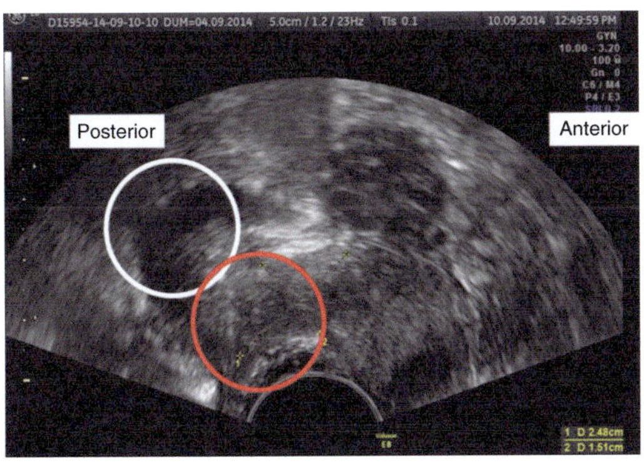

Fig. 10.13 A diabolo-like nodule as visualized using transvaginal ultrasonography. In the white circle, the rectosigmoid nodule; in the red one, the forniceal nodule

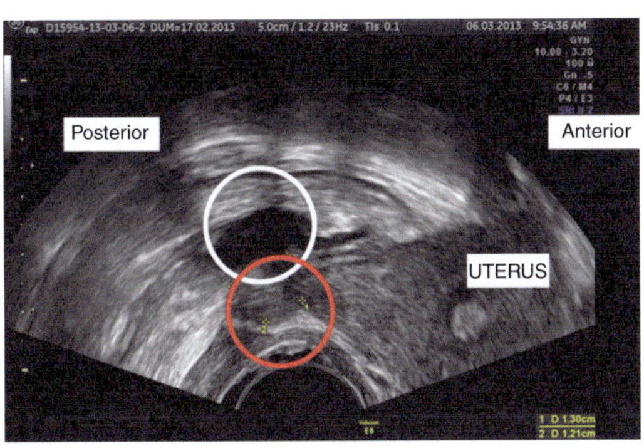

Fig. 10.14 A diabolo-like nodule as visualized using transvaginal ultrasonography. In the white circle, the rectosigmoid nodule; in the red one, the forniceal nodule

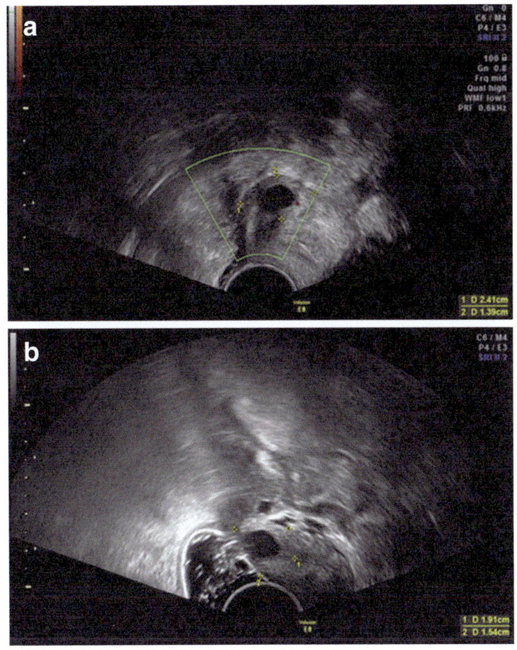

Fig. 10.15 A forniceal nodule as visualized using plain transvaginal ultrasonography (**a**) and using tenderness technique (**b**)

For vaginally located DE, the use of tenderness-guided ultrasound examination is recommended [4]. In this modality, an increased amount of ultrasound gel is inserted into the transvaginal probe cover (but using only a finger glove). This “standoff” technique creates a gap between the tip of the transvaginal probe and surrounding vaginal fornices. The transvaginal probe is gently inserted into the vagina to avoid obliteration of the gel. The gradual introduction of the probe to the level of the posterior fornix may assist to visualize lesions previously not detected. During this initial ultrasound evaluation, the patient should be asked to inform the operator about the onset and the site of any tenderness experienced during the probe’s placement in the posterior vaginal fornix. Particular attention must be noted to the indicated painful site which may reveal adjacent endometriosis lesions [21] (Fig. 10.15). Using this modality, a better visualization of the lesion has been demonstrated [21] (Videos 10.1 and 10.2). Further details are present in Chap. 14.

The use of a three-dimensional (3D) TVS is also a suggested modality. After acquiring the 3D volume, the observer can perform a virtual navigation and a 3D evaluation using the B plane with the ROI line on the left side of the 3D box and the green line curved into the center of lesion (using

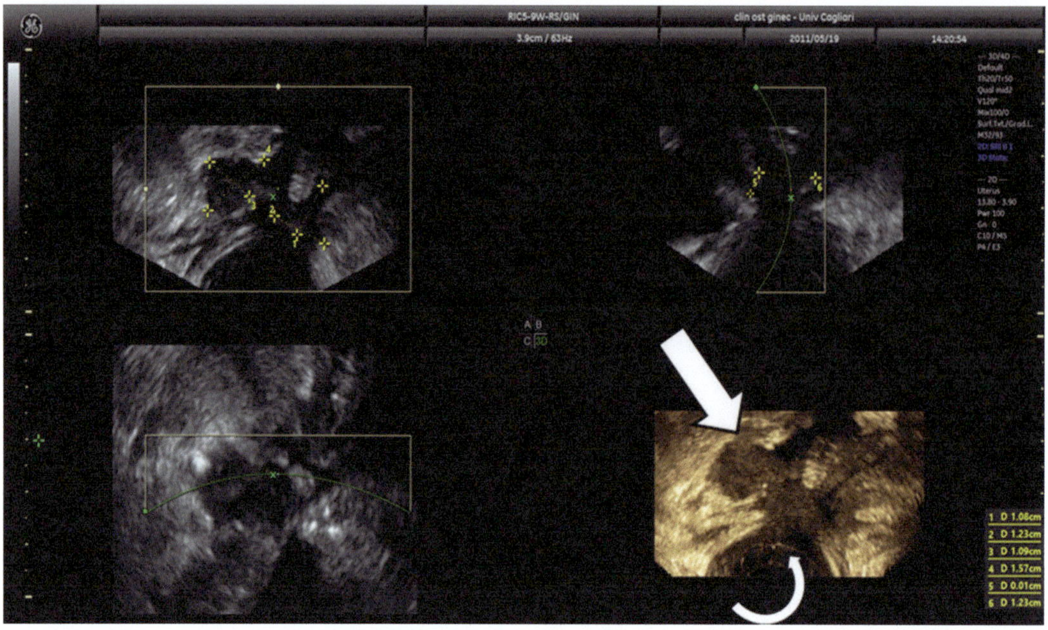

Fig. 10.16 A three-dimensional visualization of a diabolo-like nodule. The *straight arrow* indicates the rectosigmoid lesion and the *curved arrow* the forniceal nodule

a sagittal plane). Typically these lesions appear as small irregular nodules [22] (Fig. 10.16).

In the presence of suspected vaginal DE, the final recommended step for forniceal-vaginal evaluation is to perform a TVS combined with the use of either saline [23, 24] or gel [25–27] sonovaginography (see Chap. 14). Using gel sonovaginography, before the insertion of the transvaginal probe, approximately 20–50 mL of ultrasound gel is inserted into the posterior vaginal fornix by using a 20 mL plastic syringe [25–27]. The gel creates an acoustic window that allows a "standoff" view of the structures of the posterior compartment. It has been reported that using this modality gives better visualization of the lesion [25–27] (see Videos 10.3 and 10.4).

10.3 Important Technical Tip

Our advice is to use the four basic sonographic steps proposed by the IDEA consensus [5], taking note of site-specific tenderness and the dynamic evaluation of the relationship between the anterior rectal wall and the posterior vaginal fornix. In the assessment for DE lesions in the posterior compartment, our advice is to include the following information:

1. The size of DE lesion (measured in three orthogonal planes)
2. The anatomical relationship with contiguous structures
3. The possible mobility or fixation of the surrounding organs
4. The presence or absence of flow using color Doppler

The following recommendations might also be useful:

1. Perform a gradual introduction of the transvaginal probe using gentle movements and the possible addition of gel with lidocaine on the cover probe.
2. Remember the synergy between the operator and the patient especially when assessing tenderness-guided ultrasound.
3. Explore suspected vaginal DE by using gel sonovaginography. When compared to saline

sonovaginography, gel sonovaginography is less complicated to perform, requires less preparation, and produces less discomfort. Before performing gel sonovaginography, we recommend that the gel must be carefully drawn up into the syringe, ensuring there are no or only minimal air bubbles in the gel; and the syringe is filled completely, so that the plunger comes in direct contact with the gel, reducing the possibility of air pockets when instilling the gel into the vagina.

4. Report the absence of the normal sonographic anatomy.
5. Emphasize the presence of hourglass-shaped or diabolo-like nodules in the written report. This might influence the surgical planning (to proceed or not) as well as increase the surgical risks due to the associated invasiveness with such lesions.
6. Use offline 3D volumes for a virtual navigation in a suspected area which can be done to reevaluate not only the characteristics of the DE lesions but also the relationship with the surrounding organs.
7. Keep in mind that in some cases of forniceal lesions, the rectovaginal septum can be involved. This combination of lesions can be particularly difficult to remove surgically due to the proximity of the anal sphincter, and the surgeon should be advised of this.
8. Three-dimentional introital ultrasonography is another modality which can also be helpful in the assessment of rectovaginal septum DE lesions (see Chap. 14) [28].

10.4 Future Perspectives

Three-dimensional TVS may be useful since it has been demonstrated to have a significantly higher diagnostic accuracy in the diagnosis for vaginal DE with a sensitivity for posterior location (without intestinal involvement) of 87% and a specificity of 94% [22]. However, the mobility of the pelvic organs cannot be evaluated using this modality. Three-dimensional introital sonography might be an additional option, but this modality has only been evaluated for rectovaginal septum DE [28, 29].

Until now, there are no studies on rectosonography or 3D rectosonography in evaluating forniceal-vaginal DE (see Chap. 14). Transvaginal elastography may be a future tool in exploring forniceal-vaginal DE. Fusion imaging, also known as real-time virtual sonography, is a new technique that uses magnetic navigation and computer software for the synchronized display of real-time ultrasound and multiplanar reconstructed magnetic resonance imaging (MRI) images. This technique combines the advantages of both MRI and ultrasound. Fusion imaging allows better identification of the main anatomical sites of DE and has the potential to improve the performance of ultrasound and MRI examination [30].

References

1. Chapron C, Chopin N, Borghese B, Foulot H, Dousset B, Vacher-Lavenu MC, Vieira M, Hasan W, Bricou A. Deeply infiltrating endometriosis: pathogenetic implications of the anatomical distribution. Hum Reprod. 2006;21:1839–45.
2. Guerriero S, Ajossa S, Minguez JA, Jurado M, Mais V, Melis GB, Alcazar JL. Accuracy of transvaginal ultrasound for diagnosis of deep endometriosis in uterosacral ligaments, rectovaginal septum, vagina and bladder: systematic review and meta-analysis. Ultrasound Obstet Gynecol. 2015;46:534–45.
3. Vimercati A, Achilarre MT, Scardapane A, Lorusso F, Ceci O, Mangiatordi G, Angelelli G, Van Herendael B, Selvaggi L, Bettocchi S. Accuracy of transvaginal sonography and contrast-enhanced magnetic resonance-colonography for the presurgical staging of deep infiltrating endometriosis. Ultrasound Obstet Gynecol. 2012;40:592–603.
4. Guerriero S, Ajossa S, Gerada M, Virgilio B, Angioni S, Melis GB. Diagnostic value of transvaginal 'tenderness guided' ultrasonography for the prediction of location of deep endometriosis. Hum Reprod. 2008;23:2452–7.
5. Guerriero S, Condous G, Van Den Bosch T, Valentin L, Leone FPG, Van Schoubroeck D, Exacoustos C, Installè AJF, Martins WP, Abrao MS, Hudelist G, Bazot M, Alcazar JL, Gonçalves MO, Pascual MA, Ajossa s, Savelli L, Dunham R, Reid S, Menakaya U, Bourne T, Ferrero S, Leon M, Bignardi T, Holland T, Jurkovic D, Benacerraf B, Osuga Y, Somigliana E, Timmerman D. Systematic approach to sonographic evaluation of the pelvis in women with suspected endometriosis, including terms, definitions and measurements: a consensus opinion from the International Deep Endometriosis Analysis (IDEA) group. Ultrasound Obstet Gynecol. 2016;48:318.

6. Koninckx PR, Meuleman C, Demeyere S, Lesaffre E, Cornillie FJ. Suggestive evidence that pelvic endometriosis is a progressive disease, whereas deeply infiltrating endometriosis is associated with pelvic pain. Fertil Steril. 1991;55:759–65.
7. Vercellini P, Frontino G, Pietropaolo G, Gattei U, Daguati R, Crosignani PG. Deep endometriosis: definition and clinical management. J Am Assoc Gynecol Laparosc. 2004;11:153–61.
8. Anaf V, El Nakadi I, De Moor V, Chapron C, Pistofidis G, Noel JC. Increased nerve density in deep infiltrating endometriotic nodules. Gynecol Obstet Investig. 2011;71(2):112–7.
9. Matsuzaki S, Houlle C, Botchorishvili R, Pouly JL, Mage G, Canis M. Excision of the posterior vaginal fornix is necessary to ensure complete resection of rectovaginal endometriotic nodules of more than 2 cm in size. Fertil Steril. 2009;91(4 Suppl):1314–5.
10. Donnez J, Pirard C, Smets M, Jadoul P, Squifflet J. Surgical management of endometriosis. Best Pract Res Clin Obstet Gynaecol. 2004;18(2):329–48.
11. Squifflet J, Feger C, Donnez J. Diagnosis and imaging of adenomyotic disease of the retroperitoneal space. Gynecol Obstet Investig. 2002;54:43–51.
12. Del Frate C, Rossano Girometti R, Pittino M, Del Frate G, Bazzocchi M, Zuiani C. Deep retroperitoneal pelvic endometriosis: MR imaging appearance with laparoscopic correlation. Radiographics. 2006;26:1705–18.
13. Fauconnier A, Chapron C, Dubuisson JB, Vieira M, Dousset B, Bréart G. Relation between pain symptoms and the anatomic location of deep infiltrating endometriosis. Fertil Steril. 2002;78(4):719–26.
14. Chapron C, Fauconnier A, Dubuisson JB, Barakat H, Vieira M, Bréart G. Deep infiltrating endometriosis: relation between severity of dysmenorrhoea and extent of disease. Hum Reprod. 2003;18(4):760–6.
15. Vercellini P, Trespidi L, De Giorgi O, Cortesi I, Parazzini F, Crosignani PG. Endometriosis and pelvic pain: relation to disease stage and localization. Fertil Steril. 1996;65:299–304.
16. Nisenblat V, Bossuyt PMM, Farquhar C, Johnson N, Hull ML. Imaging modalities for the non-invasive diagnosis of endometriosis. Cochrane Database Syst Rev 2016;(2).
17. Noventa M, Saccardi C, Litta P, Vitagliano A, D'Antona D, Abdulrahim B, Duncan A, Alexander-Sefre F, Aldrich CJ, Quaranta M, Gizzo S. Ultrasound techniques in the diagnosis of deep pelvic endometriosis: algorithm based on a systematic review and meta-analysis. Fertil Steril. 2015;104(2):366–83.
18. Chapron C, Barakat H, Fritel X, Dubuisson JB, Breart G, Fauconnier A. Presurgical diagnosis of posterior deep infiltrating endometriosis based on a standardized questionnaire. Hum Reprod. 2005;20:507–13.
19. Fedele L, Bianchi S, Carmignani L, Berlanda N, Fontana E, Frontino G. Evaluation of a new questionnaire for the presurgical diagnosis of bladder endometriosis. Hum Reprod. 2007;22:2698–701.
20. Hudelist G, Ballard K, English J, Wright J, Banerjee S, Mastoroudes H, Thomas A, Singer CF, Keckstein J. Transvaginal sonography vs. clinical examination in the preoperative diagnosis of deep infiltrating endometriosis. Ultrasound Obstet Gynecol. 2011;37(4):480–7.
21. Guerriero S, Ajossa S, Gerada M, D'Aquila M, Piras B, Melis GB. "Tenderness-guided" transvaginal ultrasonography: a new method for the detection of deep endometriosis in patients with chronic pelvic pain. Fertil Steril. 2007;88(5):1293–7.
22. Guerriero S, Saba L, Ajossa S, Peddes C, Angiolucci M, Perniciano M, Melis GB, Alcazar JL. Three-dimensional ultrasonography in the diagnosis of deep endometriosis. Hum Reprod. 2014;29:1189–98.
23. Dessole S, Farina M, Rubattu G, Cosmi E, Ambrosini G, Nardelli GB. Sonovaginography is a new technique for assessing rectovaginal endometriosis. Fertil Steril. 2003;79:1023–7.
24. Saccardi C, Cosmi E, Borghero A, Tregnaghi A, Dessole S, Litta P. Comparison between transvaginal sonography, saline contrast sonovaginography and magnetic resonance imaging in the diagnosis of posterior deep infiltrating endometriosis. Ultrasound Obstet Gynecol. 2012;40:464–9.
25. Reid S, Winder S, Condous G. Sonovaginography: redefining the concept of a "normal pelvis" on transvaginal ultrasound pre-laparoscopic intervention for suspected endometriosis. Aust J Ultrasound Med. 2011;14:21–4.
26. Reid S, Lu C, Hardy N, Casikar I, Reid G, Cario G, Chou D, Almashat D, Condous G. Office gel sonovaginography for the prediction of posterior deep infiltrating endometriosis: a multicenter prospective observational study. Ultrasound Obstet Gynecol. 2014;44:710–8.
27. Leon M, Vaccaro H, Alcazar JL, Martinez J, Gutierrez J, Amor F, Iturra A, Sovino H. Extended transvaginal sonography in deep infiltrating endometriosis: use of bowel preparation and an acoustic window with intravaginal gel: preliminary results. J Ultrasound Med. 2014;33:315–21.
28. Pascual MA, Guerriero S, Hereter L, Barri-Soldevila P, Ajossa S, Graupera B, Rodriguez I. Diagnosis of endometriosis of the rectovaginal septum using introital three-dimensional ultrasonography. Fertil Steril. 2010;94:2761–5.
29. Pascual MA, Guerriero S, Hereter L, Barri-Soldevila P, Ajossa S, Graupera B, Rodriguez I. Three-dimensional sonography for diagnosis of rectovaginal septum endometriosis: interobserver agreement. J Ultrasound Med. 2013;32:931–5.
30. Millischer AE, Salomon LJ, Santulli P, Borghese B, Dousset B, Chapron C. Fusion imaging for evaluation of deep infiltrating endometriosis: feasibility and preliminary results. Ultrasound Obstet Gynecol. 2015;46(1):109–17.

Rectovaginal Septum Endometriosis

11

Gernot Hudelist and Kristine Aas-Eng

11.1 Introduction

The rectovaginal septum (RVS) is located in the posterior compartment of the pelvis situated retroperitoneally between the posterior wall of the vagina and the anterior part of the rectum [1]. It is a specific anatomical structure consisting of strong connective tissue between the rectum and the vagina. Histopathological studies have demonstrated that it is formed of a network of collagen and elastic fibres, small vessels, smooth muscle cells and nerve fibres predominantly deriving from the autonomic inferior hypogastric plexus [2]. It thereby connects the perineal body and endopelvic fascia (Fig. 11.1). Anatomically the RVS is described to extend from the base of the rectovaginal pouch of Douglas to the urogenital diaphragm at the top of the perineal body (Fig. 11.2) [3].

In rectovaginal endometriosis, which per definition infiltrates the RVS, the rectal wall is usually affected unlike in retrocervical endometriosis where the bowel wall is not affected by deep infiltrating disease [3]. The distinction between rectovaginal and retrocervical endometriosis is important in the surgical management since the former is often treated with bowel resection and the latter with local excision or ablation [4].

G. Hudelist (✉) · K. Aas-Eng
Department of Gynecology, Hospital St. John of God, Vienna, Austria

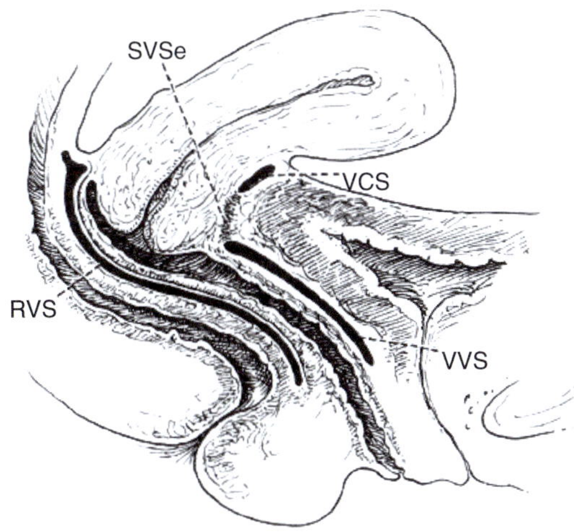

Fig. 11.1 Median sagittal section through the female pelvis showing the midline connective tissue spaces between the bladder, vagina and rectum. The vesicocervical space *(VCS)* is separated from the vesicovaginal space *(VVS)* by the supravaginal septum (SVSe). The rectovaginal space *(RVS)* is located between the rectum and the vagina, extending from the perineal body to the bottom of the cul-de-sac of Douglas (from The Global Library of Women's Medicine, free resource)

Bazot et al. defined that the RVS was affected on transvaginal ultrasound (TVS) when "a nodule or mass was found below the horizontal plane passing through the lower border of the posterior lip of the cervix (under the peritoneum)" [5]. Others similarly have defined the RVS on TVS as "the area between the rectum and the posterior vaginal wall from the level of the introitus up to a level defined by the lower border of the posterior lip of

S. Guerriero et al. (eds.), *How to Perform Ultrasonography in Endometriosis*,
https://doi.org/10.1007/978-3-319-71138-6_11

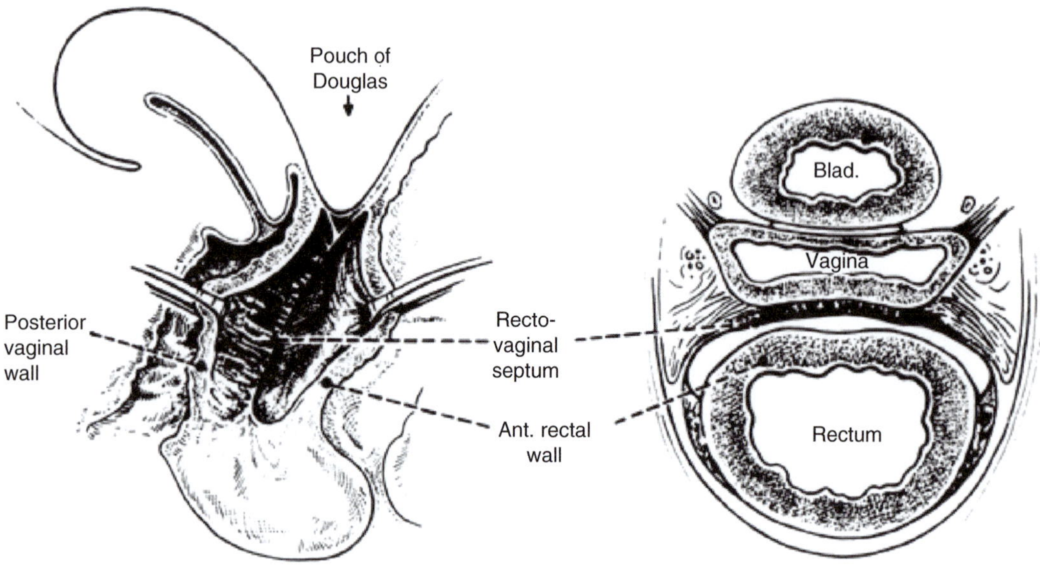

Fig. 11.2 Partly dissected rectovaginal septum extending from the pouch of Douglas to the perineal body (from The Global Library of Women's Medicine, free resource)

the cervix" [6]. The prevalence of endometriosis involving the RVS has been found to range between 6 and 52% [7, 8] in patients with suspected deep endometriosis (DE). The varying prevalence rates may be attributable to differences in sonographic definition of DE affecting the RVS but also patient populations and the sonographer's experience in TVS. RVS endometriosis does not occur solely in this anatomical compartment, i.e. the RVS, and is usually associated with endometriotic infiltration of the vagina and anterior rectal wall [9, 10], based on the presumption that it originates from these neighbouring structures [9].

TVS is regarded as the first-line tool in diagnosing DE affecting the rectum and associated structures [11, 12]. However, diagnosis of RVS nodules may be difficult which is reflected by sensitivity rates of TVS ranging between 9 and 78% [5, 6, 10]. Bazot et al. [13] compared TVS with rectal endoscopic sonography (RES) and found an improved sensitivity from 11 to 22% using RES, although the patient number was small ($n = 9$). These findings have been supported by a study comparing physical examination, TVS, RES and MRI in detecting DE [10]. Within this, physical examination and RES had similar sensitivities of 18% compared with TVS (9%) and MRI (55%).

Additional methods have been proposed to improve sensitivity rates of TVS detecting rectovaginal DE. For example, the use of 3-D TVS for RVS DE appears to reach a sensitivity of 76% and a specificity of 100% [14]. Ros et al. [15] looked at improving sensitivity of TVS in detection of rectal disease with bowel preparation from 73% without bowel preparation. Saccardi et al. [16] found saline contrast sonography, i.e. TVS with introduction of saline solution in the vagina, had better sensitivity comparable to MRI for diagnosing endometriosis of the RVS of 81% and 83%, respectively, whereas TVS without contrast had a sensitivity of 58%.

High sensitivity rates of 78% have been reported for detection of RVS endometriosis using simple vaginal examination *and* TVS when the two methods were used isolated or in a combined setting [6, 17]. However, the sensitivity for the detection of rectosigmoid lesions that often occur with RVS was higher with TVS of 90% compared to 39% vaginal examination alone. Furthermore, a modified TVS method with transvaginal "tenderness-guided" ultrasonography, which entails an acoustic window created by increasing the amount of gel to 12 mL and paying particular attention to areas that provokes pain, reached similar sensitivity for RVS nodules of 74%, specificity 88%, LR+ 6.21 and LR− 0.30 [7]. Compared to the previous studies mentioned, sensitivity rates were found to be much higher in these two studies, which may be explained by differences in patient populations and possibly the sonographers' experience. However, TVS remains the most accessible, cost-effective and well-tolerated tool in the diagnosis of RVS endometriosis with or without rectal/vaginal involvement. Ideally, a combination of clinical/visual inspection, vaginal examination and TVS may be the method of choice for accurately diagnosing RVS involvement.

11.2 How We Do It

The International Deep Endometriosis Analysis (IDEA) group proposes a four-step systematic approach to assess women with suspected endometriosis. The fourth step consists of evaluating the anterior and posterior compartment [18]. The most common sites of DE affecting the posterior compartment are the uterosacral ligaments, posterior vaginal fornix, anterior rectum/anterior rectosigmoid junction and sigmoid colon. According to the IDEA group definition, infiltration of the RVS is suspected on TVS in cases where nodular deep infiltrating disease can be visualized below the line passing along the lower border of the posterior lip of the cervix (under the peritoneum) [18] (Fig. 11.3).

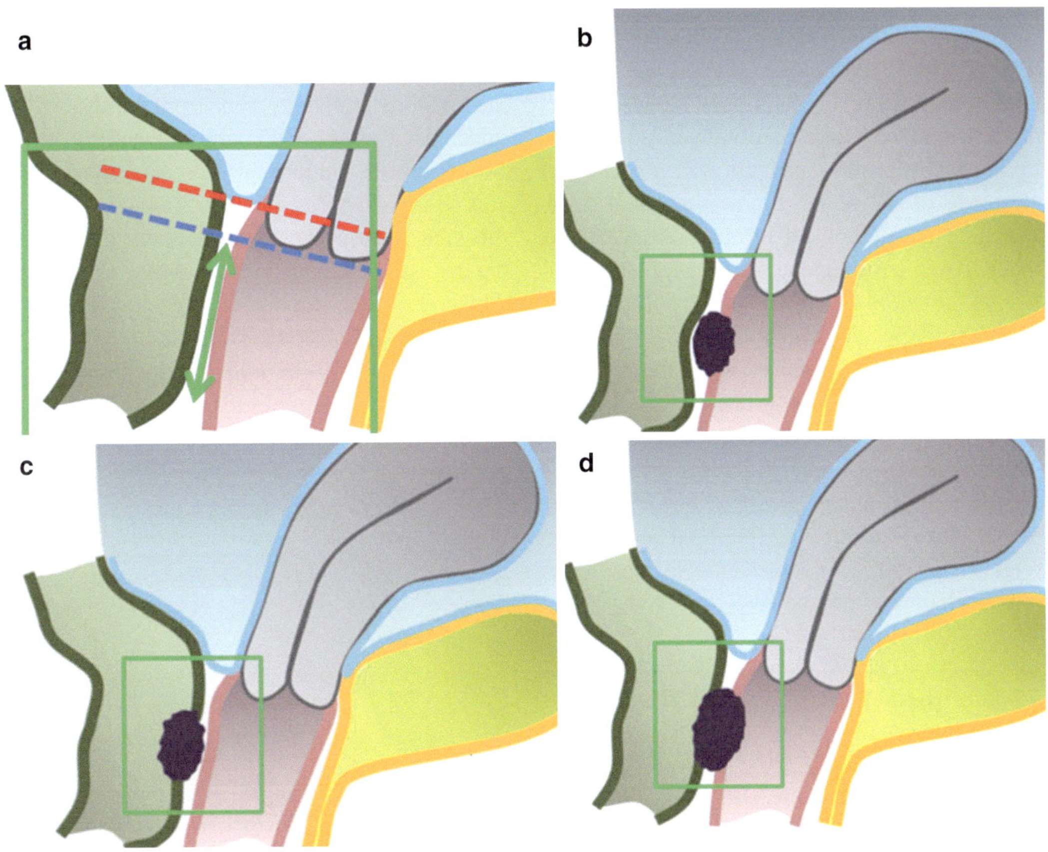

Fig. 11.3 (**a**) Schematic drawing of the RVS (double-headed *green arrow*) below (anatomically) the blue line passing along the lower border of the posterior lip of the cervix with the posterior vaginal fornix between the blue line and the red line according to the IDEA consensus (from Guerriero et al. [18] with permission). (**b–d**) Schematic drawing demonstrating DE of the RVS with predominantly vaginal involvement (**b**), rectal involvement (**c**) or both structures (**d**) (from Guerriero et al. [18] with permission)

On TVS, RVS endometriotic lesions can be described to appear isolated which is very uncommon and extremely rare. Usually, DE of the RVS involve the vaginal wall, the rectal wall or both (Fig. 11.3b, c, d). The IDEA group emphasizes the importance of locating the number, size and anatomical distribution of DE nodules in the rectovaginal septum, vaginal wall, rectovaginal nodules, rectum, rectosigmoid junction, sigmoid and uterosacral ligaments. We believe this is fundamental in planning medical and/or surgical treatment and in the follow-up of patients with DE. The RVS DE nodules should be measured in three orthogonal planes, i.e. midsagittal, anteroposterior and transverse [18]. Additionally, the estimated distance between the lower margin of the lesion and the anal verge should also be measured in the opinion of the authors due to its relevance for possible surgery.

In the author's practice, TVS and possible detection of RVS nodules in patients with DE are done without bowel preparation or other enhancement techniques. This is predominantly explained by the fact that most patients will not undergo cleansing of the bowel for personal and infrastructural reasons of our referral setting. Using the IDEA algorithm, the transvaginal probe is held in the midsagittal plane of the pelvis visualizing the uterus and cervix. Then the handle of the probe is gradually moved upwards, and at the same time, the tip of the probe is moved downwards to visualize the rectovaginal septum including neighbouring structures such as the posterior cervix and vaginal wall beginning from the introitus. Concurrently the rectal wall is thoroughly assessed for endometriotic lesions involving or separated from the RVS.

11.3 Important Technical Tips

In healthy women, the RVS appears as a thin, hyperechogenic layer between the vagina and anterior rectum, parity being associated with increasing length [19]. In the midsagittal section, the vaginal wall appears thicker compared to the RVS and usually can be visualized as iso-, partly moderate hypoechogenic layer which is in direct contact with the sonographic probe. In contrast, the anterior rectal wall, which is followed by the RVS, is visualized as an anechogenic line due to its three layers of muscle fibres and the covering mucosa which appears hyperechogenic (Fig. 11.4). In patients with DE of the posterior compartment, the endometriotic tissue infiltrating the RVS and adjacent structures such as the vagina and/or rectum usually appears as hypoechoic thickening of the posterior part of the vagina and/or anterior wall of the bowel (Fig. 11.5a–c). Rarely, cystic components of vaginal DE can be visualized as hypo- or anechogenic cystic structures which may vary in size and have smooth or irregular contours [6, 20]. Full visualization of the RVS can only be achieved by lifting the probe at the level of the vaginal introitus. The visualization of the RVS should include concomitant visualization of the rectum and vagina since these structures will most likely be affected at the same time which therefore allows better orientation and localization of disease infiltrating the RVS. DE of the RVS predominantly starts from the level of the upper third of the RVS and will extend downwards into the middle third of the vagina. As a consequence, special attention should be given to this area. In cases where bowel contents may create acoustic artefacts or may appear as possible thickening of the rectal wall suggesting rectal DE, we suggest to repeat the examination following a brief pause of 10–15 min and to possibly use bowel preparation in selected cases to increase the

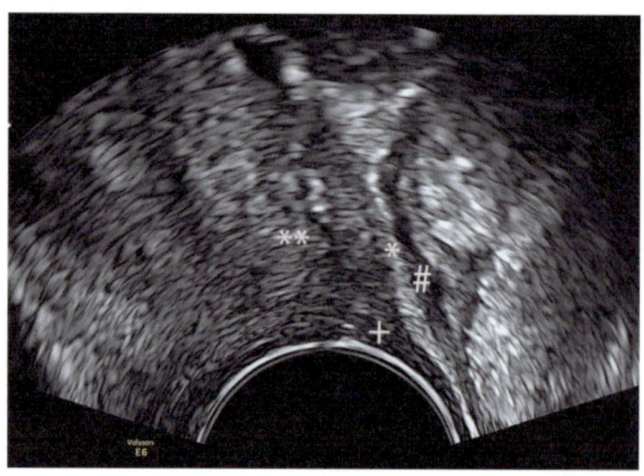

Fig. 11.4 TVS image (midsagittal section) depicting the normal sonoanatomy of the vagina appearing as moderately hypoechogenic line (+), the posterior cervical lip (**), and RVS appearing as thin and moderately hyperechogenic line (*) adjacent to the clearly hypoechogenic anterior rectal wall (#)

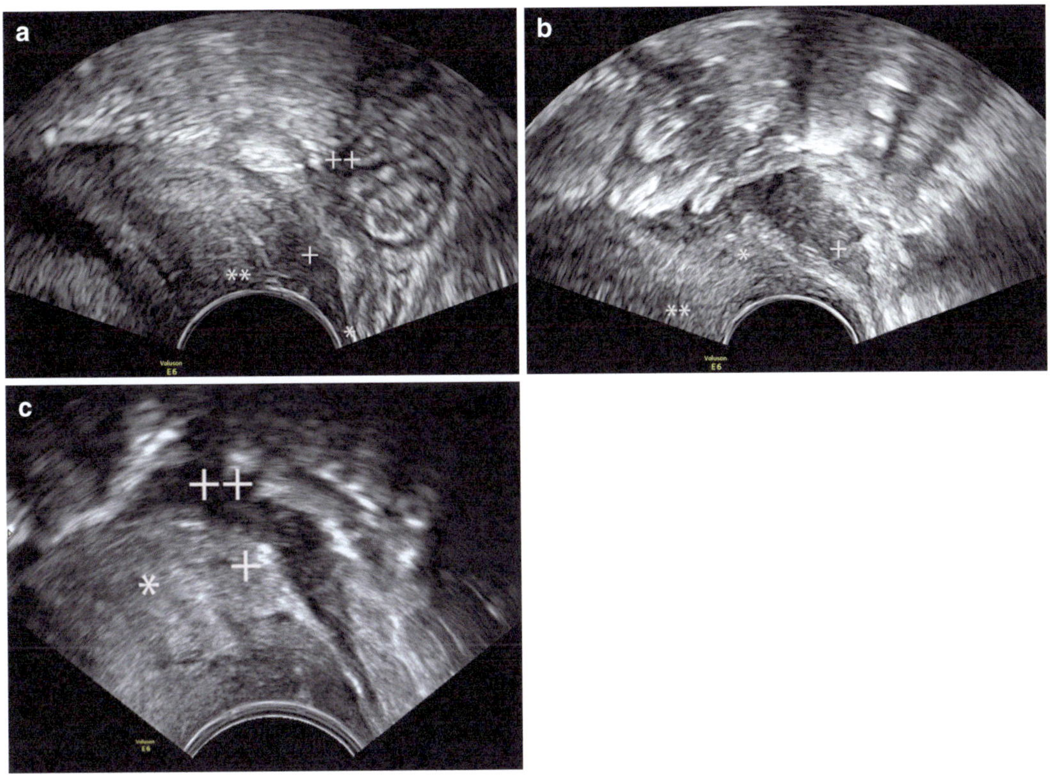

Fig. 11.5 (**a**) TVS image (midsagittal section) depicting DE of the RVS predominantly infiltrating the vagina and RVS (+) and focally the anterior rectal wall (++) which is involved above the RVS. Normal RVS (*); cervix (**). (**b**) TVS image (midsagittal section) depicting DE of the RVS predominantly infiltrating the RVS and anterior rectal wall (+) with focal infiltration of the upper vaginal fornix (*) next to the cervix (**). (**c**) TVS image (midsagittal section) depicting DE of the RVS predominantly infiltrating the vagina (+), RVS and the anterior rectal wall (++) which is involved below the level of the posterior cervical lip (*)

sonographic contrast of the vagina, RVS and rectal wall combined with a gel tip in a glove or condom covering the vaginal probe.

11.4 Future Perspectives

Over the past decade, TVS has become a standard for pre-surgical evaluation of patients with DE. In how far results of TVS influence surgical planning and practice is dependent on the grade of collaboration between the sonographer and the surgeon. In the author's practice, the ideal scenario is to perform both TVS and possible consequent surgery. TVS allows the surgeon to gain a non-invasive, in vivo image of the extent of DE prior to surgery. From the surgical point of view, it is pivotal to estimate the extent of disease laterally to pelvic sidewalls and caudally into the RVS. Lateral spread will often involve the autonomous nerve fibres and thereby increase morbidity in cases where DE is fully resected, especially in cases of bilateral inferior hypogastric nerve involvement.

DE extending deep into the RVS usually involves both the rectum and vagina. In women where surgery is considered, TVS may allow to assess the risk of rectovaginal surgery as low anterior resections with lesions with a distance less than 5–8 cm from the anal verge carry higher risks of anastomotic leaks and rectovaginal fistulas [3, 21]. The decision whether to perform protective ileostomies usually depends on the distance between the anastomosis and the anal verge, concomitant vaginal involvement and resection of vaginal DE as well as possible comorbidities of the patient. The accurate pre-surgical use of TVS to measure the distance from the anal verge to the lowermost part of the endometriotic nodule may provide this information prior to surgery and will thereby influence the surgical strategy. In addition, counselling of women with DE considering surgery may gain increasing accuracy and quality by adequate information of the extent of disease, possible surgical complications such as fistula formation and anastomotic leakage in cases of involvement of the RVS. Future studies on the accuracy of TVS regarding the extent of RVS DE and prediction of the level of bowel anastomosis in cases where rectal surgery and/or vaginal resections are performed are under way.

References

1. Chapron C, Fauconnier A, Vieira M, Barakat H, Dousset B, Pansini V, et al. Anatomical distribution of deeply infiltrating endometriosis: surgical implications and proposition for a classification. Hum Reprod. 2003;18(1):157–61.
2. Stecco C, Macchi V, Porzionato A, Tiengo C, Parenti A, Gardi M, et al. Histotopographic study of the rectovaginal septum. Ital J Anat Embryol. 2005;110(4):247–54.
3. Martin DC, Batt RE. Retrocervical, retrovaginal pouch, and rectovaginal septum endometriosis. J Am Assoc Gynecol Laparosc. 2001;8(1):12–7.
4. Kavallaris A, Kohler C, Kuhne-Heid R, Schneider A. Histopathological extent of rectal invasion by rectovaginal endometriosis. Hum Reprod. 2003;18(6):1323–7.
5. Bazot M, Thomassin I, Hourani R, Cortez A, Darai E. Diagnostic accuracy of transvaginal sonography for deep pelvic endometriosis. Ultrasound Obstet Gynecol. 2004;24(2):180–5.
6. Hudelist G, Ballard K, English J, Wright J, Banerjee S, Mastoroudes H, et al. Transvaginal sonography vs. clinical examination in the preoperative diagnosis of deep infiltrating endometriosis. Ultrasound Obstet Gynecol. 2011;37(4):480–7.
7. Guerriero S, Ajossa S, Gerada M, Virgilio B, Angioni S, Melis GB. Diagnostic value of transvaginal 'tenderness-guided' ultrasonography for the prediction of location of deep endometriosis. Hum Reprod. 2008;23(11):2452–7.
8. Exacoustos C, Malzoni M, Di Giovanni A, Lazzeri L, Tosti C, Petraglia F, et al. Ultrasound mapping system for the surgical management of deep infiltrating endometriosis. Fertil Steril. 2014;102(1):143–50. e2
9. Hudelist G, Keckstein J, Wright JT. The migrating adenomyoma: past views on the etiology of adenomyosis and endometriosis. Fertil Steril. 2009;92(5):1536–43.
10. Bazot M, Lafont C, Rouzier R, Roseau G, Thomassin-Naggara I, Darai E. Diagnostic accuracy of physical examination, transvaginal sonography, rectal endoscopic sonography, and magnetic resonance imaging to diagnose deep infiltrating endometriosis. Fertil Steril. 2009;92(6):1825–33.
11. Hudelist G, English J, Thomas AE, Tinelli A, Singer CF, Keckstein J. Diagnostic accuracy of transvaginal ultrasound for non-invasive diagnosis of bowel endometriosis: systematic review and meta-analysis. Ultrasound Obstet Gynecol. 2011;37(3):257–63.
12. Guerriero S, Ajossa S, Orozco R, Perniciano M, Jurado M, Melis GB, et al. Accuracy of transvaginal ultrasound for diagnosis of deep endometriosis in the rectosigmoid: systematic review and meta-analysis. Ultrasound Obstet Gynecol. 2016;47(3):281–9.
13. Bazot M, Malzy P, Cortez A, Roseau G, Amouyal P, Darai E. Accuracy of transvaginal sonography and rectal endoscopic sonography in the diagnosis of deep infiltrating endometriosis. Ultrasound Obstet Gynecol. 2007;30(7):994–1001.
14. Grasso RF, Di Giacomo V, Sedati P, Sizzi O, Florio G, Faiella E, et al. Diagnosis of deep infiltrating endometriosis: accuracy of magnetic resonance imaging and transvaginal 3D ultrasonography. Abdom Imaging. 2010;35(6):716–25.
15. Ros C, Martinez-Serrano MJ, Rius M, Abrao MS, Munros J, Martinez-Zamora MA, et al. Bowel preparation improves the accuracy of the transvaginal ultrasound in the diagnosis of Rectosigmoid deep infiltrating endometriosis: a prospective study. J Minim Invasive Gynecol. 2017;24:1145.
16. Saccardi C, Cosmi E, Borghero A, Tregnaghi A, Dessole S, Litta P. Comparison between transvaginal sonography, saline contrast sonovaginography and magnetic resonance imaging in the diagnosis of posterior deep infiltrating endometriosis. Ultrasound Obstet Gynecol. 2012;40(4):464–9.
17. Hudelist G, Oberwinkler KH, Singer CF, Tuttlies F, Rauter G, Ritter O, et al. Combination of transvaginal sonography and clinical examination for preoperative diagnosis of pelvic endometriosis. Hum Reprod. 2009;24(5):1018–24.
18. Guerriero S, Condous G, van den Bosch T, Valentin L, Leone FP, Van Schoubroeck D, et al. Systematic approach to sonographic evaluation of the pelvis in women with suspected endometriosis, including terms, definitions and measurements: a consensus opinion from the International Deep Endometriosis Analysis (IDEA) group. Ultrasound Obstet Gynecol. 2016;48(3):318–32.
19. Kuhn RJ, Hollyock VE. Observations on the anatomy of the rectovaginal pouch and septum. Obstet Gynecol. 1982;59(4):445–7.
20. Dessole S, Farina M, Rubattu G, Cosmi E, Ambrosini G, Nardelli GB. Sonovaginography is a new technique for assessing rectovaginal endometriosis. Fertil Steril. 2003;79(4):1023–7.
21. Bouaziz J, Soriano D. Complications of colorectal resection for endometriosis. Minerva Ginecol. 2017;69(5):477–87.

12 Rectum, Rectosigmoid, and Sigmoid Endometriosis

Manoel Orlando Goncalves, Leandro Accardo de Mattos, and Mauricio S. Abrao

12.1 Introduction

Deep intestinal endometriosis (DE) is defined as nodules infiltrating at least the muscularis propria layer [1]. Lesions with dense adhesions and/or endometriotic infiltration up to the bowel serosa are not considered DE. Statistical analysis of groups considered as reference in highly complex surgeries demonstrates that up to 50% of endometriotic patients may have intestinal involvement [2, 3].

Around 64% of the lesions are located in the rectum, 21% in the sigmoid, and 15% in the right iliac fossa (appendix, ileum, and/or cecum).

The disease may be multifocal (more than one lesion in the same segment) or multicentric (multiple lesions affecting different segments—large and small intestine, cecum, and/or appendix). Multifocality is one of the main characteristics of deep endometriosis, mainly when the intestinal tract is involved. Multifocal bowel lesions are observed in up to 30% of the patients with rectosigmoid involvement [2, 4, 5]. Likewise, resection of more than one nodule from the bowel wall is known to be more complex than resecting just one localized nodule [1, 6].

Intestinal endometriosis may cause several symptoms depending on the location, inflammatory activity, size, and related adherence process. The main complaints are cyclic:

- Painful evacuation
- Rectal bleeding
- Changes in evacuation frequency (more or less frequent)

In extreme cases, when there is significant lumen reduction, there may be subocclusive or occlusive conditions.

When the bowel is compromised in the right iliac fossa, there may be cyclic epigastric pain [7].

In some patients, there is a discrepancy between the intestinal and clinical involvement, such as:

(a) There is intestinal endometriosis without specific symptoms.
(b) There is no intestinal endometriosis, but the patient presents suggestive symptoms due to

M. O. Goncalves
Female Pelvis Diagnosis Section, Alta Laboratory, Sao Paulo, Brazil

L. A. de Mattos
Female Pelvis Diagnosis Section, DASA Laboratory, Sao Paulo, Brazil

Department of Diagnostic Imaging, Escola Paulista de Medicina, Universidade Federal de Sao Paulo (EPM-Unifesp), Sao Paulo, SP, Brazil

M. S. Abrao (✉)
Endometriosis Section, Gynecologic Division, Hospital das Clinicas HCFMUSP, Faculdade de Medicina, Universidade de Sao Paulo, Sao Paulo, Brazil

Ginecologic Division, BP—Beneficiencia Portuguesa de Sao Paulo, Sao Paulo, Brazil

S. Guerriero et al. (eds.), *How to Perform Ultrasonography in Endometriosis*, https://doi.org/10.1007/978-3-319-71138-6_12

adjacent endometriotic lesions (mainly retro- and paracervical) with or without adherence to the rectum or sigmoid.

However, one must bear in mind that intestinal pains or evacuation changes may also be caused by other diseases (e.g., neoplasias, colitis, and food intolerance).

Clinical treatments are palliative and may reduce or eliminate the symptoms without significantly reducing the size of the lesions. Surgery is the therapy of choice for symptomatic patients with deep lesions who do not improve with clinical treatment [8].

The noninvasive DE diagnosis method began approximately 20 years ago. In 1998 some authors started publishing articles using the transrectal ultrasound or rectal endoscopic sonography with good results in detecting and staging rectum and sigmoid lesions, but there are certain disadvantages: it requires the use of specific transducers, dedicated equipment, and anesthesia, and it is ineffective in other sites, mainly the anterior compartment and ovaries [9–11].

Magnetic resonance imaging was initially used to detect ovarian endometriosis; however, as of 2005 [12], specific protocols were developed to diagnose deep endometriosis. Continuous learning and further improvement of the equipment led to greater accuracy of the technique [3, 13, 14]. Specialized ultrasound examination and MRI (1.5 and 3.0 T MRI) with dedicated protocols today share the leadership in diagnosing endometriosis.

Other techniques, such as barium enema [15] and computerized tomography [16], may also be used to diagnose DE, but with significant disadvantages in terms of accuracy in detecting DE and lack of efficiency in evaluating other sites.

Transabdominal and transvaginal ultrasound (TVUS) were initially only used to examine ovarian endometrioma. However, as of 2003 [11], some researchers started publishing studies that used TVUS to diagnose deep endometriosis [14, 17, 18, 19]. Despite the variances in protocols and results among the studies, current meta-analyses demonstrate almost a consensus [20–22] that TVUS is the first-line technique to examine deep endometriosis, especially the intestinal one, and that in special groups, its efficacy might even be superior to that of the MRI in helping define the therapeutic planning.

12.2 TVUS Examination

Some basic concepts must be known in order to perform the examination:

- Terminology and anatomy:
  The distal segment of the colon is divided as follows:
  - Lower rectum: from the rectal introitus until approximately 6 cm of the anal verge (AV).
  - Middle rectum: between 6 and 12 cm of the AV.
  - Upper rectum: between 12 and 18 cm of the AV.
  - Sigmoid: more than 18 cm of the AV.
  - Rectosigmoid transition: this is the transition region between the rectum and the sigmoid, which is anatomically characterized as the ending point of the distal segment of the "taenia coli." Due to the impossibility of visualizing the "taenia" via imaging techniques, the distance of the anal verge (approximately 18 cm above the rectal introitus) is used as a criterion to locate this region (Fig. 12.1).
  - Peritoneal reflection: the rectouterine pouch's most caudal segment where the peritoneum makes a curve separating the intraperitoneal rectum from the retroperitoneal rectum. This point is approximately 7 cm above the anal verge. The reflection is visible when there is fluid in the rectouterine pouch, most often in the post-ovulation period. When the peritoneum line is not visible, the following method can be used to define the topography of the reflection: with a sagittal distal image of the colon and the transducer positioned on the anterior vaginal fornix, trace a line on the coronal axis of the inferior edge of the cervical lips [23]. Nevertheless the ideal is direct visualization of the peritoneal reflection, because the indirect method may not be precise (Fig. 12.2).

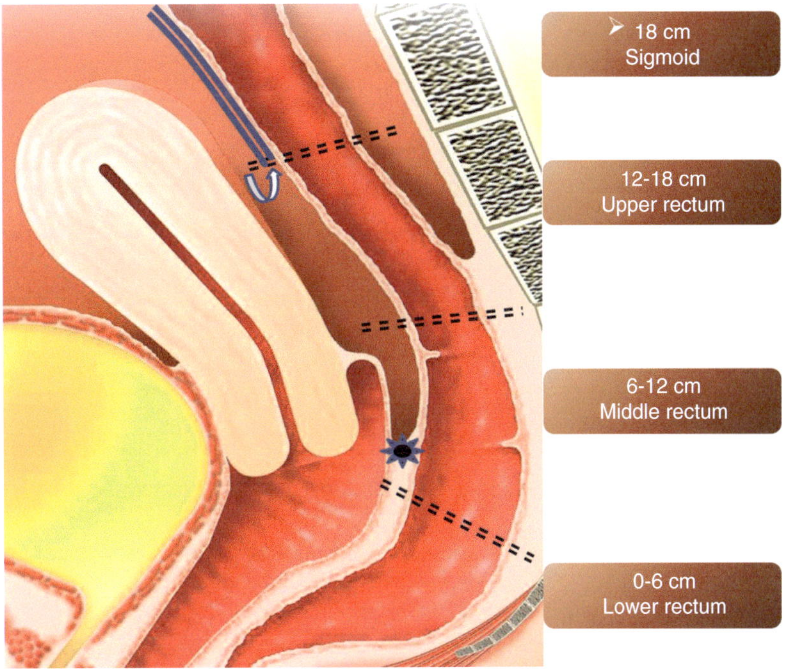

Fig. 12.1 Segments of the rectum and sigmoid. Rectosigmoid transition (*curved arrow*) at the end of "taenia coli" (*blue lines*). Peritoneal reflection (*asterisk*)

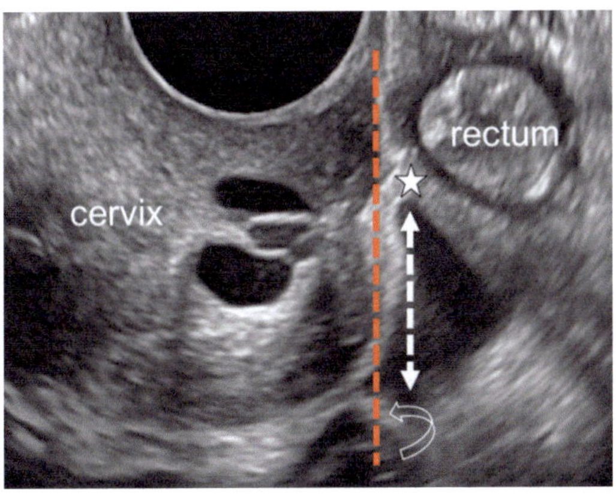

Fig. 12.2 TVUS-BP: there is approximately a 2.0 cm difference (*white line*) between the correct peritoneal reflection (*asterisk*) and the estimated one (*curved arrow*) by a line traced on the lower edge of the cervical lips (*yellow line*)

As to the compromised intestinal segment, the most important thing is to report whether the lesions are intra- or retroperitoneal, due to greater surgical difficulty if foci are located under the reflection and greater risk of postoperative fistulas, especially when a simultaneous opening of the rectum and the posterior vaginal fornix is necessary due to deep endometriotic infiltration.

- Bowel layers (Fig. 12.3)
  Beginning at the outer layer and continuing toward the inner layers:
  - Serosa: thin hyperechoic line.
  - Muscularis propria: longitudinal (external) and circular (internal). Two hypoechoic strips are separated by a fine hyperechoic line that corresponds to connective tissue.
  - Submucosa: hyperechoic strip.
  - Muscularis mucosa: hypoechoic line.
  - Mucosa: hyperechoic line.
- Aspect of the deep lesions:
  DE lesions are predominantly hypoechogenic; in addition to the glandular, stromal, and fibrosis component, the intestine's *muscularis propria* layer is significantly hypertrophic. When there is simultaneous thickening of the adjacent connecting tissue due to retrouterine endometriosis and/or significant adherences, an irregular peripheral hyperechogenic component is observed. Hyperechogenic spots and cysts are rarely seen in intestinal lesions, unlike what is observed in retrocervical and deep vaginal endometriosis.
  They tend to be nodular and fusiform in shape with somewhat irregular borders, depending

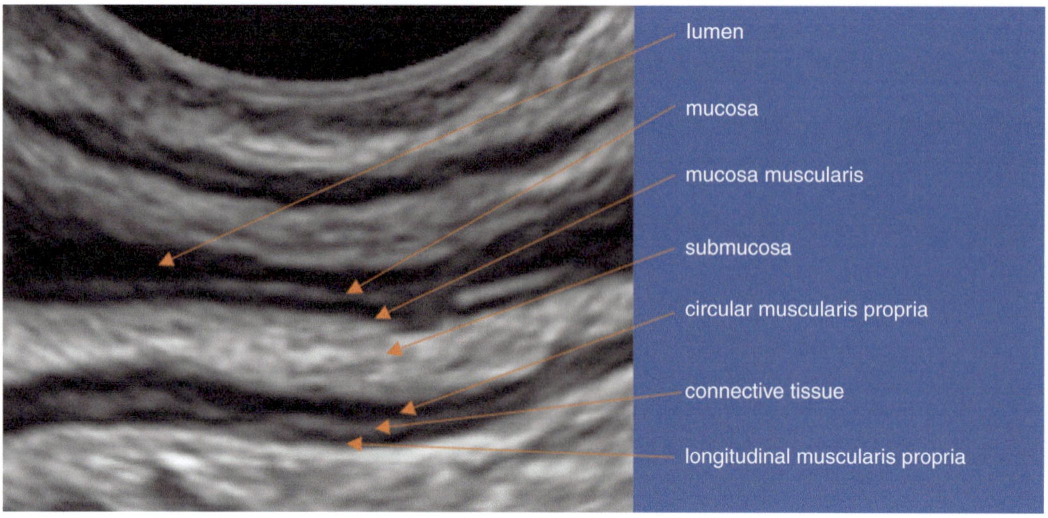

Fig. 12.3 TVUS-BP: longitudinal view of the intestine with the layers

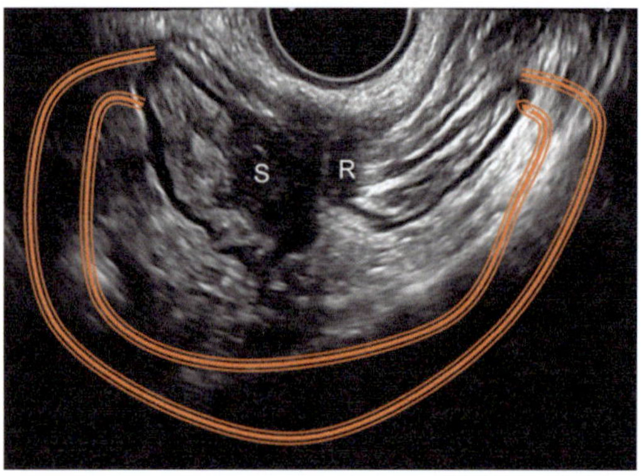

Fig. 12.4 TVUS-BP: DE in the rectum (R) and sigmoid (S) adhered to each other and forming a loop in the bowel (*yellow lines*)

on the size and degree of wall infiltration. When the lesions affect contiguous segments, the aspect may be even more bizarre (Fig. 12.4). When the intestinal endometriosis is superficial, there is only a slightly irregular thickening adhered to the loop, without alterations in the *muscularis propria* layer. Exclusive involvement of the serous membrane is more frequently caused by retrocervical or paracervical endometriosis that adheres to the intestine (Fig. 12.5)

DE is somewhat hypovascular on Doppler, and its distribution is disorderly or perpendicular to the greater axis of the loop. To our knowledge, no study has ever described any characteristic on color Doppler that may help diagnose or determine the activity level of the disease, but, in our experience, the intestinal polyps and neoplasias are more hypervascular (Fig. 12.6).

- Information about the lesions:

  Once a DE focus is detected, the following information must be given:

  – Size

    The lesions must be measured in the longitudinal, anteroposterior, and transverse axes. When the compromised segment is rectilinear, the tool to measure between two points is used; when the loop is curved ("u" shape), the trace is made manually, following the curve of the intestinal mucosa (Figs. 12.7 and 12.8). When the adjacent connecting tissue is thickened, a peripheral hyperechogenic component is observed, and when it is well defined, it must be excluded from the anteroposterior measurement of the intestinal lesion.

  – Number of lesions

    The number of lesions and the distance between them are important to define the strategy to be used in surgical cases (Fig. 12.9). Teams that receive highly complex patients have an incidence of approximately 1.5 nodules per patient with DE [24, 25].

  – Compromised circumference of the bowel

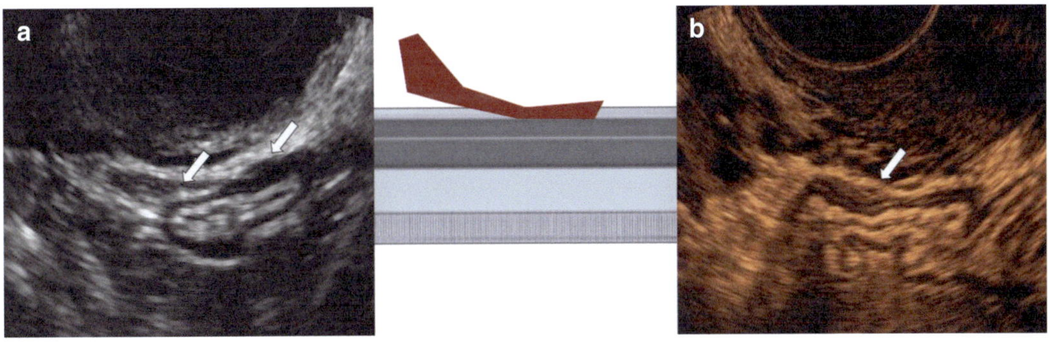

Fig. 12.5 TVUS-BP: paracervical endometriosis (**a**) adhered to and thickening the sigmoid serosa (arrows). With the use of sepia (**b**), it is easier to see that the muscular propria layer is normal

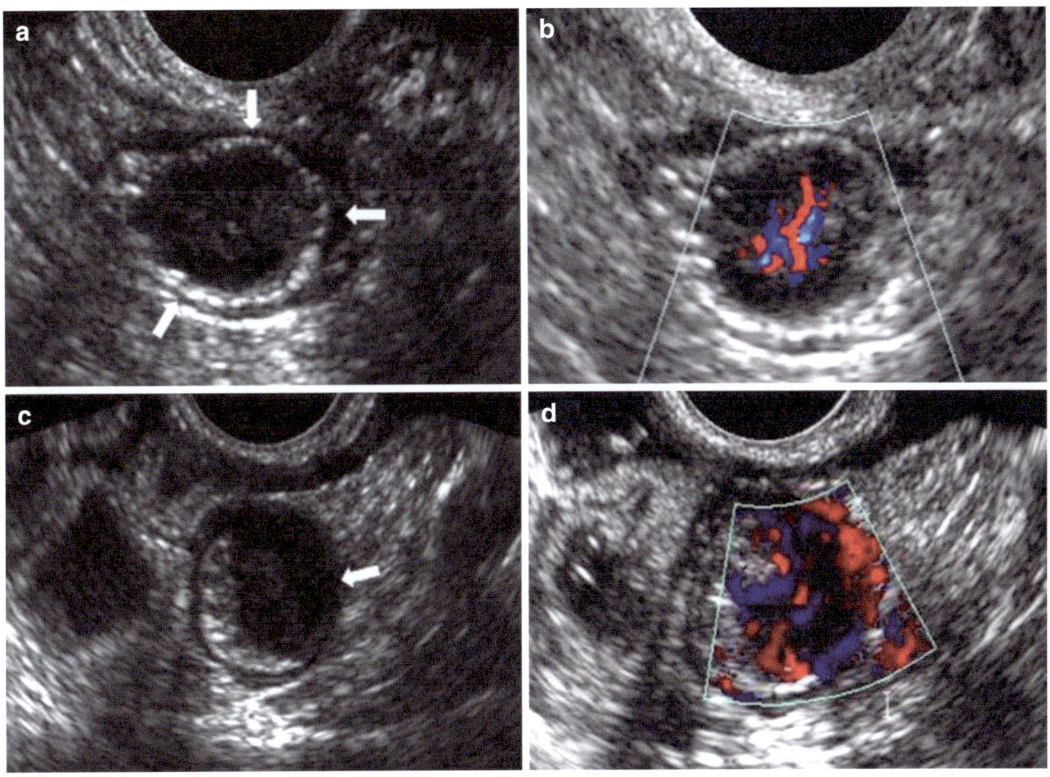

Fig. 12.6 TVUS-BP: well-delimited polyp in the intestinal lumen (**a**, **b**) completely surrounded by the wall (*arrows*). Gastrointestinal stromal tumor (**c**, **d**) that does not curve the loop's external form (*arrow*). Both protrude into the lumen and are more vascularized (**b**, **d**) and well delimited than endometriosis

The significance of the assessment of this parameter depends on the circumstance, for its usefulness resides in deciding on the surgical technique (nodulectomy or segmental resection). Most patients (approximately 80%) present lesions on the anterior wall of the rectum (up to 12 cm of the anal verge) which compromise less than 40% of the circumference. In order to estimate the percentage of the compromised circumference, the best method is to calculate the total circumference of the loop (TC) and the transverse diameter of the lesion (TD) and make the following relationship: TD/TC × 100 = % compromised (Fig. 12.8b).

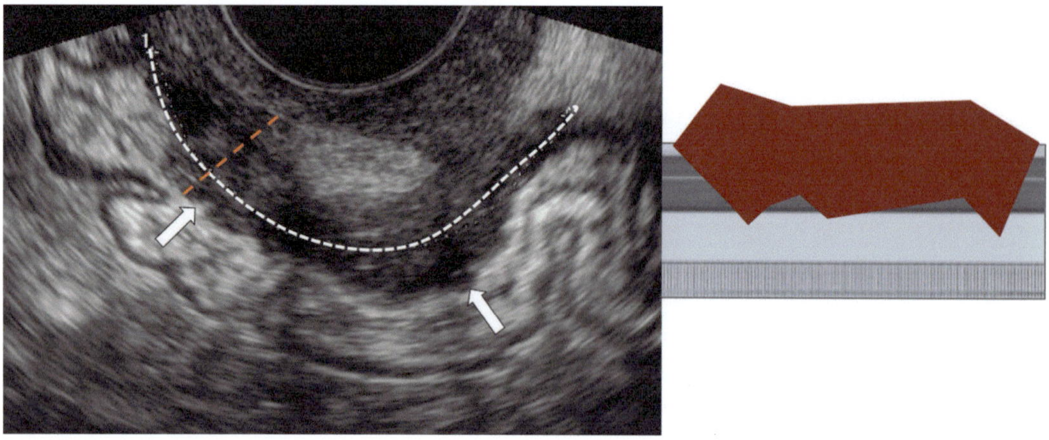

Fig. 12.7 TVUS-BP: extensive DE infiltrating the submucosa (*arrows*). Longitudinal (*white line*) and anteroposterior (yellow line) measurements

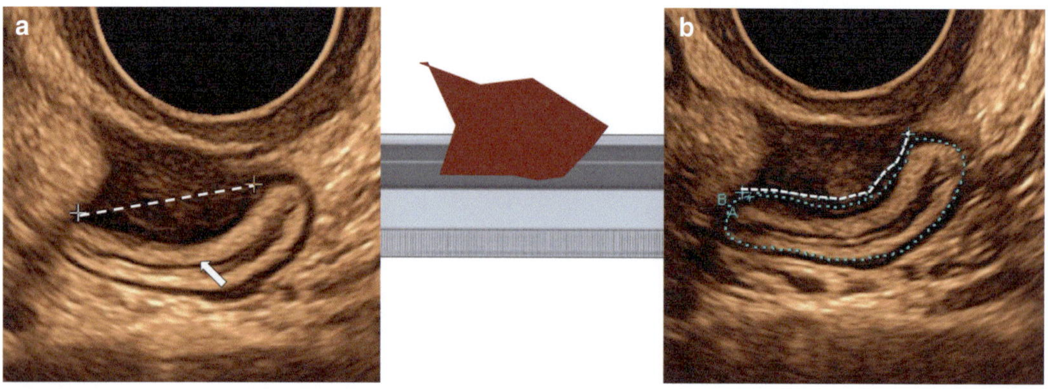

Fig. 12.8 TVUS-BP: (**a**) DE infiltrating the circular muscular layer, with normal hyperechogenic strip of the submucosa (*arrow*). (**b**) Calculation of the compromised circumference using the transverse (*white line*) and full circle (*green line*) measurements. In (**a**) we can see an underestimated measurement of the transverse axis using a straight line in a curved lesion

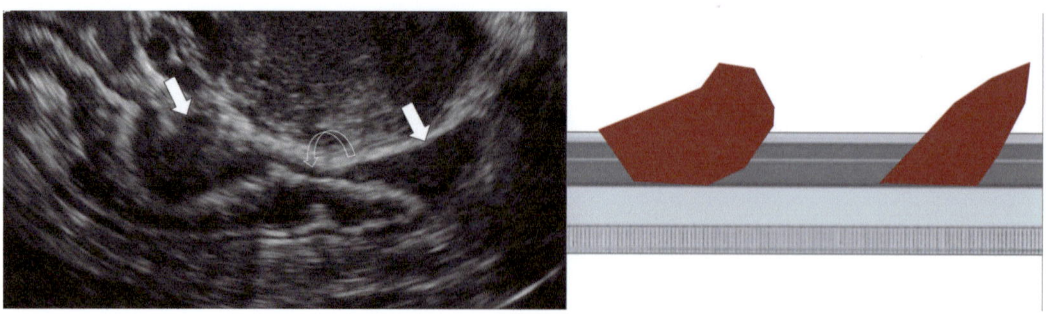

Fig. 12.9 TVUS-BP: two endometriosis lesions (*arrows*) in the same segment, separated by normal wall (curved arrow)

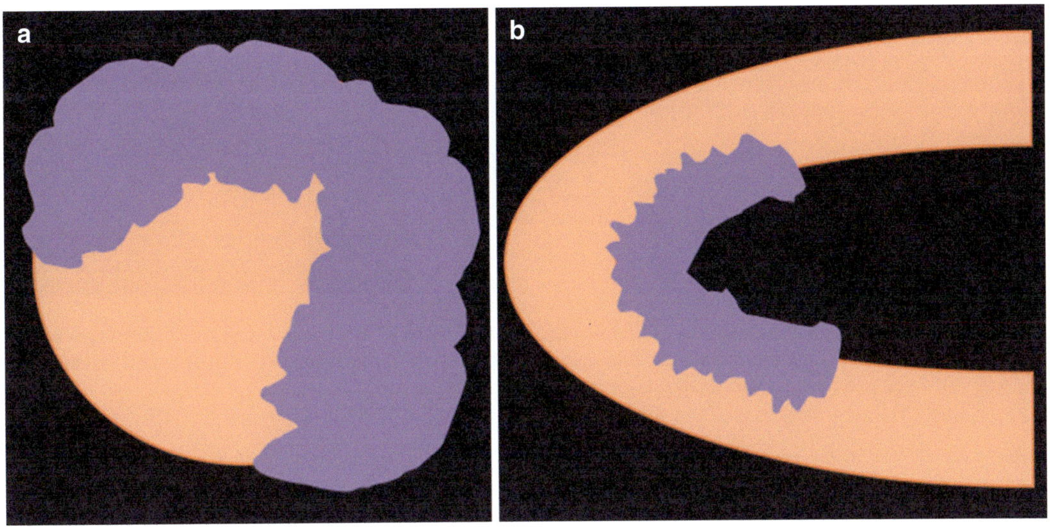

Fig. 12.10 Types of lesions that can cause stenosis. (**a**) Large lesion involving more than 50% of the circumference. (**b**) Endometriosis curving the intestine (>90°)

Abrão et al. demonstrated that when the submucosa is compromised, more than 40% of the circumference is infiltrated at the histological examination [26]. It is important to mention that this parameter is not a criterion for lumen stenosis. Significant stenosis is suggested when (Fig. 12.10):

a) The lesions compromise more than 50% of the circumference and have an anteroposterior diameter of more than 1.0 cm.
b) The DE significantly curving the compromised segment—angle greater than 90°.

   To summarize, there are morphological and measurement criteria to diagnose stenosis via TVUS; however, the subjective impression that there is little passageway for fecal content (assessed by the transversal axis of the loop) is also important. If there is doubt, other techniques may be used, such as colonoscopy, opaque enema, or CT with rectal contrast to obtain more direct and accurate information about the degree of the stenosis.

– Infiltrated intestinal layers

  There is DE when the lesion affects at least the *muscularis propria* layer. The criterion used to predict whether the lesion has infiltrated up to at least the *muscularis propria* is the existence of a nodule or hypoechoic, irregular thickening of this layer in the segment, irrespective of whether the hyperechoic strip that separates the external from the internal *muscularis propria* was interrupted (Fig. 12.8a). The criteria used to evaluate the infiltration of the submucosal layer are the existence of hypoechoic tissue originating in the serous layer and the *muscularis propria* causing partial or total interruption of the hyperechoic line corresponding to the submucosal layer (Fig. 12.11).

  When there is infiltration of several contiguous spots, the submucosal layer has a serrated aspect (Fig. 12.7). In terms of diagnosis, the submucosal and mucosal layers can be considered a single layer, since this would not impact the decision on which therapy or surgical procedure to adopt [11, 21, 25]. Hudelist and Goncalves without and with intestinal preparation, respectively, evaluated the efficiency of TVUS to determine the depth of the intestinal lesion by endometriosis (Table 12.1).

– Distance of the anal verge

  This is an important data and should be evaluated preoperatively. The surgical treatment of lower rectal lesions (defined as beginning less than 8 cm from the anal verge) is associated with a higher risk of

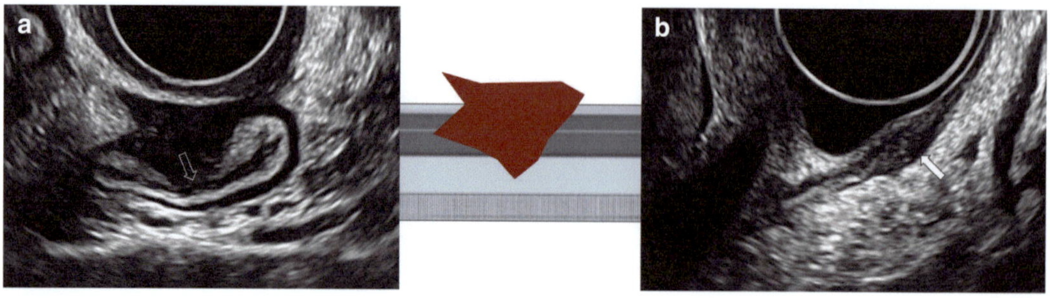

Fig. 12.11 TVUS-BP: (**a**) DE infiltrating the submucosa (arrow), characterized by interruption of the white strip of the wall. (**b**) Deep endometriosis in the posterior vaginal fornix (arrow) in the same patient, reinforcing the idea that endometriosis is almost always a multifocal disease

Table 12.1 TVUS in the evaluation of the layer infiltrated by intestinal endometriosis

	At least MP (Sens/Spec) (%)	SM/M (Sens/Spec) (%)
Goncalves 2010 with bowel preparation	100/100	83/94
Hudelist 2009 without bowel preparation	98/99	62/96

MP muscularis propria, *SM/M* submucosa/mucosa, *Sens* sensibility, *Spec* specificity

postoperative anastomotic leaks [27] and transient neurogenic bladder dysfunction [28].

It is difficult to objectively measure the distance of the anal verge via TVUS mostly because of the axis of the segment between 3 and 8 cm from the anal verge whose angle is of approximately 90° in relation to the proximal and distal segments of the rectum. This assessment is made using two parameters: the first and the second rectal curves—which are approximately 3.0 and 8.0 cm distant from the anal verge, respectively. Thus, we can estimate the distance of the lesions from the anal verge (Fig. 12.12). Obtaining this information prior to surgery also allows the surgeon to take a better strategic decision [29].

- The suprapubic and transvaginal ultrasound allows examination of at least 30–40 cm of the intestine above the anal verge.

The size, number of the lesions (if multiple - distance between them) and the compromised circumference are important information for the surgeon to determine whether to adopt the shaving, circular/linear stapler, or segmental resection technique.

To determine the best therapeutic options for patients with DE that compromises the sigmoid and/or rectum, it is important to understand the roles of clinical factors, preoperative morphologic characteristics obtained from images, surgical considerations, recurrence rate, and impact on quality of life. The analysis of all these parameters may contribute to restrain the current trend toward excessive use of laparoscopic colorectal resections [30].

12.3 Examination Technique

We always suggest the following bowel preparation prior to the ultrasound examination to detect endometriosis:

- Day before: sodium picosulfate 10 mg—oral simeticone 75 mg, oral—every 8 h
- Day of the exam: rectal enema with 120 mL of sodium diphosphate 1 h before the exam
- Two-hour fasting before the exam to reduce the possibility of intestinal peristalsis bringing feces or air from proximal intestinal segments to the rectum or sigmoid

This preparation facilitates identification of the different intestinal segments, the anal verge, and the degree of infiltration of the wall and the lesions, even when these are small or multiple.

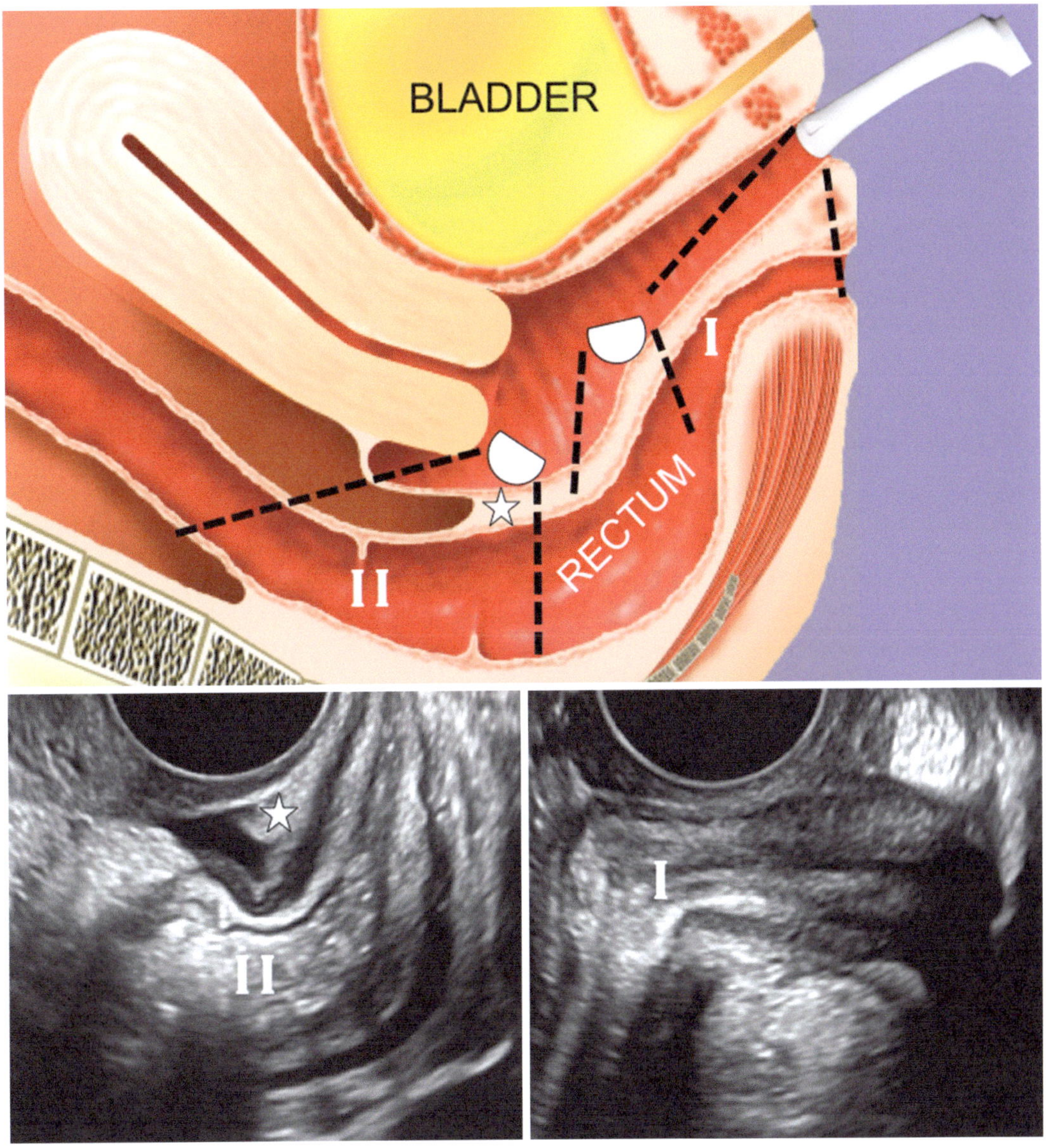

Fig. 12.12 Drawing and TVUS showing the first (at 3 cm AV) and second curves (at 8 cm AV) of the rectum. The peritoneal reflection (*asterisk*) is about 7 cm above the AV

Should there still be significant residue despite this preparation, the patient receives another unit of phosphoenema and is reevaluated after 15 or 30 min. We have performed the exam with this preparation for over 15 years and have not had any problem regarding acceptance by the patient, as long as she is previously informed about the diagnostic advantages.

It is possible to obtain good results in identifying single lesions in the rectum or sigmoid without bowel preparation. However, to our knowledge, no study has been able to identify multiple foci without bowel preparation to date. In 2010, via TVUS with prior bowel preparation, our group assessed the multiplicity of lesions in the rectum and sigmoid [25] (Table 12.2).

Table 12.2 TVUS-BP's ability to detect rectosigmoid endometriosis and estimate the existence of multifocality

	Sensitivity (%)	Specificity (%)	Accuracy (%)
Lesion detection	97	100	99
Presence of at least 2 lesions	81	99	96

Table 12.3 Comparison between the TVUS with and without bowel preparation in the diagnosis of rectosigmoid endometriosis

	Sensitivity (%)	Specificity (%)	LR+
TVUS without prior bowel preparation	73	88	6.08
TVUS with prior bowel preparation	100	99	25

LR+ likelihood ratio

Another point worth mentioning is that recent studies employing transvaginal ultrasound with prior bowel preparation have also demonstrated less learning curve time with this technique [31].

In 2017 Cristina Ros et al. [32] improved significantly the ability to detect intestinal lesions using prior bowel preparation (Table 12.3).

Several authors have proposed different protocols, such as water enema, tridimensional ultrasound, exam guided by the patient's pain, and others.

We believe that the main factors that lead to an accurate diagnosis of deep endometriosis, especially the intestinal one, are:

- Examiner's specific experience in TVUS for identification of endometriosis
- Facilitating protocols
- Examination of all sites in all patients, whether or not there are specific symptoms and even if the gynecological examination is within normality

Our team has always opted for the pelvic and transvaginal ultrasound with prior intestinal preparation in view of our belief that this is the most effective and practical method to obtain a high level of accuracy. However, each group must test the protocols proposed and found in literature and determine which has the best outcomes for them.

12.4 The Intestinal Tract Exam: Step by Step

Initiate evaluation with a suprapubic examination of the left iliac fossa [29, 33] using a high-resolution linear transducer (8–14 MHZ), the same used for breast ultrasound. We begin with transversal and longitudinal cuts of the distal descending colon and sigmoid, following them up to where possible inside the pelvis. It is usually easier to locate the sigmoid by beginning the search with transversal cuts on the lateral region of the left paracolic gutter and further complement these cuts with sagittal images.

With the same transducer, we always examine the right iliac fossa to detect lesions in the appendix, ileum, and cecum. The screening of this area begins with transversal cuts on the right paracolic gutter to identify the cecum, which is the larger loop with residue observed in this region. After locating the end of the cecum, we try to find the exit of the appendix in this region. Its emergence is often medial or central at the end of the cecum and follows inferiorly, at times "diving" into the pelvis beside the iliac vessels. When the tip or the entire appendix is in the pelvis, we must continue the evaluation while performing the transvaginal exam. The majority of the lesions are at the tip of the appendix, causing it to curve (shape of a walking cane with a curved handle). Subsequently, with transversal cuts, we move 2 or 3 cm upward to locate and follow the terminal ileum that emerges medially from the cecum (ileocecal valve). We follow the ileum until it is inferiorly possible with the linear transducer and later complement this exam by analyzing the pelvic ileal loops with the transvaginal transducer. The aspect of the lesions is similar to that observed in the rectosigmoid, and these may be single or multifocal/multicentric. When observing the lesions in the ileum and appendix, the differential diagnosis for neoplasias (mainly neuroendocrine tumors) must be borne in mind, for the aspect can be very similar to that of DE (Fig. 12.13). A safe way to differentiate them has not yet been described; however, when other foci of endometriosis are observed in the pelvis, there is very little possibility of neoplasia. In case the lesions are located only on the right iliac fossa or if in doubt, the

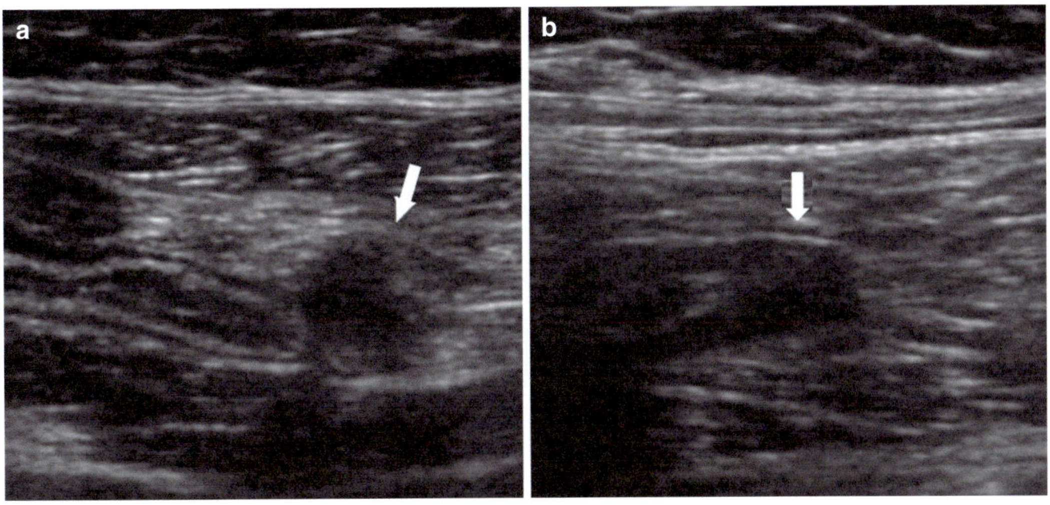

Fig. 12.13 Suprapubic ultrasound with high-resolution linear transducer: nodular thickening at the tip of the appendix (*arrows*), being endometriosis in (**a**) and carcinoid tumor in (**b**)

patient must be submitted to surgery for excision and anatomic pathological analysis.

The suprapubic examination of the loops with a high-resolution transducer is more limited when there is some content on the loops or in obese patients. Nonetheless, employment of dosed compression with the transducer and the prior bowel preparation minimize these issues.

Subsequently, the transvaginal transducer is introduced (transvaginal ultrasound with bowel preparation—TVUS-BP) and guided to the patient's sagittal axis with the beam angled downward (30–60°) to locate the rectum (Fig. 12.12).

We follow the intestine along the several segments: rectum, rectosigmoid transition, and sigmoid, along the curves. Most patients have a curve to the right and another one immediately to the left after the rectum, leading to the left adnexal region and passing beside the ipsilateral ovary (Fig. 12.14). However, there are many variations in the extension and topography of the sigmoid. This also justifies the prior bowel preparation, for it makes it easier to follow the loop.

The examiner must evaluate the largest possible rectum and sigmoid segment (usually up to 30–40 cm of the anal verge) in the longitudinal and axial axes of the bowel. Although most of the lesions are located in the anterior wall, some are more laterally located and can only be clearly seen with a transversal view. It is important to remember that endometriosis foci are seldom seen in the posterior wall of the rectum, for lesions that occupy the totality of the circumference are rare, and there are no isolated lesions on the posterior wall. We recommend at least two complete evaluations from the rectal sphincter to the proximal sigmoid. In the first evaluation, the loop is examined mainly in its longitudinal axis and, in the second, in its transversal axis. Three-dimensional transducers that allow the examiner to manually angle the beam reduce the patient's discomfort because it is thus not necessary to angle the transducer as much during transversal evaluation of the lower and middle rectum.

A normal rectosigmoid wall is 1–2 mm thick. Diffuse circumferential thickenings are related to inflammatory processes (colitis) or diverticular disease. DE is characterized by focal thickenings that begin in the most external layers (serosa and *muscularis propria*) and may infiltrate even the mucosae. In most cases, if we make a transversal cut, the thickened areas will be located in the rectum between 9 and 3 o'clock. The sigmoid presents greater variability of foci location, but the other characteristics (texture and morphology) are similar to those of the rectum.

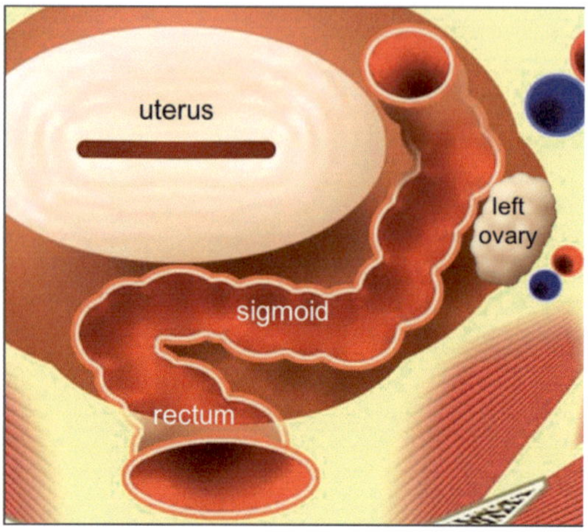

Fig. 12.14 Drawing showing one of the most frequent trajectories of the rectum and sigmoid

When the examiner suspects there is focal thickening of the wall, he must compress the transducer lightly to rectify the loop and perform visualization in several axes (transversal and longitudinal) to verify if it is not an artifact or superposition of images. False positives are more common on intestinal curves.

Once the lesion is found, all information described above must be obtained. The following is a chart with data that we attach to the report:

Distance from the anal verge	____ cm
Dimensions	Longitudinal × anteroposterior × transversal
% circumference compromised	___ %
Compromised layers	Serosa/*muscularis propria*/ submucosae
Significant stenosis	Yes/no/doubtful

When there is doubt whether the patient has significant stenosis and she will not undergo surgery, we indicate further assessments with specific exams (colonoscopy, CT with rectal contrast, or opaque enema).

If there are several lesions, each of them must be described with all the information necessary listed on a separate chart, as above. The distance between the lesions must also be measured as well as the total size of the compromised segment—including the foci and the areas that are free of endometriosis. Therefore, if a rectosigmoidectomy is indicated, the surgeon has an idea of the total segment to be excised.

The techniques adopted to resect DE vary according to each surgeon's experience and preference [34, 35]; however, generally speaking, shaving is performed when there is superficial infiltration of the bowel loop (serosa and external *muscularis propria*). In such cases, total thickness of the wall does not usually exceed 7 mm and compromises up to 30% of the circumference. For nodules less than 3 cm in length and without stenosis, a discoid resection can be performed, despite the depth of the lesion [5, 36]. Double discoid resection in the same nodule (of up to 4.0 cm) or in distinct nodules has been described [37, 38]. For nodules exceeding 3 cm in length, for multiple nodules, for compromise of more than 40% of the circumference [6], or for significant stenosis, the tendency is to perform a rectosigmoidectomy. However, more extensive and deep shavings have been described in these cases, and the surgical conduct to resect the intestinal endometriosis remains controversial and varied and depends on the experience of the surgeons and their teams.

As in other endometriotic sites, there are associated adherences. The same criteria used for other sites are adopted to evaluate the presence of adherences to the intestine, i.e., if the bowel is too close to another organ or if there are thickenings connecting it to other structures, the transducer is moved frontward and backward, pushing the organs and certifying in real time whether there is or not sliding among them.

In case of adherences in the lower posterior compartment, there may be cul-de-sac block (CSB), which is surgically defined as an adherence process that inhibits visual access of the peritoneum under the insertion of the uterosacral ligaments [39]. CSB may be partial (unilateral) or total (bilateral). CSB's most common cause is rectum adherence to the vagina and/or cervix (Fig. 12.15). It may occasionally have other causes, especially when the two ovaries are fixed retrouterine and both are adhered to the rectum or

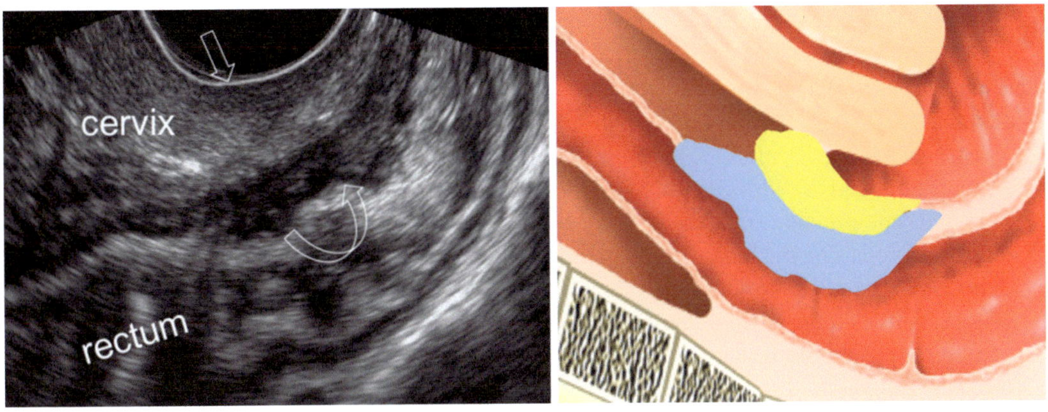

Fig. 12.15 TVUS-BP: deep endometriosis of the rectum (*curve arrow*) adherence to the posterior vaginal fornix lesion (*arrow*), causing complete Douglas cul-de-sac blockage

sigmoid. In terms of TVUS, it may be said that there is CSB when we identify a significant adherence process, usually involving the rectum and/or ovaries at the level of insertion of the uterosacral ligaments.

Some authors [23, 40] use the term sliding sign positive or negative to define if there is any sliding between the cervix and the intestine (anteverted uterus) or between the cul-de-sac and the rectosigmoid (retroverted uterus). To obtain greater exam sensitivity (as is done in the ovaries), the examiner moves the transvaginal transducer to push the uterus while pressing the anterior wall of the lower abdomen with his free hand. If there is sliding, the sign is positive and there should not be CSB. If there is no sliding, the sign is negative and suggestive of CSB [41]. Hudelist also suggest that the negative sliding sign indicates deep intestinal (rectal) endometriosis; however, certain factors, such as large uterus and large ovarian cysts located posteriorly, in addition to chronic inflammatory or adherence processes that are not related to endometriosis, may also lead to a false negative result. False positives may also occur in this maneuver since many rectal lesions do not cause a significant adherence process. Therefore, we recommend that the sliding of the structures be used as a factor solely to assess the adherence process and that diagnosis of deep endometriosis be based on the direct visualization of the lesions.

12.5 Controlling Development

As in other forms of deep endometriosis, DE has a rather slow development curve. Therefore, if there is no risk of stenosis or increased symptoms, controls may be made in 6–12 months.

In case of surgeries with resection of intestinal nodules and as long as the postoperative period presents no complications, we suggest the first control be made after 3 months. This is so because practically the entire postoperative reaction process should have already regressed during this period, and it is possible to evaluate the condition of the bowel and the related adherences/collections. Ideally, there should be no residual thickening or fluid collected in the manipulated region. Should there be parietal thickening, measurements should be made in the longitudinal, anteroposterior, and transversal axes for further control in 6–12 months. When staples are used to close the loop, it is possible to visualize them at transvaginal ultrasound and to determine if it was discoid or a segmental resection (anastomosis) and if the staples occupy only one quadrant or the total circumference of the loop in the transversal axis.

In more extensive intestinal surgeries, mainly of the rectum, it is very common to observe adherences and small quantity of fluid collected and/or septated anechoic around the loop. In general, these findings do not cause significant symptoms.

12.6 False Positives

The main causes leading to false positives in intestinal endometriosis are:

- Accentuated curves with fan-folded loops. Solution: compression maneuver with the transducer, repairing the loop.
- The sigmoid crosses the left round ligament (Fig. 12.16). Solution: rotate the transducer, and observe if the thickening extends out of the loop and heads toward the uterine horn. Unless it is compromised by endometriosis, the ligament's texture is similar to that of the uterus, unlike the DE, which, in general, is hypoechogenic.
- The tube is adjacent or adhered to the intestine. Solution: rotate the transducer, and observe if the thickening extends outside the loop. In addition, a Doppler allows detection of the typical vascularization of the tube, which is characterized by thin vessels that are parallel to the greater axis and at time have a spiral aspect. DE is quite hypovascular at Doppler; when it is present, it has a disordered aspect or is perpendicular to the greater axis of the loop.

12.7 Differential Diagnoses

Polyps: These are easily differentiated from DE due to their location in the loop's lumen and well-defined limited. They may be long with a narrow base or sessile with a wide base. Texture and vascularization vary, but, in general, they are more vascularized than DE (Fig. 12.6a, b).

Gastrointestinal stromal tumor (GIST): This is the most difficult differential diagnosis, for its nodules are hypoechogenic and quite homogeneous. However, unlike DE, they are usually round and have well-defined limits and do not curve the loop's external form. Vascularization varies but is generally more accentuated than in DE (Fig. 12.6c, d).

Adenocarcinomas: Primary neoplasias of the intestine, when observable at ultrasound, are more hyperechogenic than DE, with poorly defined limits, and they grow from the mucosae. At color Doppler, they are hypervascular and are disorderly distributed.

Should there be doubts concerning differential diagnosis, the colonoscopy is the standard exam.

12.8 Exam Time

Following the protocol we have developed, with the suprapubic evaluation of the right iliac fossa and the proximal sigmoid (linear transducer) and transvaginal, it takes us around 15–25 min to examine the intestinal sites. Some factors impact the exam time: inadequate preparation, number of detected lesions, and related adherence process. Large uteri, retroverted uterus, or ovarian cysts larger than 5 cm may also make the examination more difficult, mainly of the sigmoid, thus increasing exam time.

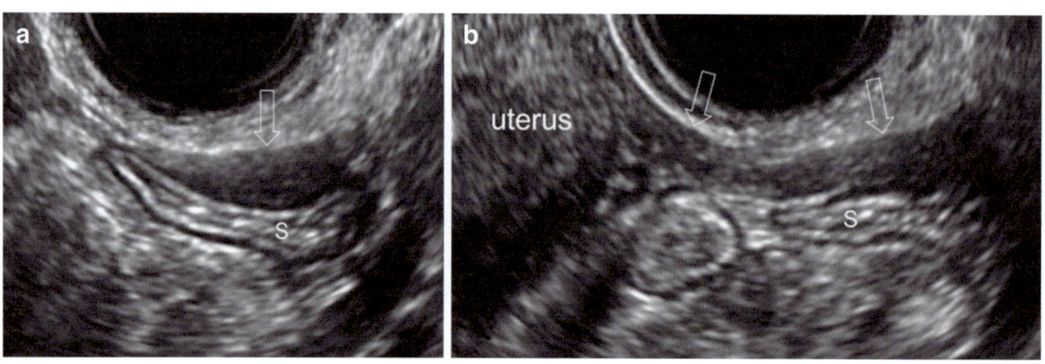

Fig. 12.16 TVUS-BP: (**a**) transversal view—apparent endometriosis (*arrow*) in the sigmoid (S) wall. (**b**) Turning the transducer, it is possible to see that it is a false lesion caused by the normal left round the ligament (*arrows*)

12.9 Important Technical Tips

- All patients with suspected endometriosis, even if they do not have intestinal symptoms, must perform bowel preparation. As in other types of deep endometriosis, the symptoms are not always exactly related to the compromised region or to the severity of the process.
- If there is fecal residue after the oral preparation and the phosphoenema, we ask the patient to be submitted to another rectal phosphoenema. If, even so, the preparation is still inadequate, we ask the patient to return the following day after a more rigorous preparation. We have had extremely rare instances in which we ask the patient to return the following day.
- Examine all possible endometriosis sites in all patients, regardless of the medical center or physical examination.
- Inform the patient about the procedure and that the discomfort is similar to that of a routine transvaginal examination. The exam does not cause significant pain, but there are factors that may increase pain, such as vaginismus, anxiety, and very large or retroverted uteri, in addition to endometriosis itself.

  Factors that may reduce pain:

  (a) Slowly introduce the vaginal transducer lubricated with gel.
  (b) If it is a 3D transducer with manual movement of the crystal, rotate the ultrasound directing it to the pouch when examining the rectum in the transversal axis.
  (c) Let the patient stretch her legs. This enables a better angle of the uterus and reduces the transducer inclination as well as allows the patient to be more relaxed.
  (d) Sedation: in general, sedation is never necessary. However, if the patient wishes, she may take a tranquilizer. Extreme cases may require sedation such as in endoscopies.
    - Use high-resolution linear transducers (10–15 MHZ) for the suprapubic intestinal examination. The conventional abdominal transducers (3–5 MHZ) or micro-convex (6–9 MHZ) does not have sufficient resolution to identify small intestinal endometriosis lesions. This examination is more difficult to perform in obese women. However, employment of dosed compression with the transducer on the abdominal wall minimizes the problem.
- Initiate the transvaginal examination by evaluating the intestine and performing a first quick screening up to the sigmoid, even if the examiner promptly identifies a focus in the rectum. In view of the light prior bowel preparation which eliminates basically the residue in the rectosigmoid, if the examiner takes too long to examine the sigmoid, content from the left colon might flow down and impair the examination. Always examine all segments in the longitudinal and transversal axes. The transversal screening must be done at the end of the examination for it causes a stronger discomfort to most of the patients.
- It is easier to follow along the intestine if the transducer is positioned in the posterior vaginal fornix. If the uterus is large or if there are large ovarian cysts, at times it is not possible to position the tip of the transducer closer to the wall of the loop. In such cases, follow the loop using the uterus or ovary as a "window" (Fig. 12.17).
- Postoperative control in up to 3 months. Bowel preparation is usually not necessary in this postoperative control unless the surgeon did not locate the intestinal lesion described prior to the surgery or supposes a significant residual focus still remains. It should be borne in mind that, in addition to the possibility of false positives and negatives at ultrasound, the surgeon not always manages to locate small and isolated sigmoid lesions, especially when there is not related adherence process.
- The initial learning curve in diagnosing DE via ultrasound is quicker than one supposes, even when we are referring to ultrasonographers that only perform pelvic examination. However, ultrasonographers experienced in abdominal ultrasonography

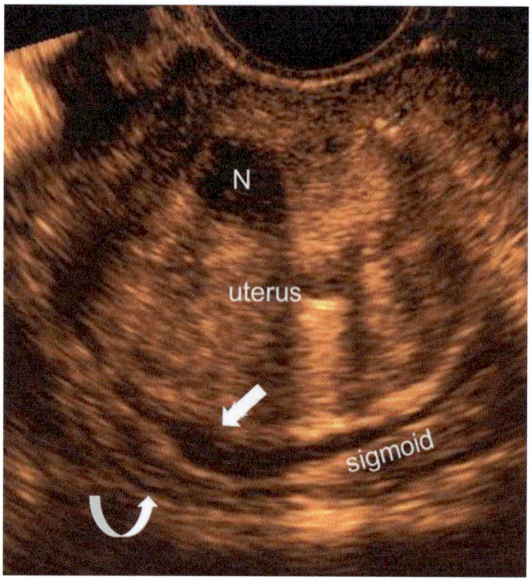

Fig. 12.17 TVUS-BP: uterus increased in volume, with fibroids (N), preventing the placement of the transducer in contact with the bowel. The sigmoid seen through the uterus, with endometriosis (arrow). The other wall is normal (curved arrow)

have an initial advantage, especially those who perform US of the hollow viscus. In any case, the basic prerequisite for quicker progress is vast experience in diagnosing gynecological pathologies.

The table below shows the results obtained by Tammaa et al. [42] in connection with the learning process to perform transvaginal ultrasound for diagnosis of rectum or sigmoid endometriosis. Summarizing:

- Approximately 40 expert-supervised examinations are necessary for the trainee to reach 60–80% of the effectiveness and efficiency of an experienced examiner.
- The learning process varies significantly among the trainees (Table 12.4).

Surgeons and imaging examiners must provide ongoing feedback in order to achieve diagnostic progress. Completed reports with the main findings of both groups and regular comparison of results are preferable, and an anatomic pathologist will have the final say in cases of discrepancy.

Table 12.4 Results of TVUS intestinal endometriosis detection obtained by trainees against the results obtained by their expert trainer (approximately 95% sensitivity and specificity in this diagnosis)

	Sensitivity (%)	Specificity (%)	LR+	LR−
Trainee 1	72	96	16.6	0.29
Trainee 2	89	95	19.6	0.12

Only 50% of the patients underwent surgery. *LR likelihood ratio*

12.10 Future Perspectives

There are currently few medical centers dedicated to the diagnosis of deep endometriosis with high levels of accuracy; thus, the first short- and medium-term perspective is that more specialized centers be created and the protocols be more homogeneous.

The greater development and spread of 3D equipment will make it possible for experts to assess this technology in advanced centers of primary health services.

Initial study on the use of fusion imaging (real-time ultrasound and multiplanar reconstructed MR images) for endometriosis was published [43]. However, these programs have still to be further developed in order to prove they can actually significantly enrich the diagnosis.

As to the ultrasound detection of deep intestinal endometriosis, the more experienced centers are close to 100% sensitivity and specificity; thus, there is little space for further progress. However, knowledge dissemination and development of new technologies are challenges still to be overcome.

12.11 Final Comments

Integration of highly trained professionals in the fields of diagnosis and treatment of endometriosis is essential for adequate therapeutic planning. In cases of surgery, this integration allows the patient to be informed on the procedure and helps build a multidisciplinary team when necessary. It is thus possible to diagnose, treat, and monitor patients in a more accurate manner while reducing costs and, most importantly, improving the patients' quality of life, not to mention increasing pregnancy possibility and reducing psychological and physical troubles caused by endometriosis.Compliance with Ethical Standards

Funding This chapter did not receive external funds.

Conflict of interest The authors certify that they have no affiliations with or involvement in any organization or entity with any financial interest.

Ethical approval This chapter is a review which does not contain any studies with human participants or animals performed by any of the authors

References

1. Chapron C, et al. Surgery for bladder endometriosis: long-term results and concomitant management of associated posterior deep lesions. Hum Reprod. 2010;25:884–9.
2. Chapron C, et al. Deeply infiltrating endometriosis: pathogenetic implications of the anatomical distribution. Hum Reprod. 2006;21:1839–45.
3. Bazot M, et al. Accuracy of magnetic resonance imaging and rectal endoscopic sonography for the prediction of location of deep pelvic endometriosis. Hum Reprod. 2007;22:1457–63.
4. Kavallaris A, Köhler C, Kühne-Heid R, Schneider A. Histopathological extent of rectal invasion by rectovaginal endometriosis. Hum Reprod. 2003;18:1323–7.
5. Remorgida V, et al. How complete is full thickness disc resection of bowel endometriotic lesions? A prospective surgical and histological study. Hum Reprod. 2005;20:2317–20.
6. Abrão MS, et al. Deep endometriosis infiltrating the recto-sigmoid: critical factors to consider before management. Hum Reprod Update. 2015;21:329–39.
7. Podgaec S, Gonçalves MO, Klajner S, Abrão MS. Epigastric pain relating to menses can be a symptom of bowel endometriosis. Sao Paulo Med J. 2008;126:242–4.
8. Garry R, Clayton R, Hawe J. The effect of endometriosis and its radical laparoscopic excision on quality of life indicators. BJOG. 2000;107:44–54.
9. Simões Abrão M, et al. Rectal endoscopic ultrasound with a radial probe in the assessment of rectovaginal endometriosis. J Am Assoc Gynecol Laparosc. 2004;11:50–4.
10. Chapron C, et al. Results and role of rectal endoscopic ultrasonography for patients with deep pelvic endometriosis. Hum Reprod. 1998;13:2266–70.
11. Bazot M, et al. Transvaginal sonography and rectal endoscopic sonography for the assessment of pelvic endometriosis: a preliminary comparison. Hum Reprod. 2003;18:1686–92.
12. Takeuchi H, et al. A novel technique using magnetic resonance imaging jelly for evaluation of rectovaginal endometriosis. Fertil Steril. 2005;83:442–7.
13. Hottat N, et al. Endometriosis: contribution of 3.0-T pelvic MR imaging in preoperative assessment—initial results. Radiology. 2009;253:126–34.
14. Abrao MS, et al. Comparison between clinical examination, transvaginal sonography and magnetic resonance imaging for the diagnosis of deep endometriosis. Hum Reprod. 2007;22:3092–7.
15. Ribeiro HS, et al. [Double-contrast barium enema in the diagnosis of intestinal deeply infiltrating endometriosis]. Rev Bras Ginecol Obstet. 2008;30:400–5.
16. Biscaldi E, Ferrero S, Remorgida V, Rollandi GA. Bowel endometriosis: CT-enteroclysis. Abdom Imaging. 2007;32:441–50.
17. Hudelist G, et al. Combination of transvaginal sonography and clinical examination for preoperative diagnosis of pelvic endometriosis. Hum Reprod. 2009;24:1018–24.
18. Guerriero S, et al. Diagnostic value of transvaginal 'tenderness-guided' ultrasonography for the prediction of location of deep endometriosis. Hum Reprod. 2008;23:2452–7.
19. Exacoustos C, et al. OC19.04: Sonographic evaluation of posterior deep pelvic endometriosis: endovaginal-, transrectal- and vaginosonography to assess the extension of the disease. Ultrasound Obstet Gynecol. 2005;26:340–1.
20. Piketty M, et al. Preoperative work-up for patients with deeply infiltrating endometriosis: transvaginal ultrasonography must definitely be the first-line imaging examination. Hum Reprod. 2009;24:602–7.
21. Hudelist G, Tuttlies F, Rauter G, Pucher S, Keckstein J. Can transvaginal sonography predict infiltration depth in patients with deep infiltrating endometriosis of the rectum? Hum Reprod. 2009;24:1012–7.
22. Nisenblat V, et al. Combination of the non-invasive tests for the diagnosis of endometriosis. Cochrane Database Syst Rev. 2016;(7):CD012281.
23. Guerriero S, et al. Systematic approach to sonographic evaluation of the pelvis in women with suspected endometriosis, including terms, definitions and measurements: a consensus opinion from the International Deep Endometriosis Analysis (IDEA) group. Ultrasound Obstet Gynecol. 2016;48:318–32.
24. Chapron C, et al. Anatomical distribution of deeply infiltrating endometriosis: surgical implications and proposition for a classification. Hum Reprod. 2003;18:157–61.
25. Goncalves MO, Podgaec S, Dias JA Jr, Gonzalez M, Abrao MS. Transvaginal ultrasonography with bowel preparation is able to predict the number of lesions and rectosigmoid layers affected in cases of deep endometriosis, defining surgical strategy. Hum Reprod. 2010;25:665–71.

26. Abrão MS, et al. Endometriosis lesions that compromise the rectum deeper than the inner muscularis layer have more than 40% of the circumference of the rectum affected by the disease. J Minim Invasive Gynecol. 2008;15:280–5.
27. Ruffo G, et al. Laparoscopic colorectal resection for deep infiltrating endometriosis: analysis of 436 cases. Surg Endosc. 2010;24:63–7.
28. Dousset B, et al. Complete surgery for low rectal endometriosis: long-term results of a 100-case prospective study. Ann Surg. 2010;251:887–95.
29. Goncalves MO, Dias JA Jr, Podgaec S, Averbach M, Abrão MS. Transvaginal ultrasound for diagnosis of deeply infiltrating endometriosis. Int J Gynaecol Obstet. 2009;104:156–60.
30. Acien P, et al. Is a bowel resection necessary for deep endometriosis with rectovaginal or colorectal involvement? Int J Womens Health. 2013;5:449–55.
31. Young SW, et al. Initial accuracy of and learning curve for transvaginal ultrasound with bowel preparation for deep endometriosis in a US Tertiary Care Center. J Minim Invasive Gynecol. 2017;24(7):1170–6. https://doi.org/10.1016/j.jmig.2017.07.002.
32. Ros C, et al. Bowel preparation improves the accuracy of transvaginal ultrasound in the diagnosis of rectosigmoid deep infiltrating endometriosis: a prospective study. J Minim Invasive Gynecol. 2017;24(7):1145–51. https://doi.org/10.1016/j.jmig.2017.06.024.
33. Young SW, et al. Sonographic evaluation of deep endometriosis: protocol for a US radiology practice. Abdom Radiol (NY). 2016;41:2364–79.
34. Panebianco V, et al. [Low anterior resection of the rectum using mechanical anastomosis in intestinal endometriosis]. Minerva Chir. 1994;49:215–7.
35. Duepree HJ, et al. Laparoscopic resection of deep pelvic endometriosis with rectosigmoid involvement. J Am Coll Surg. 2002;195:754–8.
36. de Almeida A, Fernandes LF, Averbach M, Abrão MS. Disc resection is the first option in the management of rectal endometriosis for unifocal lesions with less than 3 centimeters of longitudinal diameter. Surg Technol Int. 2014;24:243–8.
37. Pereira RMA, et al. Use of circular stapler for laparoscopic excision of rectosigmoid anterior wall endometriosis. Surg Technol Int. 2008;17:181–6.
38. Kondo W, et al. Surgical techniques for the treatment of bowel endometriosis. J Minim Invasive Gynecol. 2015;22:S131.
39. Revised American Society for Reproductive Medicine classification of endometriosis: 1996. Fertil Steril. 1997;67:817–21.
40. Reid S, et al. Prediction of pouch of Douglas obliteration in women with suspected endometriosis using a new real-time dynamic transvaginal ultrasound technique: the sliding sign. Ultrasound Obstet Gynecol. 2013;41:685–91.
41. Hudelist G, et al. Uterine sliding sign: a simple sonographic predictor for presence of deep infiltrating endometriosis of the rectum. Ultrasound Obstet Gynecol. 2013;41:692–5.
42. Tammaa A, et al. Learning curve for the detection of pouch of Douglas obliteration and deep infiltrating endometriosis of the rectum. Hum Reprod. 2014;29:1199–204.
43. Millischer A-E, et al. Fusion imaging for evaluation of deep infiltrating endometriosis: feasibility and preliminary results. Ultrasound Obstet Gynecol. 2015;46:109–17.

Other Locations of Deep Endometriosis

13

Stefano Guerriero, Silvia Ajossa, Ornella Comparetto, Camilla Ronchetti, Virginia Zanda, Bruno Piras, Alba Piras, and Valerio Mais

13.1 Introduction

While pelvic endometriosis is defined as lesions of the fallopian tubes, ovaries, and local peritoneum, extrapelvic endometriosis refers to endometriotic implants found elsewhere in the body [1]. The extrapelvic implantation of endometrial tissue has been described in virtually every organ, system, and tissue in the body [2]. The true prevalence of extrapelvic endometriosis is unknown because of a lack of well-defined epidemiological studies; in fact, only surgical and gynecological case reports are reported. Many diagnostic methods have been proposed, but none of them represents the gold standard. The role of ultrasonography has been proposed and recognized only in some locations [1].

The multiple localization of endometriosis in combination with the wide range of its clinical expressions should raise the clinical suspicion in every woman with cyclical symptoms in extrapelvic organs. There are currently no accepted classification systems for extrapelvic endometriosis, although in 1989, Markham et al. [3] proposed a classification system that divided extragenital endometriosis into four different classes including a class "I" involving the intestinal tract, a class "U" involving the urinary system, a class "L" involving the lung and thoracic cavity, and a class "O" involving "all other sites." However, this classification remains underused in the literature. In the present chapter, we will describe only the localizations in which the use of ultrasound has been reported, in particular:

(a) Abdominal wall endometriosis
   - Laparotomy scar endometriosis (most frequent)
   - Umbilical (0.5–1% of all cases of extragenital endometriosis)
   - Inguinal canal or canal of Nuck endometriosis
   - Rectus abdominis muscles
(b) Abdominal organs
   - Lower abdomen (endometriosis of the appendix)
   - Upper abdomen (hepatic and diaphragmatic endometriosis)

13.2 Abdominal Wall Endometriosis

Abdominal wall endometriosis is defined as the presence of ectopic endometrium located at the

---

Electronic Supplementary Material The online version of this chapter (https://doi.org/10.1007/978-3-319-71138-6_13) contains supplementary material, which is available to authorized users.

S. Guerriero (✉) · S. Ajossa · O. Comparetto
C. Ronchetti · V. Zanda · B. Piras · A. Piras · V. Mais
Department of Obstetrics and Gynecology, University of Cagliari, Policlinico Universitario Duilio Casula, Monserrato, Cagliari, Italy
e-mail: gineca.sguerriero@tiscali.it; gineca.sajossa@tiscali.it; camilla.ronchetti@fastwebnet.it; zavirgi@tiscali.it; valerio.mais@alice.it

S. Guerriero et al. (eds.), *How to Perform Ultrasonography in Endometriosis*,
https://doi.org/10.1007/978-3-319-71138-6_13

abdominal wall structures. It is a predominantly iatrogenic condition. Many cases of abdominal wall endometriosis occur after laparoscopy or laparotomy involving the uterine cavity. Most cases of abdominal wall endometriosis occur as a result of closure to cesarean-section scars, but some lesions are not a consequence of the previous surgery. The extremely high incidence of a history of previous cesarean section in the abdominal wall endometriosis group suggests that the endometrium during pregnancy may have certain characteristics that make transplantation and implantation particularly successful [1].

Symptoms of abdominal wall endometriosis include a growing, painful, tender mass that may increase in size and become more painful during menses. Cyclical bleeding can occur at the site of the lesion [4]. The success rate of medical therapy has been reported to be low, offering only temporary relief of symptoms often followed by recurrence after cessation of the drug. Wide surgical excision therefore is the treatment of choice [4].

13.2.1 Scar Endometriosis

This condition is caused by the dissemination of endometrial tissue into a wound at the time of surgery. The deposits can involve uterine scar, abdominal musculature, or subcutaneous tissue. Endometriosis has been reported in scars originated after cesarean section, in episiotomy scar after delivery, and in consequence of procedures involving contact with endometrial tissue, such as hysterectomy, ectopic pregnancies, salpingostomies, and those performed during the first half of pregnancy [5].

Reported incidences vary around 3.5% of women who had a gynecological intervention [5] and could be present in approximately 0.8% of all women who had cesarean deliveries. The occurrence of endometriosis in the episiotomy scar is less frequent than in scars of the abdominal wall [4]. Cesarean section might be the first risk factor for the development of scar endometriosis. This high risk can be explained by the higher exposure of endometrial cells to the subcutaneous tissue during the procedure [5]. Unfortunately this condition is often misdiagnosed since endometriosis may occur from 6 months to several years after surgery, the pain is often not cyclic, and not always there is a palpable mass. The sonographic finding of a solid mass in the abdominal wall is not pathognomonic for endometriosis, but if located close to a cesarean section scar, it should be considered in the differential diagnosis (Figs. 13.1, 13.2, and 13.3) (Videos 13.1, 13.2, 13.3, 13.4, and 13.5) [4].

13.2.2 Villar's Nodule

Umbilical endometriosis, also known as Villar's nodule, is a rare occurrence and is often a result of iatrogenic seeding in surgical scars (Fig. 13.4). Umbilical endometriosis in the absence of any prior abdominal or uterine surgery is an even rarer clinical entity [6]. Umbilical endometriosis has been reported in more than 100 cases and was first described by Villar in 1886. The umbilicus represents the location of 0.5–1% of extrapelvic endometrioses [7].

It may appear during active menstrual life as a small, firm, bluish-pink mass in the umbilical area, with a diameter varying from a few millimeters to 6 cm. It may cause pain, swelling, or tenderness mainly in the premenstrual period. Sometimes secretion or some bleeding may occur through the umbilical skin, concomitant with menses; for this reason, it is often called the "menstruating tumor." Umbilical endometriosis frequently exists as a solitary lesion without accompanying pelvic disease [7] (Figs. 13.5, 13.6, and 13.7) (Videos 13.6 and 13.7).

13.2.3 Inguinal Endometriosis or Canal of Nuck Endometriosis

The canal of Nuck is an evagination of the parietal peritoneum that accompanies the round ligament through the inguinal ring into the inguinal canal. Endometriosis in the inguinal region was first reported by Cullen in 1896, and the incidence of this localization of endometriosis in women was found to be 0.6% [8]. Direct extension of endometrial

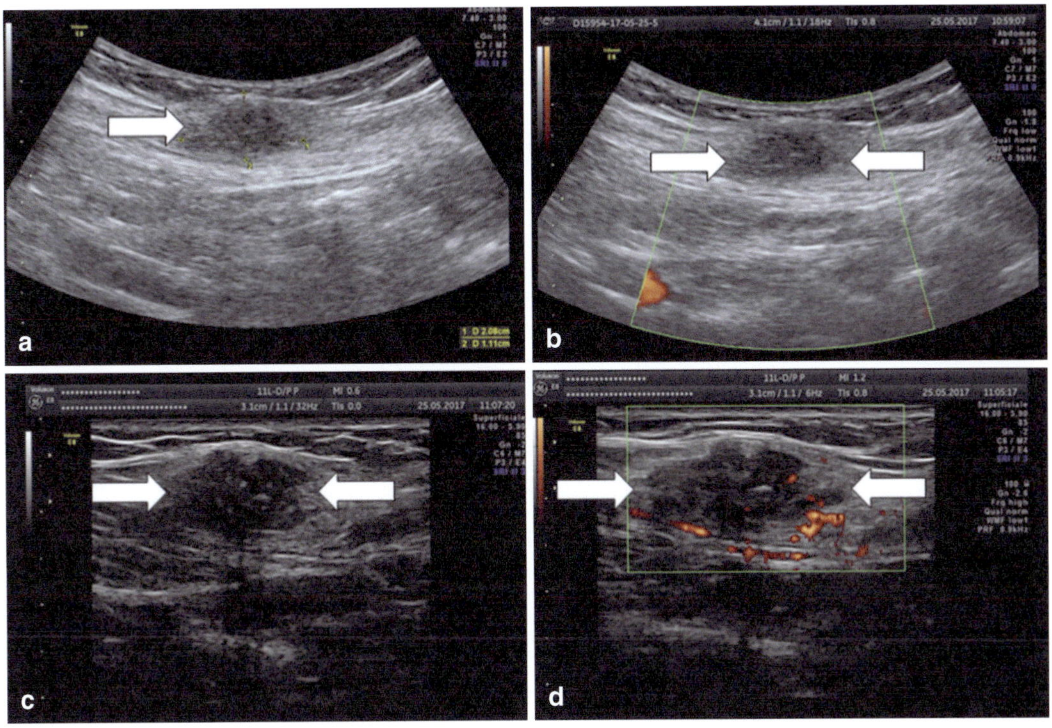

Fig. 13.1 Some ultrasonographic images of scar endometriosis (*straight arrows*) in a 32-year-old woman with a cesarean section 6 years before. In the pictures (**a**) and (**b**), the nodule visualized using convex probe and, in the pictures (**c**) and (**d**), using linear probe. The resolution is better in (**c**) and (**d**) due to higher frequencies with a more detailed and sensitive color Doppler evaluation (**d**)

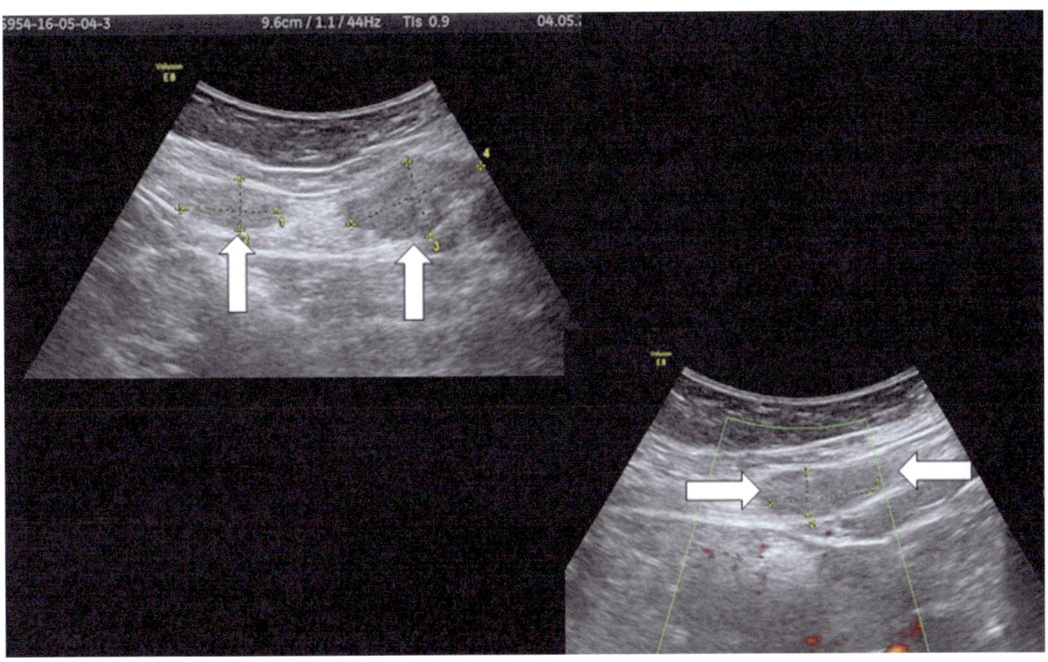

Fig. 13.2 Ultrasonographic images of two nodules of scar endometriosis (*straight arrows*) in a 39-year-old woman with a previous cesarean section 6 years before

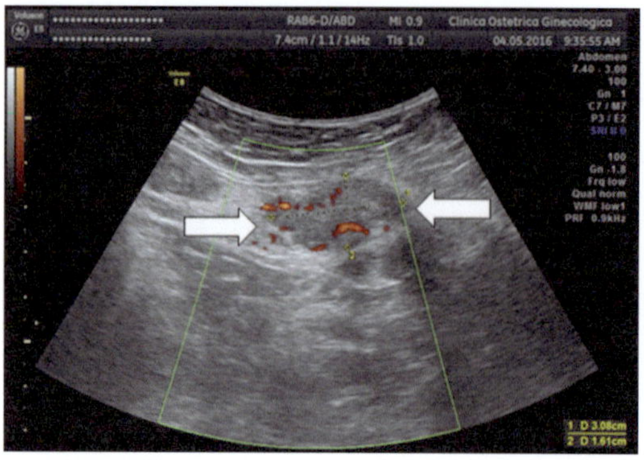

Fig. 13.3 Color Doppler ultrasonographic images (*straight arrows*) of a scar endometriosis in a 39-year-old woman with one previous cesarean section 6 years before

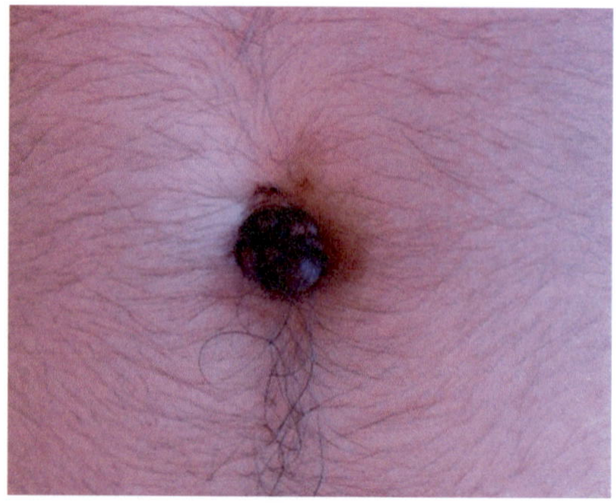

Fig. 13.4 The typical appearance of Villar's nodule

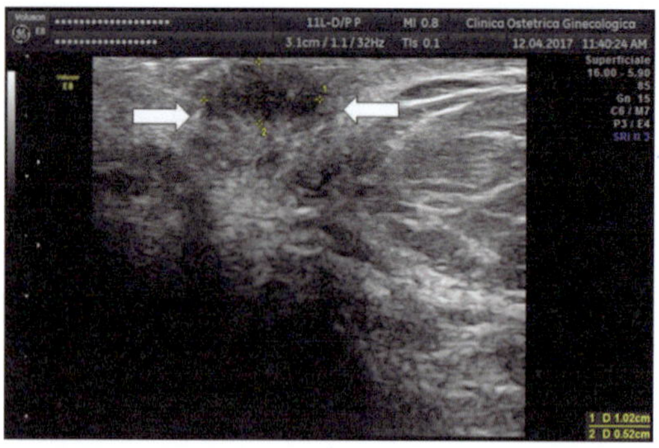

Fig. 13.5 The ultrasonographic appearance of Villar's nodule (*straight arrows*) in a 33-year-old woman without previous abdominal surgery

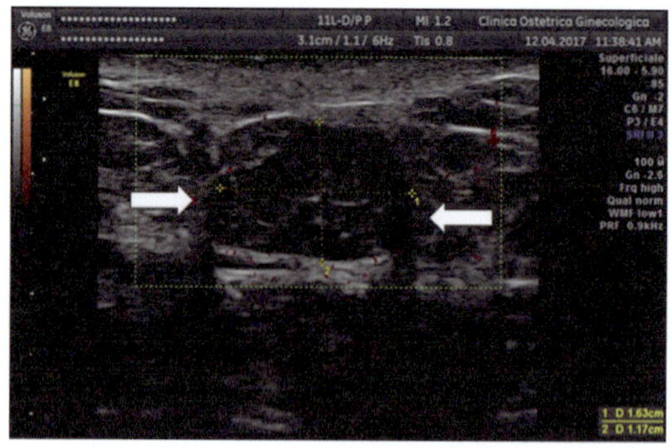

Fig. 13.6 A more detailed visualization (due to a better focalization) of Villar's nodule (*straight arrows*) of Fig. 13.5. The solid appearance is more evident

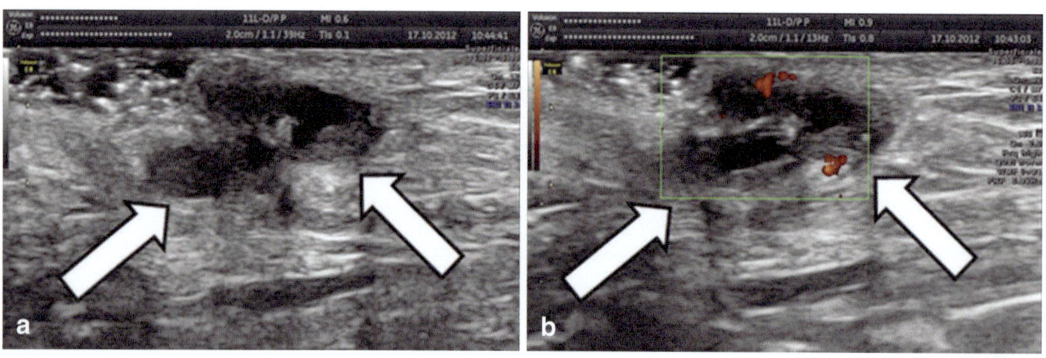

Fig. 13.7 The ultrasonographic appearance of Villar's nodule (*straight arrows*) using B-mode (**a**) and color Doppler (**b**) in a 20-year-old woman without previous abdominal surgery. In this case, the ultrasonographic appearance was more cystic than solid

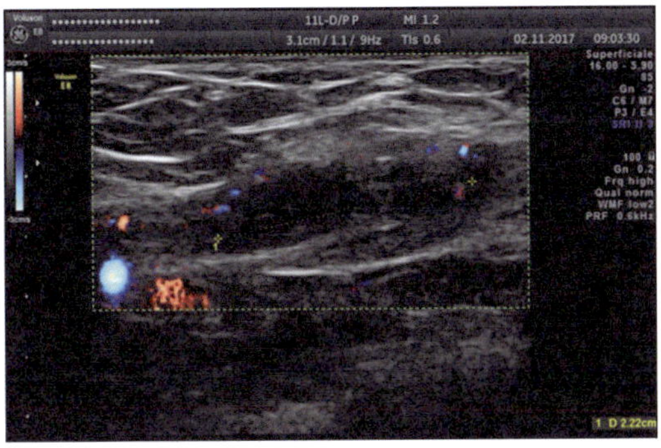

Fig. 13.8 Sonographic features of right inguinal endometriosis presenting as a cystic mass with internal septa, hypoechoic content, and few peripheral color spots located in inguinal area

tissue along the round ligament is a possible pathogenesis of inguinal endometriosis because, occasionally, it will remain patent, creating a link between the peritoneal cavity and the inguinal canal [9] (Fig. 13.8) (Video 13.10). More than 90% of inguinal endometriosis cases are right sided and often associated with an inguinal hernia. Common symptoms associated with inguinal endometriosis are inguinal pain and the presence of an inguinal mass, which sometimes becomes enlarged during the menstrual period [8].

13.2.4 Rectus Abdominis Endometriosis

Endometriosis involving the rectus abdominis muscle is a very rare occurrence. Up to the present, only 18 cases with lesions contained entirely within the rectus abdominis muscle were clearly documented in medical literature with only four cases as a primary location [10] (Figs. 13.9, 13.10, and 13.11) (Videos 13.8 and 13.9).

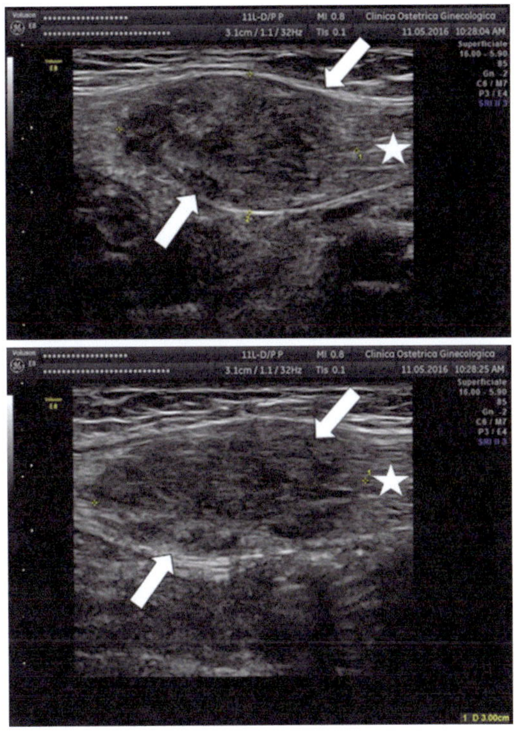

Fig. 13.9 The ultrasonographic appearance of a *rectus abdominis endometriosis* (*straight arrows*) in a 30-year-old woman with one previous cesarean section 4 years before. The muscular layer (star)

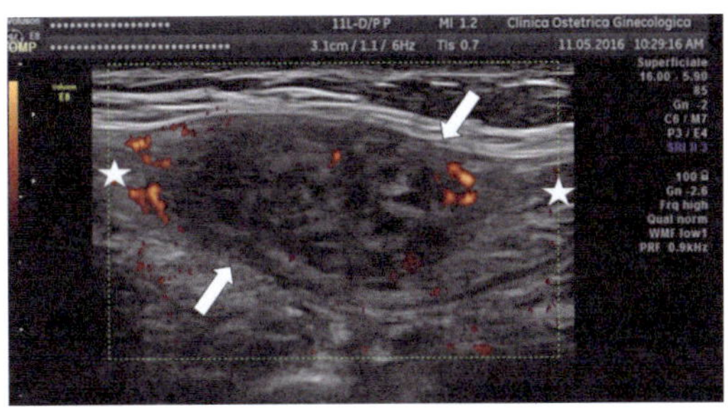

Fig. 13.10 The power Doppler ultrasonographic appearance of a *rectus abdominis endometriosis* (*straight arrows*) in a 30-year-old woman with one previous cesarean section 4 years before. The muscular layer (*star*)

13.2.5 Intra-abdominal Endometriosis

Endometriosis can be located in every organ of the abdomen. Case reports include findings of extrapelvic endometriosis in the appendix, inside liver parenchyma, and diaphragm muscle. Interestingly, the spleen, with its important immunologic functions, has not been a site of reported endometriosis [1].

13.2.6 Endometriosis of the Appendix

Endometriosis of the appendix is a rare condition. It may be asymptomatic or present as acute

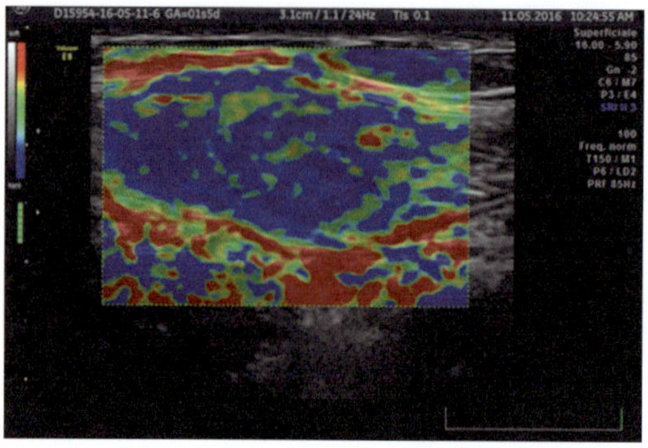

Fig. 13.11 The sonoelastographic appearance of a *rectus abdominis endometriosis* (*straight arrows*) in a 30-year-old woman with one previous cesarean section 4 years before

appendicitis, lower gastrointestinal bleeding, intestinal perforation, or intestinal obstruction from intussusception. Appendiceal endometriosis can be diagnosed histopathologically. The mucosa of the appendix is never affected, and usually glandular tissue, endometrial stroma, and hemorrhage are observed in the muscular and seromuscular layers [11].

13.2.7 Hepatic Endometriosis

Hepatic endometriosis is one of the rarest localizations of extrapelvic endometriosis; only 22 cases have been reported so far in the literature. The pathogenesis of hepatic endometriosis is unclear with vascular-lymphatic dissemination having a potential role. Although ultrasound, computerized tomography (CT), and magnetic resonance imaging (MRI) are helpful, no typical image of endometriosis cyst has been described, so the final diagnosis can be made only by histological evaluation [12].

13.2.7.1 Differential Diagnosis and Transformation

Endometriosis of the abdominal wall may be difficult to diagnose; it is often mistaken both clinically and by diagnostic imaging for other abnormal conditions such as a suture granuloma, an incisional hernia, or primary or metastatic cancer [4]. The diagnosis of hepatic endometriosis can be difficult with the differential diagnosis including both benign conditions, such as echinococcal cyst, abscess, hematoma, cystadenoma, and malignant cystic neoplasms, such as cystadenocarcinoma or metastatic disease [12]. The differential diagnosis of appendicular endometriosis should include diverticular disease, colorectal carcinoma, inflammatory bowel disease, carcinoid tumors, benign intramural neoplasm, occult intra-abdominal metastases, mesenteric neoplasm, and pelvic abscess [13].

Malignant transformation has been reported in approximately 1% of endometriosis cases, and most frequently this transformation takes place at the ovary, accounting for about 80% of the endometriosis-associated malignancies [14]. Malignant transformation of endometriosis occurring in surgical abdominal scar is very rare: clear cell histology accounts for only 4.5% of extragonadal endometriosis-associated malignancies while representing the most common histotype in case of parietal localization [15]. A series of 23 cases of endometriosis associated with clear cell carcinoma (CCC) arising within cesarean section scar are reported in the literature [16]. Despite the rarity of this condition, the number of reported cases has increased over time likely due to a higher attention focused on this disease but also to the increased rate of cesarean sections and uterine surgeries documented over time. Careful collection and evaluation of patient history would be important to have a high index of suspicion for endometriosis-associated malignancy. These masses usually reach very large dimensions before the diagnosis is made [16].

13.3 How We Do It

1. *Importance of history and concomitant assumption of oral contraceptives*
   A detailed clinical history should be taken for all women with suspected endometriosis, with particular emphasis on symptoms. The following should be noted specifically: previous myomectomy or cesarean delivery (the main cause of this extrapelvic endometriosis lesions), previous surgery for endometriosis, family history

of endometriosis, previous nonsurgical treatment for endometriosis (type, duration, effect), the kind of pain (chronic and acute pelvic pain more or less related with the menstruation), and concomitant use of oral contraceptives because there can be a delay in diagnosis due to partial resolution of symptoms. The onset and duration of symptoms should be noted and, if possible, the intensity of the pain recorded by asking the patient to use a visual analog scale or investigating it with a 0–10 narrative numeric rating scale [17].

2. *Kind of probe to be used in case of suspicion of extrapelvic deep endometriosis*

   Transabdominal sonography using a linear transducer (5.0–13.0 MHz) is mandatory in detecting, locating, and characterizing abdominal wall endometriosis [18]. If possible, depending of the deepness of lesion, linear superficial probe should be useful to guide the surgical removal and repair.

3. *Typical ultrasonographic findings*

   At ultrasound examination, abdominal wall endometriosis shows features similar to those of deep infiltrating pelvic endometriosis but different from those of ovarian endometrioma. The nodules appear solid with ill-defined outer borders (Figs. 13.1, 13.2, 13.3, 13.4, 13.5, 13.6, 13.7, 13.9, 13.10, and 13.11). It is necessary to evaluate the appearance of the margins (smooth, irregular, or frankly spiculated) [18]. A cystic lesion is present in few cases (Villar and Nuck nodules) (Fig. 13.7). The echotexture should be evaluated and compared with that of adjacent normal subcutaneous tissue. On ultrasound, scar endometriosis usually appears as an inhomogeneous hypoechoic roundish nodule with fibrotic changes (in the form of hyperechoic spots or strands), a peripheral hyperechoic ring, spiculated margins, and a single vascular pedicle entering the mass at the periphery (Figs. 13.1, 13.2, and 13.3) [19].

   Sonographic features of inguinal endometriosis are variable. It could present as a solid mass, a cystic mass (Fig. 13.8) (Video 13.10), or a combined cystic and solid mass. Some cystic masses have internal septa and could appear hypoechoic or hyperechoic [7]. Usually few peripheral color Doppler spots are present (Fig. 13.8) (Video 13.10).

4. *Modality of evaluation of localization*

The operator should note not only the presence of the lesion but also the number of lesions, the localization (right, left, and median, at the level of the umbilicus, or at the right/left inguinal canal), the depth (superficial, in the subcutaneous fat tissue or involving the muscle layer or between these two layers also evaluating the relationship with the fascia), and the relationship with the scar of a previous cesarean section. In addition, the operator should evaluate the dimensions of the lesions recording the three orthogonal diameters. Power Doppler sonography, with a pulse repetition frequency of 500–750 Hz, is useful to assess the vascularity of all lesions (Figs. 13.1, 13.3, and 13.7) (Videos 13.3, 13.7, and 13.9). Excessive vascularization is related to the neoplastic transformation and is mandatory for the differential diagnosis.

13.4 Important Technical Tips

1. Use of the highest possible frequency to better define the border of the lesion and the vascularization (Fig. 13.1).
2. Suggest to the women to move her legs alternatively during the scan to better identify the muscular layer (Videos 13.8 and 13.9).
3. Evaluate multifocality because multiple lesions are possible.
4. Perform a concomitant TV evaluation using the International Deep Endometriosis Analysis (IDEA) protocols [17] to exclude other associated endometriotic lesions. As a matter of fact, the purpose of performing an ultrasound examination in a woman with diagnosis of extrapelvic endometriosis and with suspected pelvic endometriosis is to try to explain underlying symptoms, map the disease location, and assess the severity of disease prior to medical therapy or surgical intervention. This examination should be carried out in every woman with extrapelvic endometriosis, even

if there are no symptoms of pelvic endometriosis, and according to the IDEA consensus that proposes four basic sonographic steps when examining women with suspected or known endometriosis [17].

13.5 Future Perspectives

Although hormonal therapy may be a useful initial approach for reducing symptoms and for decreasing the size of larger cutaneous lesions prior to planned surgical excision [20], surgery for extragenital endometriosis clearly improves outcome through relief of symptoms, improved quality of life, increased fertility rates, and reduced recurrences [21]. Recently a new therapeutic method has been proposed for the treatment of abdominal wall endometriosis: ultrasound (US)-guided high-intensity-focused ultrasound (HIFU) ablation. This technique appears to be safe and effective for the treatment of abdominal wall endometriosis in 21 cases reported in the literature [22].

Three-dimensional (3D) sonography appears to be a quick, easy, specific, and noninvasive tool in the diagnosis and presurgical approach of extrapelvic endometriosis. The 3D reconstruction clearly showed the irregular shapes and borders of the endometriotic nodule and gave a more exact analysis of the surrounding tissue (Figs. 13.12, 13.13, 13.14, and 13.15). Moreover, the depth of infiltration through the facial plane can easily be shown. Preoperative evaluation of the dimension, volume, and infiltration of the abdominal wall endometriotic mass could be very useful to estimate how large the excision will be in order to use a mesh prosthesis [23].

MRI may be an addition technique for the evaluation of endometriosis before surgery especially

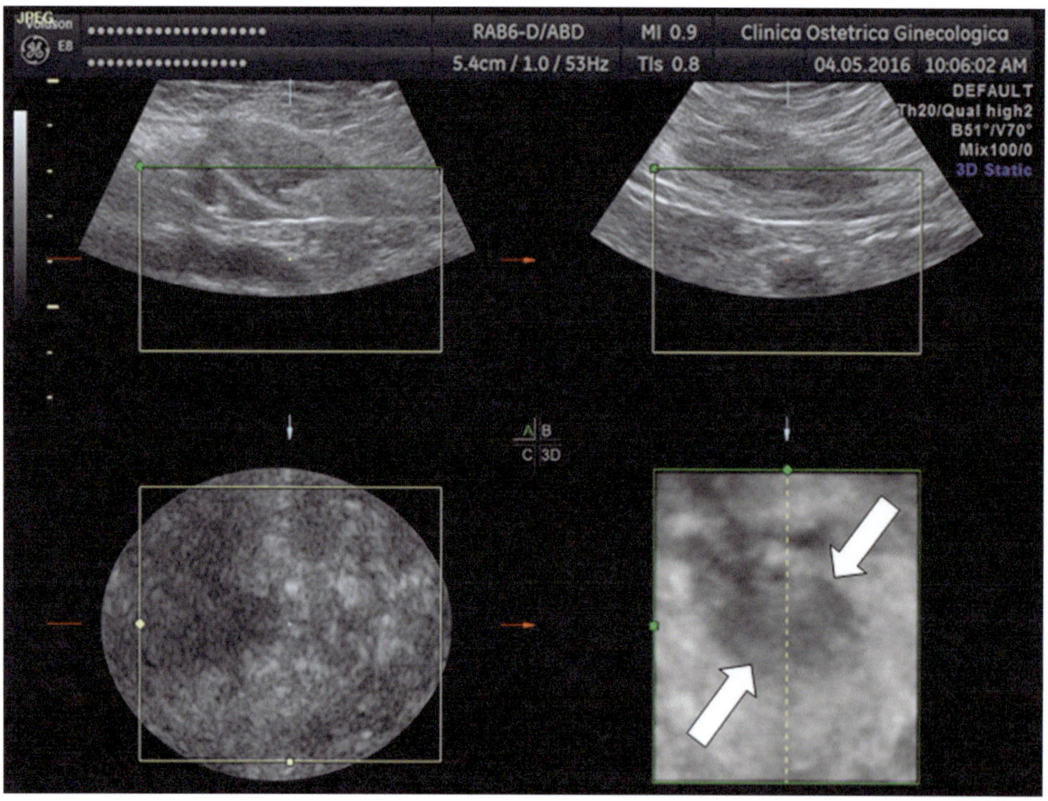

Fig. 13.12 Three-dimensional ultrasonographic appearance of a scar endometriosis (*straight arrows*) in a 39-year-old woman with one previous cesarean section 6 years before

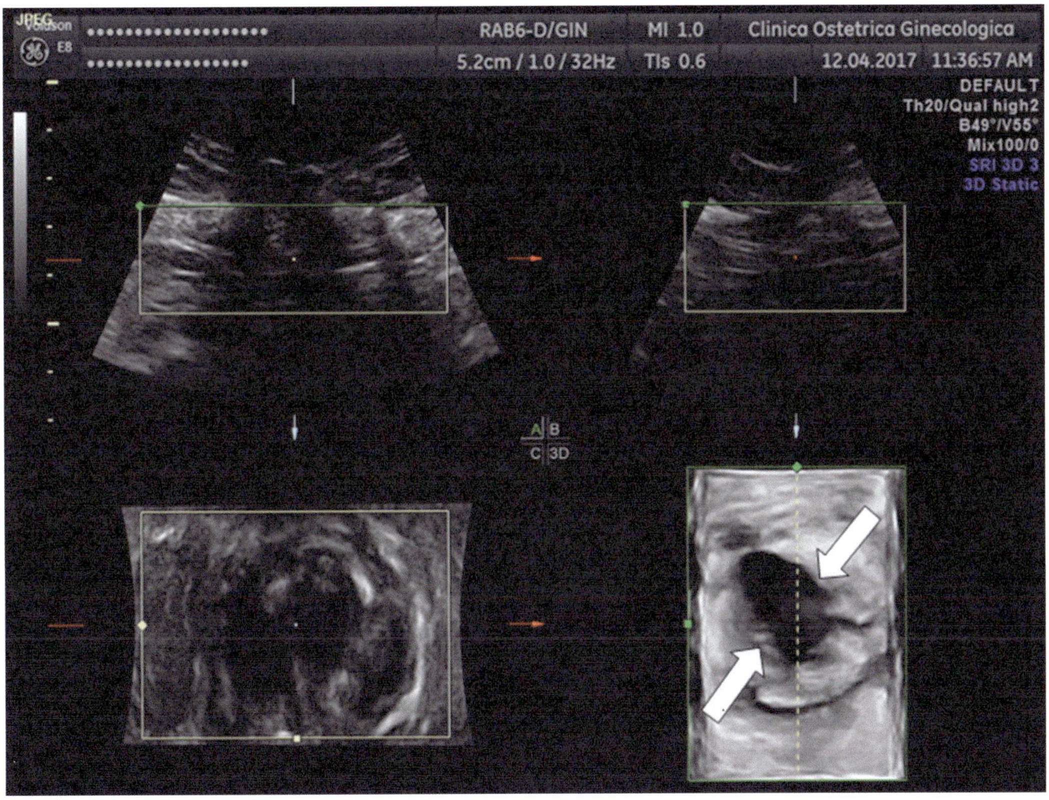

Fig. 13.13 Three-dimensional ultrasonographic appearance of a scar endometriosis (*straight arrows*) in a 32-year-old woman with a cesarean section 6 years before

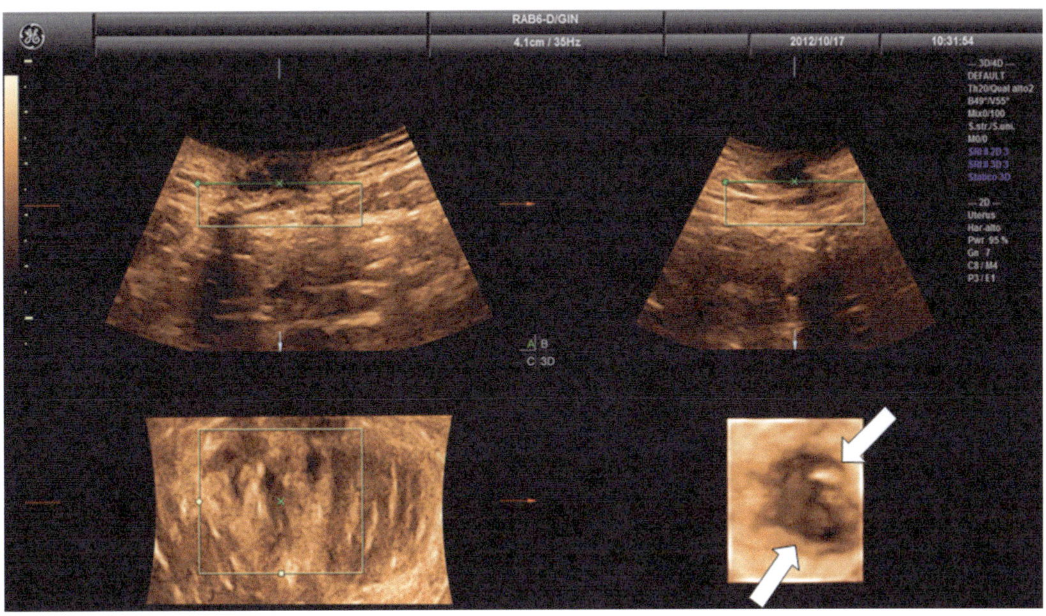

Fig. 13.14 Three-dimensional ultrasonographic appearance of Villar's nodule (*straight arrows*) in a 20-year-old woman without previous abdominal surgery

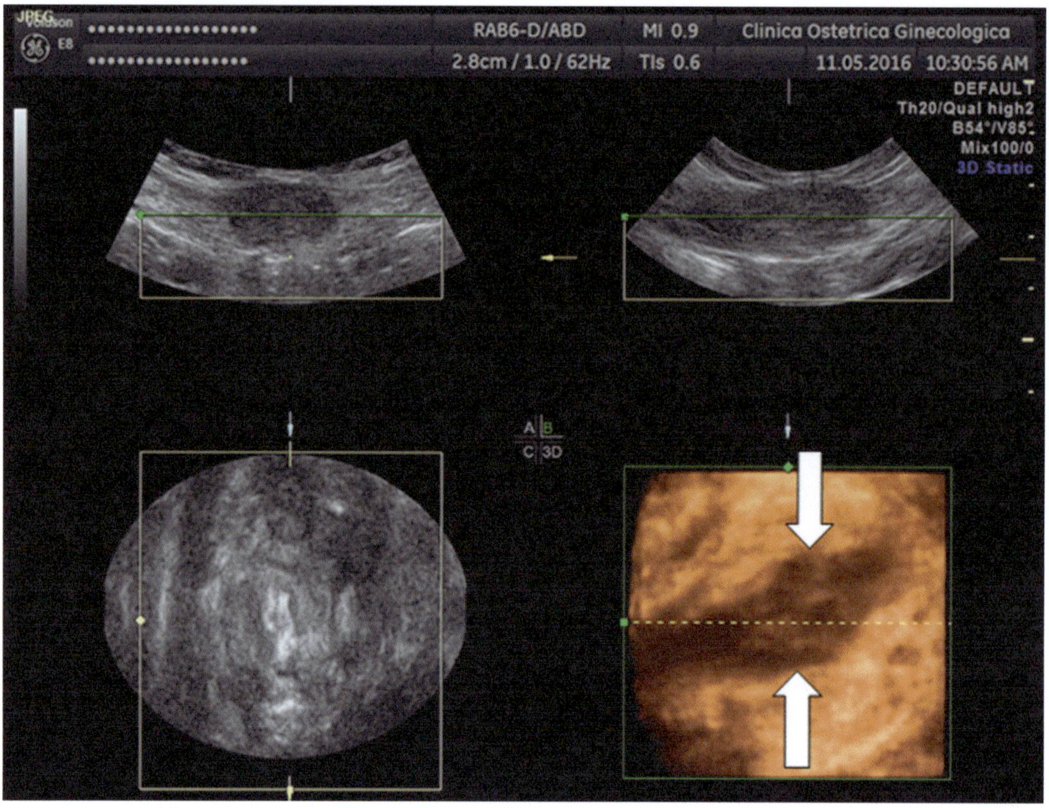

Fig. 13.15 Three-dimensional ultrasonographic appearance of a *rectus abdominis endometriosis* (*straight arrows*) in a 30-year-old woman with one previous cesarean section 4 years before

in controversial cases as it can confirm the diagnosis of endometriosis and rule out other diseases. MRI has shown a sensitivity and specificity of greater than 90% in the detection of endometriomas, with its main limitation being the detection of small (<3 mm) peritoneal implants. The addition of fat-saturated T1-weighted imaging has improved diagnostic accuracy in the evaluation of both endometriomas and peritoneal disease by narrowing the dynamic range, increasing lesion conspicuity, and differentiating lipid-containing ovarian masses from those containing blood [24].

References

1. Jubanyik KJ, Comite F. Extrapelvic endometriosis. Obstet Gynecol Clin North Am. 1997; 24(2):411–40.
2. Jenkins S, Olive DL, Haney AF. Endometriosis: pathogenetic implications of the anatomic distribution. Obstet Gynecol. 1986;67:335–8.
3. Markham SM, Carpenter SE, Rock JA. Extrapelvic endometriosis. Obstet Gynecol Clin North Am. 1989;16:193–219.
4. Hensen JH, Van Breda Vriesman AC, Puylaert JB. Abdominal wall endometriosis: clinical presentation and imaging features with emphasis on sonography. AJR Am J Roentgenol. 2006;186(3):616–20.
5. Nominato NS, Prates LF, Lauar I, Morais J, Maia L, Geber S. Caesarean section greatly increases risk of scar endometriosis. Eur J Obstet Gynecol Reprod Biol. 2010;152(1):83–5.
6. Krantz AM, Dave AA, Margolin DJ. A case of umbilical endometriosis: Villar's nodule. Cureus. 2016;8(12):e926.
7. Dessy LA, Buccheri EM, Chiummariello S, Gagliardi DN, Onesti MG. Umbilical endometriosis, our experience. In Vivo. 2008;22:811–5.
8. Yang DM, Kim HC, Ryu JK, Lim JW, Kim GY. Sonographic findings of inguinal endometriosis. J Ultrasound Med. 2010;29:105–10.
9. Wang CJ, Chao AS, Wang TH, Wu CT, Chao A, Lai CH. Challenge in the management of endometriosis in the canal of Nuck. Fertil Steril. 2009;91(3):936.e9–11.
10. Giannella L, La Marca A, Ternelli G, Menozzi G. Rectus abdominis muscle endometriosis: case report and review of the literature. J Obstet Gynaecol Res. 2010;36(4):902–6.

11. Yoon J, Lee YS, Chang HS, Park CS. Endometriosis of the appendix. Ann Surg Treat Res. 2014;87(3):144–7.
12. De Riggi MA, Fusco F, Marino G, Izzo A. Giant endometrial cyst of the liver: a case report and review of the literature. G Chir. 2016;37(2):79–83.
13. Basso MP, Christiano AB, Oliveira ALC, Cunrath GS, Netinho JG. Appendicular endometriosis as a cause of chronic abdominal pain alone in the right iliac fossa: case report and literature review. J Coloproctol. 2012;32(1):80–3.
14. Van Gorp T, Amant F, Neven P, Vergote I, Moerman P. Endometriosis and the development of malignant tumors of the pelvis. A review of the literature. Best Pract Res Clin Obstet Gynaecol. 2004;18:349–71.
15. Stevens EE, Pradhan TS, Chak Y, Lee YC. Malignant transformation of endometriosis in a cesarean section abdominal wall scar: a case report. J Reprod Med. 2013;58(5–6):264–6.
16. Ferrandina G, Palluzzi E, Fanfani F, Gentileschi S, Valentini AL, Mattoli MV, Pennacchia I, Scambia G, Zannoni G. Endometriosis-associated clear cell carcinoma arising in caesarean section scar: a case report and review of the literature. World J Surg Oncol. 2016;14:300.
17. Guerriero S, et al. Systematic approach to sonographic evaluation of the pelvis in women with suspected endometriosis, including terms, definitions and measurements: a consensus opinion from the International Deep Endometriosis Analysis (IDEA) group. Ultrasound Obstet Gynecol. 2016;48:318–32.
18. Savelli L, Manuzzi L, Di Donato N, Salfi N, Trivella G, Ceccaroni M, Seracchioli R. Endometriosis of the abdominal wall: ultrasonographic and Doppler characteristics. Ultrasound Obstet Gynecol. 2012;39(3):336–40.
19. Francica G. Reliable clinical and sonographic findings in the diagnosis of abdominal wall endometriosis near cesarean section scar. World J Radiol. 2012;4(4):135–40.
20. Ling CM, Lefrebre G. Extrapelvic endometriosis: a case report and review of the literature. J Soc Obstet Gynaecol Can. 2000;22(2):97–100.
21. Veeraswamy A, Lewis M, Mann A, Kotikela S, Hajhosseini B, Nezhat C. Extragenital endometriosis. Clin Obstet Gynecol. 2010;53(2):449–66.
22. Wang Y, Wang W, Wang L, Wang J, Tang J. Ultrasound-guided high-intensity focused ultrasound treatment for abdominal wall endometriosis: preliminary results. Eur J Radiol. 2011;79(1):56–9. https://doi.org/10.1016/j.ejrad.2009.12.034. Epub 2010 Feb 8.
23. Picard A, Varlet MN, Guillibert F, Srour M, Clemenson A, Khaddage A, Seffert P, Chene G. Three dimensional sonographic diagnosis of abdominal wall endometriosis: a useful tool? Fertil Steril. 2011;95(1):289.e1–4.
24. Gougoutas CA, Siegelman ES, Hunt J, Outwater EK. Pelvic endometriosis: various manifestations and MR imaging findings. AJR Am J Roentgenol. 2000;175(2):353–8.

14 Modified Ultrasonographic Techniques

Simone Ferrero,
Umberto Leone Roberti Maggiore, Fabio Barra,
and Carolina Scala

14.1 Introduction

Over the last 10 years, transvaginal ultrasonography (TVS) has become the first-line investigation in women with suspicion of deep endometriosis (DE) [1]. In fact, TVS has good diagnostic performance, and it has several advantages compared with other imaging techniques due to its high diffusion among gynecologists, the relatively low cost, the low discomfort for the patients, and the fact that it does not require the use of radiation. Based on this background, the International Deep Endometriosis Analysis (IDEA) group recently described a systematic approach to the examination of patients with suspicion of DE [2].

A frequent criticism to TVS is that its diagnostic accuracy in patients with DE is dependent on the experience of the sonographer. Improvement in the diagnostic accuracy of TVS may be obtained using a series of modified sonographic techniques based on the introduction of saline solution or gel in the vagina and/or rectum. These techniques, named "enhanced" or "modified" TVS, may be useful when the findings of TVS are inconclusive or when the sonographers have limited experience in the diagnosis of DE. In fact, the distention of the vagina and/or rectum may enhance the visualization of DE lesions.

The most common modified TVS techniques will be described in this chapter.

Electronic Supplementary Material The online version of this chapter (https://doi.org/10.1007/978-3-319-71138-6_14) contains supplementary material, which is available to authorized users.

S. Ferrero (✉) · U. L. R. Maggiore · F. Barra
C. Scala
Academic Unit of Obstetrics and Gynecology, Ospedale Policlinico San Martino, Genoa, Italy

Department of Neurosciences, Rehabilitation, Ophthalmology, Genetics, Maternal and Child Health (DiNOGMI), University of Genoa, Genoa, Italy
e-mail: simone.ferrero@unige.it

14.2 Tenderness-Guided Transvaginal Ultrasonography

Tenderness-guided transvaginal ultrasonography (tg-TVS) is based on the principle of creating an acoustic window between the transvaginal probe and the surrounding vaginal structures by increasing the amount of gel introduced inside the probe cover [3]. In addition, during the exam, the patients are asked to indicate which points felt tender under gentle pressure of the probe, and particular attention is paid by the sonographer to identify endometriotic nodules in these areas [3].

S. Guerriero et al. (eds.), *How to Perform Ultrasonography in Endometriosis*,
https://doi.org/10.1007/978-3-319-71138-6_14

14.2.1 Technique

Twelve milliliter of ultrasound gel are introduced into the probe cover (usually a finger from a latex glove) instead of the usual 3–4 mL. The probe is gently inserted in the vagina in order to minimize the risk of squeezing out the gel. The exam starts with the evaluation of the vaginal wall at the level of the posterior vaginal fornix that can be examined with a sliding up-and-down movement of the probe. The patient is requested to inform the operator about the onset and site of any tenderness experienced during the probe's pressure in the posterior fornix. When tenderness is evoked, the sliding movement is stopped, and particular attention is paid to the painful site via gentle pressure with the probe's tip for the detection of endometriotic nodules [3]. Deep endometriotic nodules appear as hypoechoic linear thickening or nodules/masses with or without regular contours [4].

The usual time required to perform tg-TVS in patients with suspected DE is about 15–20 min; however, less time is required when the exam is negative [3, 5].

14.2.2 Diagnostic Performance

A prospective study including 50 women with suspected rectovaginal endometriosis (31 with DE at surgery) investigated the accuracy of tg-TVS in the diagnosis of DE [3]. The study showed that this technique has a good to excellent diagnostic performance with specificity of 95% (95% CI, 78–100%) and sensitivity of 90% (95% CI, 80–93%); the positive predictive value was 97% (95% CI, 85–100%), the negative predictive value was 86% (95% CI, 70–90%), the positive likelihood ratio (LR+) was 17.2, the negative likelihood ratio (LR−) was 0.1, and the kappa value was 0.86 (95% CI, 0.56–0.91). This diagnostic performance was subsequently confirmed in another prospective study including 88 women (72 with DE) [5]. With respect to the vaginal walls, the sensitivity was 91% (95% CI, 79–97%), the specificity 89% (95% CI, 81–93%), the LR+ 8.2, and an LR− 0.09. For endometriosis of rectovaginal septum, the sensitivity was 74% (95% CI, 64–80%), the specificity 88% (95% CI, 4–8%), the LR+ 6.2, and the LR− 0.3. For other locations (uterosacral ligaments, rectosigmoid, anterior pouch, and bladder), the sensitivity was lower (ranging from 67 to 33%) with a comparable specificity. More recently, a prospective study including 59 patients with clinical suspicion of DE (30 patients with surgical diagnosis of rectosigmoid endometriosis) compared the diagnostic accuracy of magnetic resonance imaging (MRI) and tg-TVS in diagnosing rectosigmoid endometriosis [4]. There was no significant difference in the sensitivity and specificity of MRI and tg-TVS in identifying rectosigmoid involvement. In particular, the specificity, sensitivity, and LR+ and LR− of tg-TVS were 86%, 73%, 5.317, and 0.309, respectively.

14.3 Sonovaginography

Sonovaginography (SVG) consists of TVS combined with the introduction of saline solution or gel into the posterior vaginal fornix to improve the visualization of vaginal and rectovaginal septum DE. On regular TVS, these nodules may escape detection primarily because of the close proximity of these structures to the transvaginal transducer [6]. The increased clarity on gel sonovaginography is achieved because the instilled gel causes standoff and partial distension of vaginal walls.

14.3.1 Technique

SVG was first described by Dessole et al. in 2003 [7]. Immediately before the exam, the patients are asked to partially empty the bladder in order to leave a small amount of urine within to enhance the examination of the anterior vaginal wall and of the vesicovaginal septum [7]. After the patient seat in the gynecological position, the gynecological bed is slightly tilted in anti-Trendelenburg position to avoid saline solution reflux from the vagina during the exam. A 24-mm Foley catheter is introduced into the vagina, and its balloon is inflated using 5–6 mL of saline solution. A limitation of this technique is that an operator and an assistant are required to perform each exam [7]. The operator uses the right hand to handle the transvaginal probe and the left hand to close the vaginal channel, narrowing the minor labia with the dorsal surface of the forefinger and the middle finger. This maneuver is necessary to avoid the reflux of saline solution from the vagina during the exam. The assistant injects 200–400 mL of saline solution through a Foley catheter [7].

Other authors described the use of a purpose-designed hydraulic ring (Colpo-Pneumo Occluder, CooperSurgical, Berlin, Germany) that is placed at the base of the transvaginal probe and is inflated with approximately 40 mL of saline solution in order to prevent the escape of the 60–120 mL of saline that is subsequently injected into the vagina using a Foley catheter [8]. The saline solution in the vagina creates an acoustic window between the transvaginal probe and the surrounding structures; furthermore, it distends the vaginal walls [7, 8]. This technique improves the visualization of the vaginal walls, vaginal fornix, uterosacral ligaments, pouch of Douglas, rectovaginal septum, and vesicovaginal septum. During the exam, the transvaginal probe is not in contact with the uterine cervix; the scan is performed by sliding the probe back and forward, longitudinally and transversally, with up, down, and angled movements around the cervix, which was used as a reference point. The endometriotic lesions appear as hypoechoic, irregular structures.

SVG is well tolerated, and the intensity of pain perceived by the patients is similar to that reported during TVS [7].

Other techniques to perform SVG have been described. SVG can be performed by inserting into the posterior vaginal fornix a condom attached to a saline giving set. The transvaginal probe is then introduced into the vagina superior to the condom which is resting against the posterior vaginal wall. Once the transvaginal probe is in situ, the condom is filled with 200–400 mL of normal saline to enhance the visualization of the retrocervical area, the posterior fornix, the posterior vaginal wall, and the rectovaginal septum [9]. In the original study describing this technique, the SVG was performed during general anesthesia just prior to laparoscopy [9]; the bladder was emptied by using a urinary catheter, and the patient was slightly tilted in anti-Trendelenburg position.

A modified SVG technique consists in the simple introduction of 20 mL [6, 10, 11] or 50 mL [12] of ultrasound gel into the posterior vaginal fornix using a syringe prior to performing TVS in the office setting. The gel should be loaded carefully into the syringe to decrease the presence of air bubbles/pockets within the gel. Recently, Sibal described in details a technique to minimize the presence of air bubbles within the filled syringe [6]. An assistant should hold the bottle of gel with its mouth facing downward. The syringe is introduced into the lower part of the inverted bottle. Then, instead of pulling the plunger out to fill the syringe, as is the usual practice, the plunger is held steady in position, and the barrel (outer sleeve) is slowly pushed farther up into the inverted bottle of gel to fill the syringe with 20 mL of gel. The syringe must be filled completely, so that the plunger comes in direct contact with the gel, thus further decreasing the possibility of air pockets when instilling the gel into the vagina. Some gel is usually sticking onto the external surface of the syringe, and it can be used as a lubricant when the syringe is introduced into the vagina. Subsequently, the gel-lubricated tips of index and middle fingers of the gloved right hand are introduced into the vagina. The syringe, held in the gloved left hand, is held such that its tip lies in the groove above and between the index and middle fingers. The syringe is introduced into the vagina, directed by the fingers of the right hand in the vagina (Fig. 14.1). The fingers of the right hand are then removed, and the syringe is gently pushed farther inside along the posterior vaginal wall such that there is enough of it outside to grip and push the plunger to introduce the gel into the vagina. The syringe must be inserted far enough into the vaginal canal such that the gel fills the posterior fornix completely [11]. The syringe is then withdrawn. A 20-mL volume of gel is thus placed in the upper vagina mainly in the posterior fornix. The transvaginal transducer is gently introduced into the vagina, carefully observing the vaginal side walls for any abnormalities as the probe is gradually advanced upward. It is important to assess the lower vagina initially before assessing the upper vagina and cervix because once the transducer is pushed up, the gel gets displaced, and withdrawing and reinserting the transducer result in air bubbles getting into the vaginal gel, causing suboptimal imaging, in addition to loss of gel volume in the upper vagina.

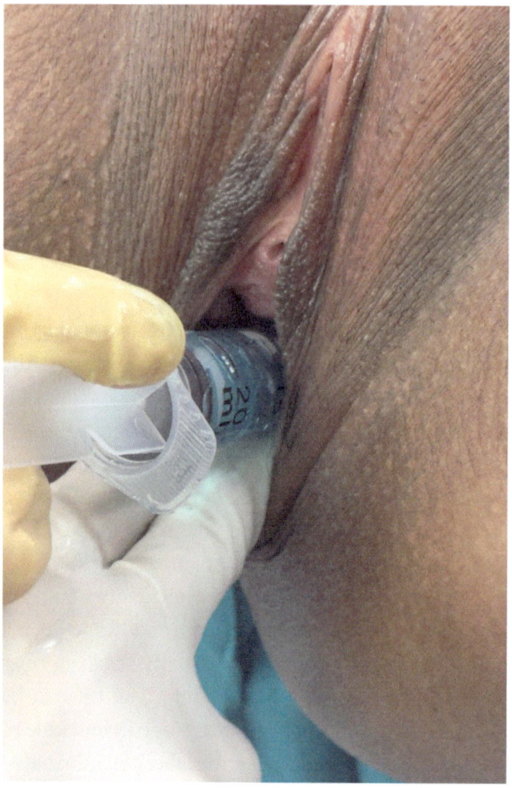

Fig. 14.1 Sonovaginography with gel. The syringe completely filled with gel is held in the left hand. It is introduced into the vagina such that its tip lies in the groove above and between the index and middle fingers

The ultrasound gel distends the vagina and allows the anatomical contours of the inner vagina to be clearly visualized (Figs. 14.2 and 14.3). The main advantage of using gel instead of saline as a distention medium during SVG is that gel SVG requires only one operator to insert the gel and perform the examination [10, 11].

Some authors reported the use of bowel preparation prior to SVG: an oral laxative (sodium picosulfate, ten drops by mouth) the night before the examination and a rectal enema

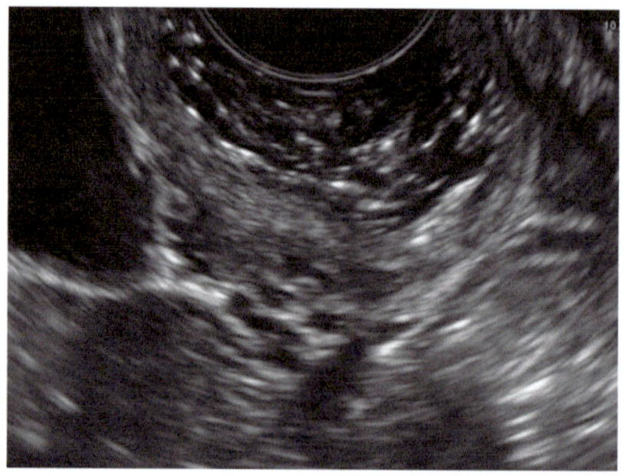

Fig. 14.2 Sonovaginography with gel. The ultrasound gel distends the vagina and facilitates the visualization of the anatomical contours of the inner vagina

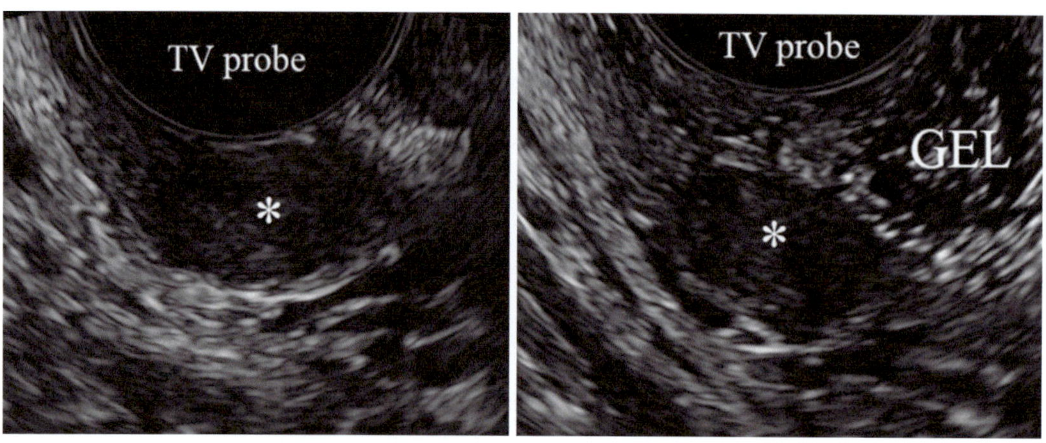

Fig. 14.3 Sonovaginography with gel. On the left, a vaginal nodule (*asterisk*) can be observed by transvaginal ultrasonography; on the right, the visualization of the nodule is enhanced by sonovaginography with gel. *TV probe* transvaginal probe

(120 mL of sodium diphosphate) 1–2 h before the examination [12].

14.3.2 Diagnostic Performance

A preliminary prospective study including 46 women scheduled for surgery because of recto-vaginal endometriosis showed that SVG (200–400 mL of saline solution in the vagina) diagnoses rectovaginal endometriosis more accurately than TVS. The diagnostic performance of SVG in detecting rectovaginal endometriosis was sensitivity 90.6%, specificity 85.7%, PPV 93.5%, and NPV 80.0% [7]. In a prospective pilot study including 33 women with suspected endometriosis, SVG (a condom attached to a saline giving set inserted in the posterior vaginal fornix) was performed immediately before laparoscopy under general anesthesia [9]. The sensitivity, specificity, positive predictive value, and negative predictive value for SVG in the prediction of rectovaginal endometriotic nodules were 75%, 94.7%, 75%, and 94.7%. Another study performed by the same authors showed that SVG (10–20 mL of ultrasound gel into the vagina) has sensitivity of 100%, specificity of 91.7%, NPV of 70%, and PPV of 100% in diagnosing DE of the posterior compartment [10]. A multicenter prospective study including 189 women with clinical suspicion of endometriosis investigated the accuracy of SVG (20 mL of ultrasound gel into the vagina) in diagnosing posterior DE [11]. For the prediction of posterior compartment DE overall (anterior rectum, rectosigmoid, uterosacral ligaments, rectovaginal septum, and/or vagina), the sensitivity was 86%, specificity was 93%, PPV was 83%, and NPV was 94%. For the prediction of bowel endometriosis, the sensitivity was 88.4%, specificity was 93.2%, PPV was 79.2%, and NPV was 96.5%. Specificity was high for all locations, but sensitivity varied depending on location (being as high as 88% for bowel nodules, but as low as 18% in the posterior vaginal wall and rectovaginal septum). A prospective study including 51 patients with DE (50 mL of ultrasound gel into the vagina after bowel preparation) reported a sensitivity of 100%, a specificity of 93%, and LR+ of 14.0 for rectosigmoid involvement. The sensitivity, specificity, LR+, and LR− for vaginal involvement were 60%, 98%, 30.0, and 0.41. The sensitivity, specificity, LR+, and LR− for retrocervical involvement were 84%, 96%, 19.4, and 0.16 [12].

A prospective study including 54 women compared clinical evaluation, TVS, SVG (60–120 mL of saline solution), and MRI in the diagnosis of posterior DE [8]. SVG correctly identified 43 (93.5%) cases of posterior DE, presenting higher accuracy than the other techniques. SVG had a sensitivity of 93.5%, a specificity of 87.5%, a PPV of 97.7%, a NPV of 70.0%, a LR+ of 7.47, and a LR− of 0.07 in diagnosing posterior DE. There was no significant difference in the pain perceived by the patients during TVS and SVG.

14.4 Rectal Water Contrast Transvaginal Ultrasonography

Rectal water contrast transvaginal ultrasonography (RWC-TVS) is based on the concept of distending the rectosigmoid colon by using saline solution while performing ultrasonography [13]. The aim of this exam is to facilitate the identification of rectosigmoid endometriotic nodules and the assessment of their characteristics during TVS.

14.4.1 Technique

A bowel preparation is advisable before the exam. In some studies, patients were asked to drink four doses of a granular powder dissolved in 1000 mL of water per dose on the day before the exam [14]. However, in common clinical practice, bowel preparation consists of a rectal enema performed within few hours before the ultrasonography to eliminate the feces present in the rectosigmoid colon [15–17].

A 6-mm (18 Ch) flexible catheter is inserted through the anal os into the rectal lumen up to a 15–20-cm distance from the anus (Fig. 14.4). A gel infused with lidocaine may be used to minimize the discomfort due to the passage of the catheter. After the connection of a 50-mL syringe to the catheter, warm sterile saline solution is slowly injected inside the rectosigmoid under ultrasonographic control. Hundred milliliter of saline solution are infused continuously at the beginning of the procedure; subsequently, additional saline solution (up to 350 mL) is injected as requested by the ultrasonographer depending on the distensibility of the intestinal wall (Fig. 14.5). During the examination, a Klemmer forceps may be placed on the catheter to prevent backflow of the saline solution through the catheter when the solution was not being injected. Usually, there is no significant leakage of saline solution into the space between the catheter and the anus. The exam is performed both during and following saline injection. The use of the water contrast allows to dynamically evaluate the endometriotic lesions.

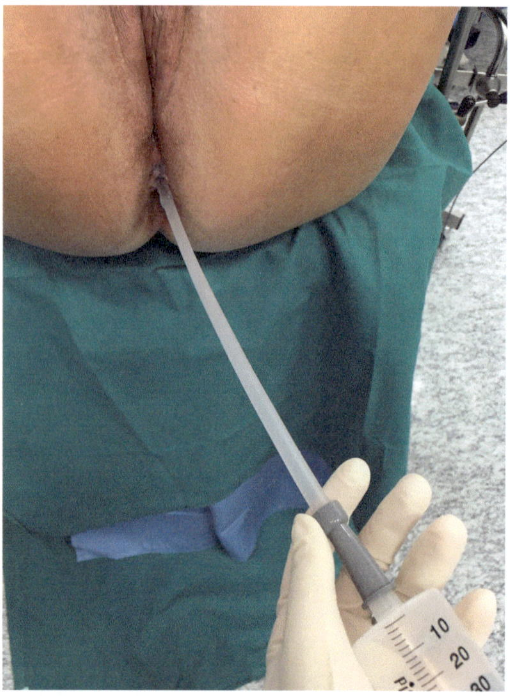

Fig. 14.4. A 6-mm (18 Ch) catheter is inserted through the anal os into the rectal lumen

After a sagittal scan of the uterine cervix is obtained with the transvaginal probe, the sonographer focuses on the anterior and lateral sides of the rectosigmoid, where deep endometriotic nodules are usually located. As in traditional TVS, at RWC-TVS the normal layers of the rectosigmoid can be evaluated. The serosa appears as thin hyperechoic line, the muscularis propria is hypoechoic with the longitudinal smooth muscle (outer) and circular smooth muscle (inner) separated by a faint thin hyperechoic line, the submucosa is hyperechoic, and the mucosa is hypoechoic. In RWC-TVS, the interface between the lumen and the mucosal layer is hyperechoic (Fig. 14.6) [16]. Rectosigmoid endometriotic nodules appear as a thickening of the hypoechoic muscularis propria or as rounded or triangular

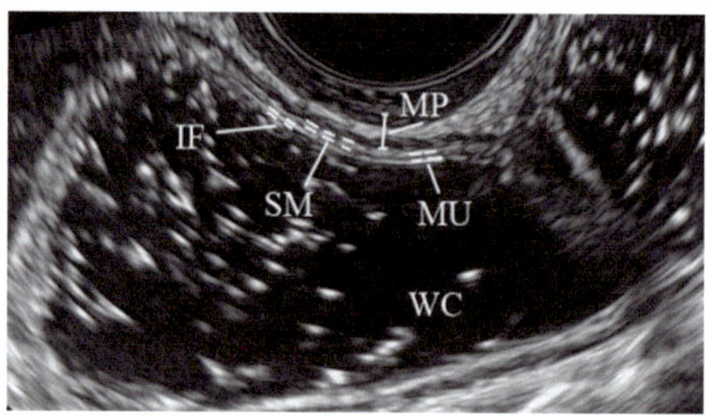

Fig. 14.6 Rectal water contrast transvaginal ultrasonographic image showing normal rectal wall. The various layers can be recognized: muscularis propria (MP), submucosa (SM), and mucosa (MU). The interface (IF) between the lumen and the mucosal layer is hyperechoic. The rectum is dilated by saline solution (WC)

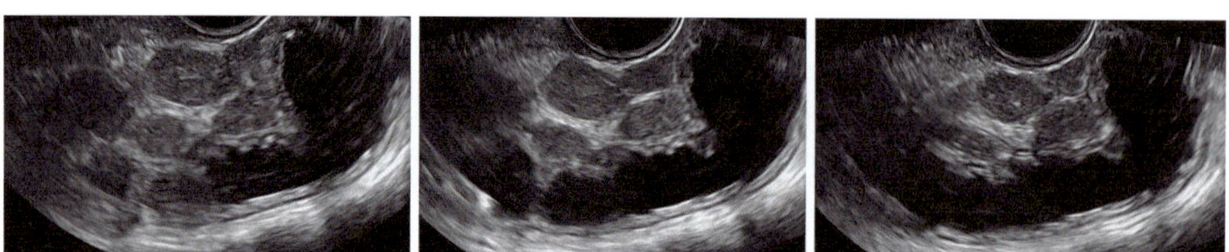

Fig. 14.5 Progressive distention of the rectosigmoid colon during rectal water contrast transvaginal ultrasonography

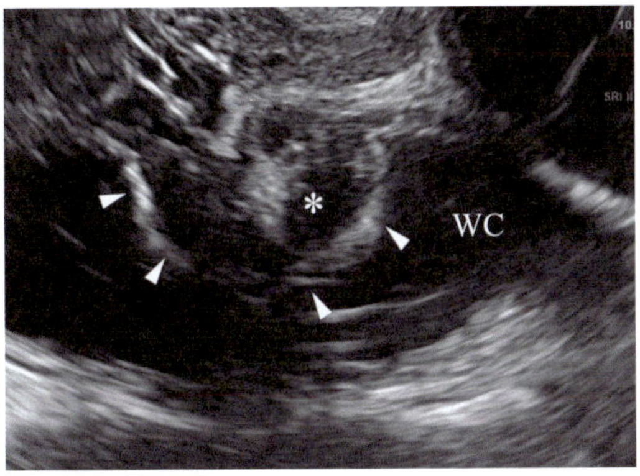

Fig. 14.7 Rectal water contrast transvaginal ultrasonography shows a rectal endometriotic nodule (*asterisk*). The hyperechoic submucosa is not infiltrated (*arrowheads*). The rectum is dilated by saline solution (WC)

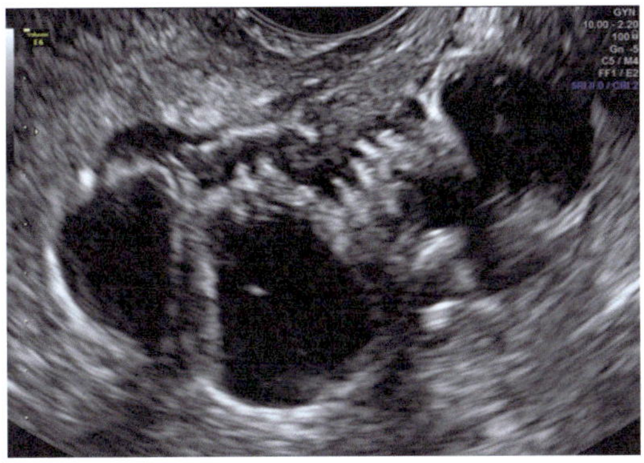

Fig. 14.8 Rectal water contrast transvaginal ultrasonography shows a rectal endometriotic nodule. The nodule has prominent spikes toward the bowel lumen that are enhanced by the distention of the rectum ("Indian headdress" or "moose antler" sign)

hypoechoic nodules, with or without hyperechoic foci with blurred margins. The endometriotic nodule replaces the normal appearance of the muscularis propria; retraction and adhesions are often present (Figs. 14.7, 14.8, and 14.9).

The time required to perform RWC-TVS is about 15–20 min [16]. RWC-TVS is usually well tolerated [14–16, 18], and it is always carried out without the need of local or general anesthesia.

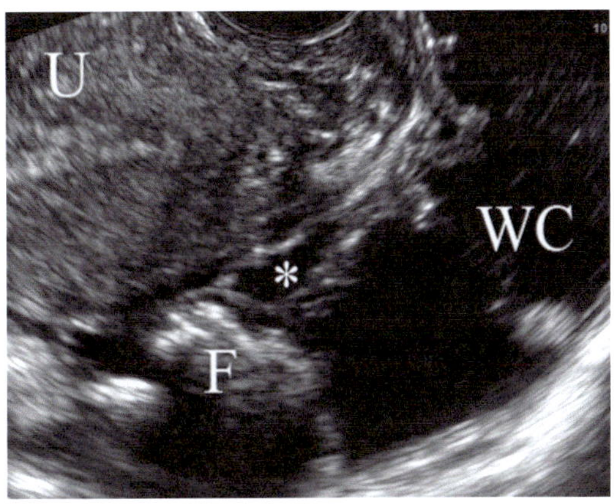

Fig. 14.9 Rectal water contrast transvaginal ultrasonography shows a retrocervical endometriotic nodule (largest diameter 15.5 mm) infiltrating the muscular layer of the rectum. The rectum is dilated by saline solution (WC); feces (F) can be observed in the rectum. *U* uterus

14.4.2 Diagnostic Performance

Several studies investigated the diagnostic performance of RWC-TVS in diagnosing rectosigmoid endometriosis and compared RWC-TVS with other imaging techniques used for the diagnosis of colorectal endometriosis.

The use of RWC-TVS for the diagnosis of rectosigmoid endometriosis was originally described in a prospective study including 35 patients with rectovaginal endometriosis [19]. The exam showed good diagnostic performance (Table 14.1), but it underestimated the depth of infiltration in nodules reaching the submucosa. Subsequently, the same authors compared the performance of TVS and RWC-TVS in diagnosing intestinal infiltration in women with suspicion of rectovaginal endometriosis [14]. RWC-TVS was more accurate than TVS in diagnosing intestinal infiltration, but patients reported more pain with this technique than TVS (Figs. 14.10 and 14.11, and Video 14.1).

A prospective study including 61 patients with suspected rectosigmoid endometriosis demonstrated that RWC-TVS and transrectal sonography (TRS) have the same accuracy in the diagnosis of rectosigmoid endometriosis [17]. Furthermore, in the same study, the authors showed that RWC-TVS and barium enema are equally effective in the detection of a significant intestinal stenosis (≥50% of the lumen) due to endometriosis [17] (Videos 14.1 and 14.2, Fig. 14.12).

Table 14.1 Performance of RWC-TVS in diagnosing rectosigmoid endometriosis

Authors	Study population	Patients with rectosigmoid endometriosis at surgery/histology	Accuracy	Sensitivity	Specificity	PPV	NPV	LR+	LR−
Valenzano Menada et al., 2008 [19]	35	21	94.3% (80.8–99.3)	100% (83.9–100.0)	85.7% (57.2–98.2)	91.3% (74.4–97.4)	100%	7.00 (1.94–25.26)	–[a]
Valenzano Menada et al. [14]	90	29	98.9% (94.0–100.0)	95.7% (78.1–99.9)	100.0% (94.6–100.0)	100.0%	98.5% (90.8–99.8)	–[b]	0.04 (0.01–0.30)
Bergamini et al. [17]	61	51	95.1% (86.3–99.0)	96.1% (86.5–99.5)	90.0% (55.5–99.8)	98.0% (88.4–99.7)	81.8 (53.2–94.7)	9.61 (1.50–61.73)	0.04 (0.01–0.17)
Ferrero et al. [18]	96	48	95.8% (89.7–98.9)	93.8% (82.8–98.7)	97.9% (88.9–100.0)	97.8% (86.6–99.7)	94% (84.0–97.9)	45.00 (6.46–313.41)	0.06 (0.02–0.19)
Leone Roberti Maggiore et al. [16]	286	151	94.8% (92.2–97.4)	92.7% (87.3–96.3)	97.0% (93.0–99.2)	97.2% (93.0–99.2)	92.3% (86.6–96.1)	31.29 (11.90–82.25)	0.08 (0.04–0.13)
Ferrero et al. [15]	70	40	94.3% (88.9–99.7)	92.5% (78.6–98.4)	96.7% (82.9–99.9)	97.4% (86.2–99.9)	90.6% (75.0–98.0)	27.8 (4.03–191.01)	0.08 (0.03–0.23)

PPV positive predictive value, *NPV* negative predictive value, *LR+* positive likelihood ratio, *LR−* negative likelihood ratio
[a]LR− could not be calculated because of the absence of false-negative cases
[b]LR+ could not be calculated because of the absence of false-positive cases

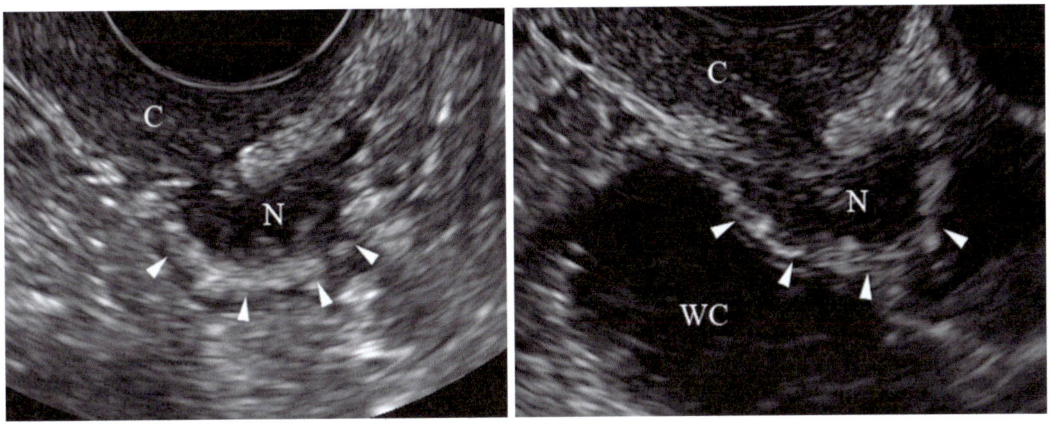

Fig. 14.10 Rectal hypoechoic endometriotic nodule with blurred margins and hyperechoic foci on transvaginal ultrasonography (on the *left*) and rectal water contrast transvaginal ultrasonography (on the *right*). The arrowheads indicate the submucosa that is not infiltrated by the endometriotic nodule. *C* uterine cervix, *N* nodule, *WC* water contrast. The same nodule is shown in Video 14.1

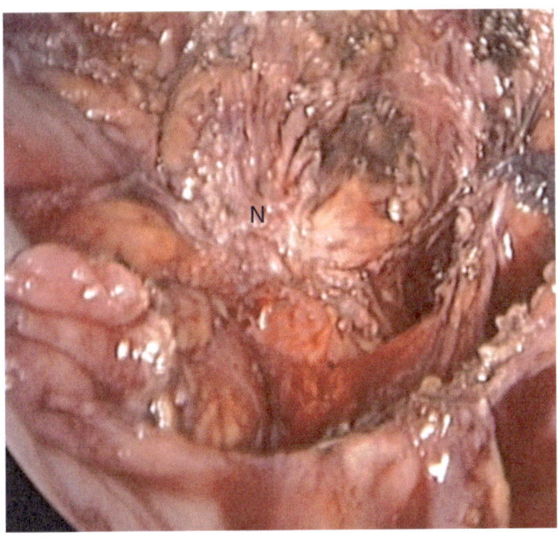

Fig. 14.11 Laparoscopic image of the rectal nodule (N) shown in Fig. 14.10 and Video 14.1

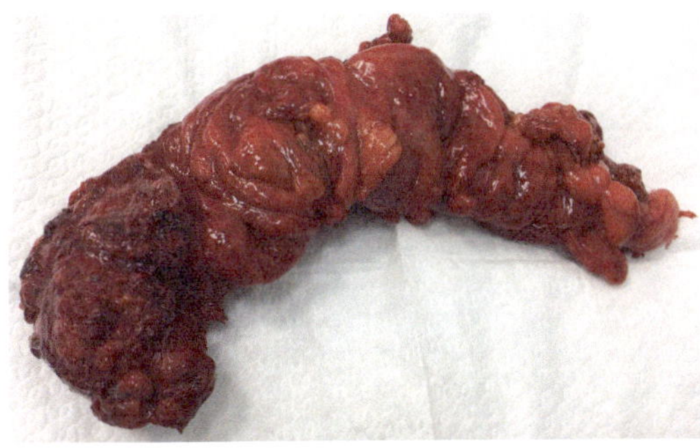

Fig. 14.12 The resected rectal specimen shown in Video 14.2

Another prospective study demonstrated that RWC-TVS and multidetector computerized tomography enema (MDCT-e) have similar accuracy in diagnosing rectosigmoid endometriosis [18]. Both exams underestimated the size of the endometriotic nodules compared to histology; however, the underestimation was greater for RWC-TVS than for MDCT-e. In addition, in both imaging techniques, the underestimation was greater for nodules with diameter $\geq$ 30 mm. RWC-TVS and MDCT-e had similar accuracy in diagnosing multifocal rectosigmoid endometriosis. RWC-TVS was better tolerated by the patients compared with MDCT-e.

A large prospective study including 286 patients of reproductive age with clinical suspicion of rectosigmoid endometriosis compared the accuracy of RWC-TVS and magnetic resonance enema (MR-e) in the diagnosis of rectosigmoid endometriosis [16]. The two techniques had similar accuracy in the diagnosis of rectosigmoid endometriosis, but the accuracy of RWC-TVS was superior to that of MR-e in the detection of infiltration of the mucosal layer. A similar intensity of pain was perceived by the patients during RWC-TVS and MR-e.

A recent prospective study compared the performance of RWC-TVS and computed tomographic colonography (CTC) in diagnosing rectosigmoid endometriosis [15]. The results of imaging techniques were compared with surgical and pathologic findings. Out of 70 patients with clinical suspicion of rectosigmoid endometriosis, 40 patients (57.1%) had surgical diagnosis of rectosigmoid endometriosis. There was no significant difference in the accuracy of RWC-TVS and CTC in the diagnosis of rectosigmoid endometriosis. Both techniques similarly estimated the length (midsagittal diameter) of the endometriotic nodules independently from their location in the low rectum, upper rectum, or rectosigmoid. CTC was significantly more precise than RWC-TVS in estimating the distance between the lower margin of the rectosigmoid nodule and the anal verge. RWC-TVS was significantly more accurate than CTC in in diagnosing multifocal rectosigmoid endometriosis. Patients perceived less pain during RWC-TVS than during CTC.

The major limitation of RWC-TVS is that it allows diagnosing only rectosigmoid nodules because lesions located above the sigmoid are beyond the field that can be explored by TVS. CTC has the advantage of investigating the whole bowel allowing diagnosing multicentric lesions (i.e., right colon, ileon, ileocecal junction, or appendix), and, thus, these two techniques may be combined to obtain a preoperative assessment of the whole colon.

14.5 Three-Dimensional Rectosonography

Three-dimensional rectosonography (3D-RSG) is a modification of the RWC-TVS technique that is mainly based on the acquisition of 3D images when a rectosigmoid nodule is identified at TVS.

14.5.1 Technique

In the original description of the 3D-RSG technique, the patients slowly inject themselves with 120 mL of warm water into the rectum using a 60-mL syringe with conical tip [20]. Several 3D acquisitions are obtained by using a 3D transvaginal transducer. The structures of interest visualized during the 3D acquisition are the uterosacral ligaments, vaginal apex, rectovaginal septum, rectosigmoid colon, and rectum. These images allow to provide a better characterization of the nodules, including measurement of the diameters in three planes, determination of the volume, the anatomic extension, and whether the nodules cause bowel stenosis [21]. Each time, several 3D TVUS acquisitions of the posterior compartment are performed, especially when intestinal infiltration is suspected. After acquisition, the multiplanar display shows a sagittal view, an axial plane, and a coronal plane. The coronal plane could not have been obtained with conventional 2D sonography. Several 3D image programs are used for offline analysis. The virtual organ computer-aided analysis (VOCAL) mode is used to assess the volume of the DE, and the tomographic ultrasound imaging (TUI) mode provides series of slices through any one of these planes (Fig. 14.13). The TUI display is modified to provide the maximum of number of slices in the region of interest (ROI) and allows to obtain a better appreciation of intestinal wall infiltration. At the end of the procedure, the surface mode is used to reconstruct the endometriotic nodule entirely, in a kind of virtual colonoscopy that allows to assess the intestinal stenosis caused by the nodule.

A colorectal preparation is used before the procedure, a rectal enema is administered twice (at 2 h and 1 h) before the procedure [21]. In case of inadequate bowel preparation, the procedure may require to be postponed [21].

14.5.2 Diagnostic Performance

So far, 3D-RSG was used to investigate posterior DE in only one series of 50 patients [20, 21]. Eighteen of the 20 intestinal nodules (90%) were identified among 19 patients by 3D-RSG. No intestinal lesions were observed by 3D-RSG in 31 patients. When MRI was used as reference technique, the diagnostic performance of 3D-RSG was sensitivity 95%, specificity 97%,

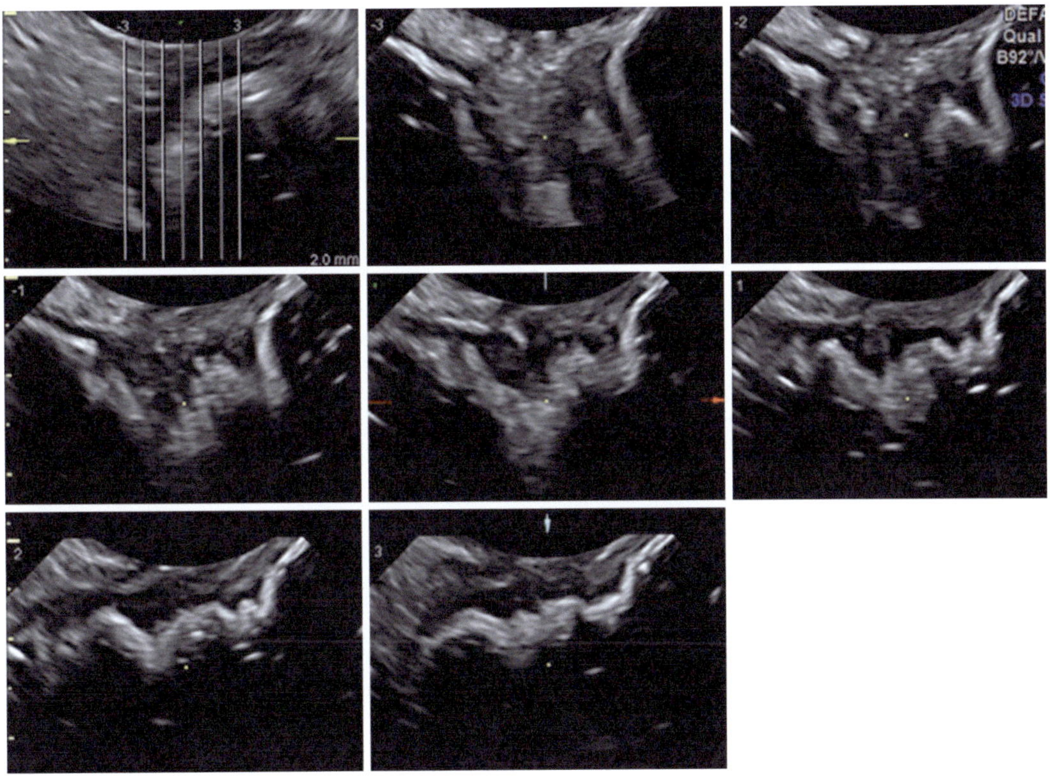

Fig. 14.13 Tomographic ultrasound images obtained during rectal water contrast transvaginal ultrasound. This series of slices can provide information regarding the extent of infiltration of intestinal wall by endometriotic nodule

PPV 95%, NPV 97%, positive likelihood ratio 30.3, and negative likelihood ratio 0.05.

14.6 Future Perspective

In patients with suspicion of DE, if the initial scan reveals lesions in a determined area, it is unlikely that additional testing is required because of the high specificity of TVS [22]. In a meta-analysis, Guerriero et al. found that enhanced approaches are not more accurate than plain TVS for this diagnosis of rectosigmoid endometriosis [23]. Modified ultrasonographic techniques should be used when the result of TVS are inconclusive or if it is felt additional information on the features of DE should be obtained [24]. However, a limitation of TVS is that it depends on the examiner's ability and experience; therefore, modified ultrasonographic techniques could be an option for those operators who do not achieve good results with TVS. The selection of a particular modified ultrasonographic technique depends on the skill and experience of the sonographer as well as the TVS findings [24]. For example, SVG significantly improves the visualization of the anterior and posterior vaginal fornices. Similarly, RWC-TVS may improve the visualization of rectosigmoid nodules when the sonographers are learning to image the posterior compartment.

An advantage of modified ultrasonographic techniques compared with other imaging modalities (such as MRI) is that they cause low pain or discomfort for the patient and they can be performed directly by the gynecologists at low cost. Furthermore, these techniques can also be performed as a dynamic test because the operator can assess the changes in the position of endometriotic nodules compared to the position of the pelvic organs (such as the bowel and bladder) and assess their infiltration. Nowadays, the major challenge in the imaging diagnosis of endometriosis remains the detection of superficial lesions. Future studies should assess whether modified ultrasonographic techniques can allow the detection of superficial endometriotic lesions.

References

1. Piketty M, Chopin N, Dousset B, Millischer-Bellaische AE, Roseau G, Leconte M, et al. Preoperative work-up for patients with deeply infiltrating endometriosis: transvaginal ultrasonography must definitely be the first-line imaging examination. Hum Reprod. 2009;24(3):602–7.
2. Guerriero S, Condous G, Van den Bosch T, Valentin L, Leone FP, Van Schoubroeck D, et al. Systematic approach to sonographic evaluation of the pelvis in women with suspected endometriosis, including terms, definitions and measurements: a consensus opinion from the International Deep Endometriosis Analysis (IDEA) group. Ultrasound Obstet Gynecol. 2016;48(3):318–32.
3. Guerriero S, Ajossa S, Gerada M, D'Aquila M, Piras B, Melis GB. "Tenderness-guided" transvaginal ultrasonography: a new method for the detection of deep endometriosis in patients with chronic pelvic pain. Fertil Steril. 2007;88(5):1293–7.
4. Saba L, Guerriero S, Sulcis R, Pilloni M, Ajossa S, Melis G, et al. MRI and "tenderness guided" transvaginal ultrasonography in the diagnosis of recto-sigmoid endometriosis. J Magn Reson Imaging. 2012;35(2):352–60.
5. Guerriero S, Ajossa S, Gerada M, Virgilio B, Angioni S, Melis GB. Diagnostic value of transvaginal 'tenderness-guided' ultrasonography for the prediction of location of deep endometriosis. Hum Reprod. 2008;23(11):2452–7.
6. Sibal M. Gel sonovaginography: a new way of evaluating a variety of local vaginal and cervical disorders. J Ultrasound Med. 2016;35(12):2699–715.
7. Dessole S, Farina M, Rubattu G, Cosmi E, Ambrosini G, Nardelli GB. Sonovaginography is a new technique for assessing rectovaginal endometriosis. Fertil Steril. 2003;79(4):1023–7.
8. Saccardi C, Cosmi E, Borghero A, Tregnaghi A, Dessole S, Litta P. Comparison between transvaginal sonography, saline contrast sonovaginography and magnetic resonance imaging in the diagnosis of posterior deep infiltrating endometriosis. Ultrasound Obstet Gynecol. 2012;40(4):464–9.
9. Reid S, Bignardi T, Lu C, Lam A, Condous G. The use of intra-operative saline sonovaginography to define the rectovaginal septum in women with suspected rectovaginal endometriosis: a pilot study. Australas J Ultrasound Med. 2011;14(3):4–9.
10. Reid S, Winder S, Condous G. Sonovaginography: redefining the concept of a "normal pelvis" on transvaginal ultrasound pre-laparoscopic intervention for suspected endometriosis. Australas J Ultrasound Med. 2011;14(2):21–4.
11. Reid S, Lu C, Hardy N, Casikar I, Reid G, Cario G, et al. Office gel sonovaginography for the prediction of posterior deep infiltrating endometriosis: a multicenter prospective observational study. Ultrasound Obstet Gynecol. 2014;44(6):710–8.
12. Leon M, Vaccaro H, Alcazar JL, Martinez J, Gutierrez J, Amor F, et al. Extended transvaginal sonography in deep infiltrating endometriosis: use of bowel preparation and an acoustic window with intravaginal gel: preliminary results. J Ultrasound Med. 2014;33(2):315–21.
13. Rubin C, Kurtz AB, Goldberg BB. Water enema: a new ultrasound technique in defining pelvic anatomy. J Clin Ultrasound. 1978;6(1):28–33.
14. Valenzano Menada M, Remorgida V, Abbamonte LH, Nicoletti A, Ragni N, Ferrero S. Does transvaginal ultrasonography combined with water-contrast in the rectum aid in the diagnosis of rectovaginal endometriosis infiltrating the bowel? Hum Reprod. 2008;23(5):1069–75.
15. Ferrero S, Biscaldi E, Vellone VG, Venturini PL, Leone Roberti Maggiore U. Computed tomographic colonography vs rectal water-contrast transvaginal sonography in diagnosis of rectosigmoid endometriosis: a pilot study. Ultrasound Obstet Gynecol. 2017;49(4):515–23.
16. Leone Roberti Maggiore U, Biscaldi E, Vellone VG, Venturini PL, Ferrero S. Magnetic resonance enema vs rectal water-contrast transvaginal sonography in diagnosis of rectosigmoid endometriosis. Ultrasound Obstet Gynecol. 2017;49(4):524–32.
17. Bergamini V, Ghezzi F, Scarperi S, Raffaelli R, Cromi A, Franchi M. Preoperative assessment of intestinal endometriosis: a comparison of transvaginal sonography with water-contrast in the rectum, transrectal sonography, and barium enema. Abdom Imaging. 2010;35(6):732–6.
18. Ferrero S, Biscaldi E, Morotti M, Venturini PL, Remorgida V, Rollandi GA, et al. Multidetector computerized tomography enteroclysis vs. rectal water contrast transvaginal ultrasonography in determining the presence and extent of bowel endometriosis. Ultrasound Obstet Gynecol. 2011;37(5):603–13.
19. Menada MV, Remorgida V, Abbamonte LH, Fulcheri E, Ragni N, Ferrero S. Transvaginal ultrasonography combined with water-contrast in the rectum in the diagnosis of rectovaginal endometriosis infiltrating the bowel. Fertil Steril. 2008;89(3):699–700.
20. Philip CA, Bisch C, Coulon A, de Saint-Hilaire P, Rudigoz RC, Dubernard G. Correlation between three-dimensional rectosonography and magnetic

resonance imaging in the diagnosis of rectosigmoid endometriosis: a preliminary study on the first fifty cases. Eur J Obstet Gynecol Reprod Biol. 2015;187:35–40.

21. Philip CA, Bisch C, Coulon A, Maissiat E, de Saint-Hilaire P, Huissoud C, et al. Three-dimensional sonorectography: a new transvaginal ultrasound technique with intrarectal contrast to assess colorectal endometriosis. Ultrasound Obstet Gynecol. 2015;45(2):233–5.
22. Guerriero S, Ajossa S, Minguez JA, Jurado M, Mais V, Melis GB, et al. Accuracy of transvaginal ultrasound for diagnosis of deep endometriosis in uterosacral ligaments, rectovaginal septum, vagina and bladder: systematic review and meta-analysis. Ultrasound Obstet Gynecol. 2015;46(5):534–45.
23. Guerriero S, Ajossa S, Orozco R, Perniciano M, Jurado M, Melis GB, Alcazar JL. Accuracy of transvaginal ultrasound for diagnosis of deep endometriosis in the rectosigmoid: systematic review and meta-analysis. Ultrasound Obstet Gynecol. 2016;47(3):281–9.
24. Hoyos LR, Johnson S, Puscheck E. Endometriosis and imaging. Clin Obstet Gynecol. 2017;60(3):503–16.

Additional Radiological Techniques (MRI)

15

Federica Schirru, Stefano Guerriero, and Luca Saba

15.1 Introduction

Endometriosis is a chronic, oestrogen-dependent inflammatory disease affecting approximately 5–10% of women of reproductive age [1–12]. Radiology plays a key role in the diagnostic process in evaluating staging of the disease and in the accurate preoperative planning [13–19]. Sonography (two-dimensional and three-dimensional US) is the first-line approach for the evaluation of endometriosis but has suboptimal results in detecting extrapelvic implants and has a reduced sensitivity for endometrial plaques. On the other hand, MRI allows for highly accurate assessment of pelvic and extrapelvic lesions, deep endometriosis and adhesions, thus taking a central role in diagnosis and staging, suggesting a proper surgical treatment [7].

Taking into account the wide variety of clinical manifestations, the multifocal distribution of lesions, the involvement of gynaecological and non-gynaecological sites and the difficulties in diagnosis as well in the planning of surgical treatment, endometriosis is considered an extremely complex pathology.

F. Schirru · L. Saba (✉)
Department of Radiology, University of Cagliari, Policlinico Universitario Duilio Casula, Monserrato, Cagliari, Italy
e-mail: lucasaba@tiscali.it

S. Guerriero
Department of Obstetrics and Gynecology, University of Cagliari, Policlinico Universitario Duilio Casula, Monserrato, Cagliari, Italy
e-mail: gineca.sguerriero@tiscali.it

15.2 How We Do It

15.2.1 Imaging of Endometriosis: General Concepts

An early diagnosis of endometriosis is necessary for a proper management of the disease and an adequate planning of the surgical treatment which should be as conservative as possible in order to preserve the reproductive capacity of patients [20]. There are several imaging techniques that allow to identify and characterize [21–27] with high sensitivity and specificity the disease, in particular ultrasonography and magnetic resonance imaging. However, in many cases, imaging diagnosis remains challenging.

As already described in the previous chapters, ultrasonography (US) undoubtedly represents the first-line approach in the study of endometriosis by means of its high sensitivity and specificity as well as its low cost. However, it has limitations regarding the field of view, which is inadequate to evaluate any extrapelvic endometrial implant and the dependence by operator ability [22]. Therefore, when US is not sufficient to make a conclusive diagnosis or to banish any doubt, other imaging methods are performed.

MRI is usually performed in the most difficult cases and for an optimal presurgery planning. It is considered an excellent technique for diagnosing and assessing endometriosis according to its high spatial resolution, high space/contrast

S. Guerriero et al. (eds.), *How to Perform Ultrasonography in Endometriosis*,
https://doi.org/10.1007/978-3-319-71138-6_15

resolution, a wide field of view and an excellent tissue characterization. Moreover, it allows both to detect endometrial implants hidden by adhesions and to recognize lesions located in an extrapelvic site. In addition, MRI, also with the use of contrast material, permits to distinguish deep pelvic endometriosis from other pelvic inflammatory conditions or to solve differential diagnosis problems, for instance, between benign and malignant ovarian masses or with other malignancies of the pelvic organs [7, 8, 23–25]. In literature, there is no general agreement on the use of US rather than MRI. In general, papers published by gynaecologists support US diagnostic superiority, while those published by radiologists emphasize the value of MRI [22]. However, the most recent meta-analyses have shown that additional examinations, especially MRI, are recommended in symptomatic patients with negative US findings [22, 26]. Moreover, MRI is also suggested as a second-line approach in preoperative workup of deep pelvic endometriosis in patients with unclear US [22]. The value of MRI can further grow and improve by means of an intense collaboration between radiologists and gynaecologists.

The Computed Tomography (CT) has a marginal role in the assessment of endometriosis because it lacks both sensitivity and specificity, and often findings are nonspecific and nondiagnostic. However, CT might be useful in evaluating any complications of endometriosis, such as intestinal obstruction, hydronephrosis consequent to ureteral compression, hemoperitoneum and acute abdomen secondary to the rupture of an endometrioma [27].

15.2.2 Magnetic Resonance Imaging Technique

Recently (in December 2016), the European Society of Urogenital Radiology (ESUR) has published guidelines for optimal MRI protocols and imaging interpretation in endometriosis. These are based on a careful and detailed review of the most recent literature and on the consensus opinion between experts from the Female Pelvic Imaging working group of the European Society of Urogenital Radiology (EPI-ESUR). Recommendations have been proposed in guidelines for indication for MRI, technical requirements, patient preparation and MRI acquisition protocols [22].

15.2.2.1 Indications for MRI in Endometriosis

In the literature, there is no common agreement on the use of US rather than MRI, and there are no publications for executing MRI in pelvic endometriosis. Common indications for pelvic MRI are evaluation of pelvic pain and infertility or assessment of adnexal mass; however, in many ESUR centres, the most frequent reason that leads to MRI is the staging of deep pelvic endometriosis (90% of cases). Therefore, considering the most recent meta-analyses (as mentioned in the previous paragraph), guidelines suggest that [22]:

- MRI should be considered the second-line approach in evaluation of pelvic endometriosis, especially in symptomatic patients with negative US findings.
- MRI is recommended before surgery for preoperative workup of pelvic endometriosis.

15.2.2.2 Technical Requirements

1.5-T or 3.0-T System and Array Type

Guidelines do not provide any recommendations regarding the use of 1.5-T magnet rather than 3.0-T magnet; both are considered valid for studying endometriosis, but there are no sufficient comparing studies in literature [22]. The increased spatial resolution, due to the improved signal-to-noise ratio of 3.0-T MRI versus 1.5-T, allows to identify smaller lesions of DPE and surface implants by showing adhesions and peritoneal irregularities [28–30]. However, due to the increased image heterogeneity at 3.0-T system, negative effects on fat-saturation techniques (which are very useful in the imaging study of the disease) may occur [29, 31]. Therefore, more comparative studies are needed for a more accurate evaluation of the two systems and for choosing what is the better one in the assessment of endometriosis.

Both with 1.5-T magnet and with 3.0-T, pelvic phased-array coils are recommended by guidelines for DPE evaluation [22]. These assure a high signal-to-noise ratio, high spatial resolution with anatomical detail accuracy and improved tissue characterization. For such reasons, pelvic phased-array coils should be used for the study of pelvis. Although some authors have described a higher diagnostic accuracy of endoluminal coils in evaluating the invasion and the infiltration depth within the rectal wall or bladder, their use seems limited by the small field of view and the pain related to their positioning. Moreover, the use of the endovaginal coil prevents endoluminal filling with ultrasound gel, which is a useful tool for improving the visualization of the vagina and rectal wall [32].

Timing of MRI Examination

The timing of MRI examination is controversial and, in fact, there is not a common agreement. Some authors have argued that there is no greater diagnostic accuracy of MRI performed during the menstrual cycle since the signal or the size of endometriosis nodules do not significantly change with menses [27]. In a recent paper, Menni et al. have suggested that MRI should be performed in the first 12 days after the beginning of patient's last menstrual period. In fact, during this phase, endometrial haemorrhagic foci are best detected because of the maximum hyperintense signal of blood products in the T1-weighted images [7]. In conclusion, guidelines do not recommend a specific timing, related to the menstrual cycle, of MRI examination in the evaluation of DPE [22].

Patient Preparation: Fasting, Bowel Preparation, and Bladder Emptying

Adequate patient preparation is necessary to obtain high-quality images, and, despite this, no general consensus is found on patient preparation before MRI examination. The MRI protocol should be chosen and tailored according to the principal indication, and it will be different depending on whether endometriosis or an anterior mass have to be evaluated.

Fasting before the onset of MRI is recommended by guidelines, but its length is variable (3, 4 or 6 h) [22]. It is useful in order to reduce intestinal peristalsis.

Bowel preparation is advocated as "best practice" for the detection of DPE. Several studies suggest an intestinal preparation that involves the use of oral laxatives on the day before the examination or a bowel enema with water. In addition, it is recommended that patients undergo a dietary preparation with a low-residue regimen on the day before and the day of examination [22, 33].

There is a common agreement on the importance of an adequate bladder distension in order to achieve a precise detection of endometrial implants. A moderately filled or full bladder allows to modify the angle of uterine anteversion; in this manner, the visualization of pelvic anatomical structures is improved with a consequent better detection of small endometrial implants sited in the vesicouterine pouch or anterior to it. Another advantage of having a moderately full bladder is the reduction of motion artefacts (due to the intestinal peristalsis) because the sigma and the adjacent small intestine loops are displaced superiorly. For all these reasons, a moderately full bladder is recommended in the evaluation of DPE, and, in general, patients are instructed to not empty the bladder 1 h before the examination [22]. In contrast, an empty or overfilled bladder might compromise the evaluation of anatomic structures, resulting in a worst detection of lesions. In addition, the overfilled bladder may be the cause of motion artefacts due to the activity of the detrusor muscle [8, 24, 34].

Patient Position

MRI should be performed with the patient in the supine position; however, the prone position may be considered an option in claustrophobic patients in order to reduce stress, anxiety and distress [22].

Antiperistaltic Agent

Antispasmodic agents (e.g. hyoscine-*N*-butylbromide, glucagon) are recommended in the evaluation of DPE, as they reduce motion artefacts caused by bowel and uterine peristalsis [22, 32].

Vaginal and Rectal Opacification

There is some discrepancy in the literature regarding the improvement of diagnostic accuracy and image interpretation obtained through the vaginal or rectal opacification. Filling the vaginal or the rectum cavity with sterile ultrasound gel or with water has the aim to distend these cavities; this improves the visualization and differentiation of the various anatomical structures that are close to each other [32]. Besides, the patient's discomfort and the onset of motion artefacts for rectosigmoid colon spasm limit the clinical practice of rectal opacification [35]. So, both vaginal and rectal opacification are considered an option in the evaluation of deep endometriosis [22].

15.2.2.3 MRI Protocol

There is a large variability concerning the protocols used for the study of endometriosis. However, guidelines recommend the use of 2D-T2-weighted sequences in three planes (axial, sagittal and oblique), T1-weighted sequences with and without fat suppression and half-Fourier single shot turbo-spin-echo acquisition. No recommendations are provided regarding the use of diffusion-weighted imaging and susceptibility-weighted imaging [22].

T2-weighted sequences are considered the best sequences for detecting pelvic endometriosis as they are able to provide accurate assessment of both localization and extension of the implants, as well as their relationships with the surrounding structures. Sequences should be acquired on the axial (from Renal hila to the pubic bone), coronal and oblique planes [32, 36]. The coronal oblique images (perpendicular to the long axis of the uterine corpus) improve the evaluation of possible adenomiosis, implants within the lower sigma or the upper third rectal wall and adhesions between all these structures and the uterus. Instead, the axial oblique images (perpendicular to the long axis of the cervical canal or along the uterosacral ligaments) improve the evaluation of uterosacral ligament implants and the parametric involvement [32, 37, 38].

T1-weighted sequences with and without fat suppression are considered the "gold standard" sequences in diagnosis of endometrioma, allowing to differentiate it from haemorrhagic cysts or fatty content cysts [39, 40]. They are useful for the evaluation of the signal of normal anatomical structures and the characterization of uterine and ovary lesions. In particular, the suppression of fat signal permits to better highlight the hyperintense signal of haemorrhagic foci of endometrial lesions, even if small [7].

Half-Fourier acquisition single shot turbo-spin-echo acquisition (HASTE; also known as single-shot fast-spin echo (SSFSE)) is recommended for the evaluation of uterine peristalsis; in fact, it has been observed that in patients with endometriosis, uterine peristalsis is reduced during the periovulatory phase, thus favouring infertility [39–41]. Moreover, these sequences provide kinematic images that also allow to detect pelvic adhesions [42].

Due to its ability to characterize tissues and cellularity, *diffusion-weighted imaging (DWI)* with quantitative assessment of the diffusion coefficient (ADC) plays an important role in MR imaging, especially in the field of pelvic oncology [43]. However, there are no sufficient studies to determine the diagnostic accuracy of DWI in evaluating endometriosis and its utility in differentiating benign lesions from malignant ones. Balaban et al. has demonstrated that endometrioma has lower ADC values, at all b values, compared with those of haemorrhagic ovarian cysts [44]. Diffusion tensor imaging (DTI) is a particular application of DWI which could be useful in evaluating patients with endometriosis and suspected involvement of the sacral nerve roots [45].

Susceptibility-weighted imaging (SWI) are able to detect small amounts of haemorrhage and blood products which distort the local magnetic field and may be less visible on other MRI sequences. According to this, SWI is sensitive in the diagnosis of extraovarian endometriosis, in particular abdominal wall endometriosis [46, 47].

The Use of Intravenous Contrast-Enhanced MRI

In general, the use of contrast medium is often reserved for specific cases and therefore depends on the indication to MRI examination. The presence of mural nodules in an endometrioma is the main indication because of the strong suspect of malignant transformation. It can also be useful to distinguish an endometrioma from a lutean ovarian cyst or a tubo-ovarian abscess or to distinguish endometriosis from pelvic inflammatory disease [23, 48].

15.2.3 MR Imaging Features of Endometriosis

Endometriosis has three different clinical patterns of manifestation, which can occur alone or coexist:

- Ovarian endometrioma
- Peritoneal endometriosis (with or without adhesions)
- Deep endometriosis

15.2.4 Ovarian Endometrioma

Endometrioma is described as an ovarian peculiar pseudocyst lined by functioning endometrial-like tissue composed of a highly vascularized stroma and a surface epithelium. Its content is a dense dark fluid, consisting of high concentrations of degenerated blood products accumulated over successive menstrual cycles. Because of this aspect, endometrioma is also called "chocolate cysts". In case of larger endometriomas, it could be possible to observe clots, thin septa, "haematocrit effect", fluid levels or peripheral nodules (due to clots) [27, 33, 49].

Endometriomas can be either single or multiple, bilateral (in more than 50% of cases), unilocular or multilocular. In case of inter-ovarian adhesions, a particular condition called "kissing ovaries" can be observed [50, 51].

15.2.4.1 MRI Findings

Since endometrioma may contain variable amounts of blood breakdown products, proteins and fluids, its appearance on MR imaging can be variable [52].

Usually, it appears as a cystic mass with a homogeneous hyperintense signal on T1-weighted images ("lightbulb-like" brightness), which is due to the high concentrations of paramagnetic haemoglobin in blood degradation products. On T2-weighted images, the lesion is characterized by intermediate-to-low signal. A typical feature of endometrioma is the "T2-shading" sign, which consists of a low signal (T2 shortening) affecting variable portions of the cyst (small portions or the entire cyst). In particular, the phenomenon ranges from a homogeneous complete absence of signal to different gradations of decreased signal intensity on T2-weighted sequences [53–55]. The dependence of signal intensity to the high concentration of protein and iron within the cyst, due to recurrent haemorrhages, reflects the chronic nature of endometrioma. It is important to highlight that any signal loss on T2-weighted images is highly specific for endometrioma, regardless of the degree of signal loss [21].

Recently, Corwin et al. have describe an MRI finding called "T2 dark spots", found in some cases of haemorrhagic cystic ovarian lesions. "T2 dark spots" are defined as markedly hypointense foci within the cyst on T2-weighted images with or without T2 shading. They may be located within the cyst, often against the cyst wall, but not within the cyst wall itself [56].

Another important feature is the presence of multiple endometriotic cysts. This seems related to the fact that cysts undergo repeated rupture because of the hormonal stimulation resulting in internal bleeding. The bilateralism and multiplicity of hyperintense on T1-weighted adnexal cysts can be considered a valid diagnostic criterion to distinguish the endometrioma from other haemorrhagic lesions, even greater specificity than the T1 signal hyperintensity alone [49, 57].

Chemical-selective T1-weighted fat-saturated sequences are very useful for the diagnosis of endometriosis. In fact, the saturation of the fat improves the contrast resolution among non-fat-containing T1-hyperintense structures, making possible to detect even very small endometriomas. Moreover, the loss of fat signal is advantageous in characterization of T1-hyperintense adnexal lesions, allowing, for instance, the differentiation between endometrioma and mature cystic teratoma [53, 55]. It should also be emphasized that chemical-selective T1-weighted fat-saturated sequences are preferred to short-tau inversion recovery (STIR) sequences because, in the latter, signal loss is not a finding specific for fat. Indeed, both haemorrhagic cysts and endometriomas may have a relaxation time similar to those of fat, thus mimicking a mature cystic teratoma [20, 57] (Fig. 15.1).

The use of contrast medium is reserved for specific cases, firstly in the suspicious of malignant transformation of endometrioma. In general, on post-contrast sequences, the peripheral low signal intensity rim (the thick fibrous wall of the cyst) may show intense contrast enhancement [49].

On DWI imaging, most part of endometrioma shows restricted diffusion and low ADC values, but this finding is not specific. In fact, both benign endometrioma and haemorrhagic ovarian cysts, as well as endometrial implants or benign mature

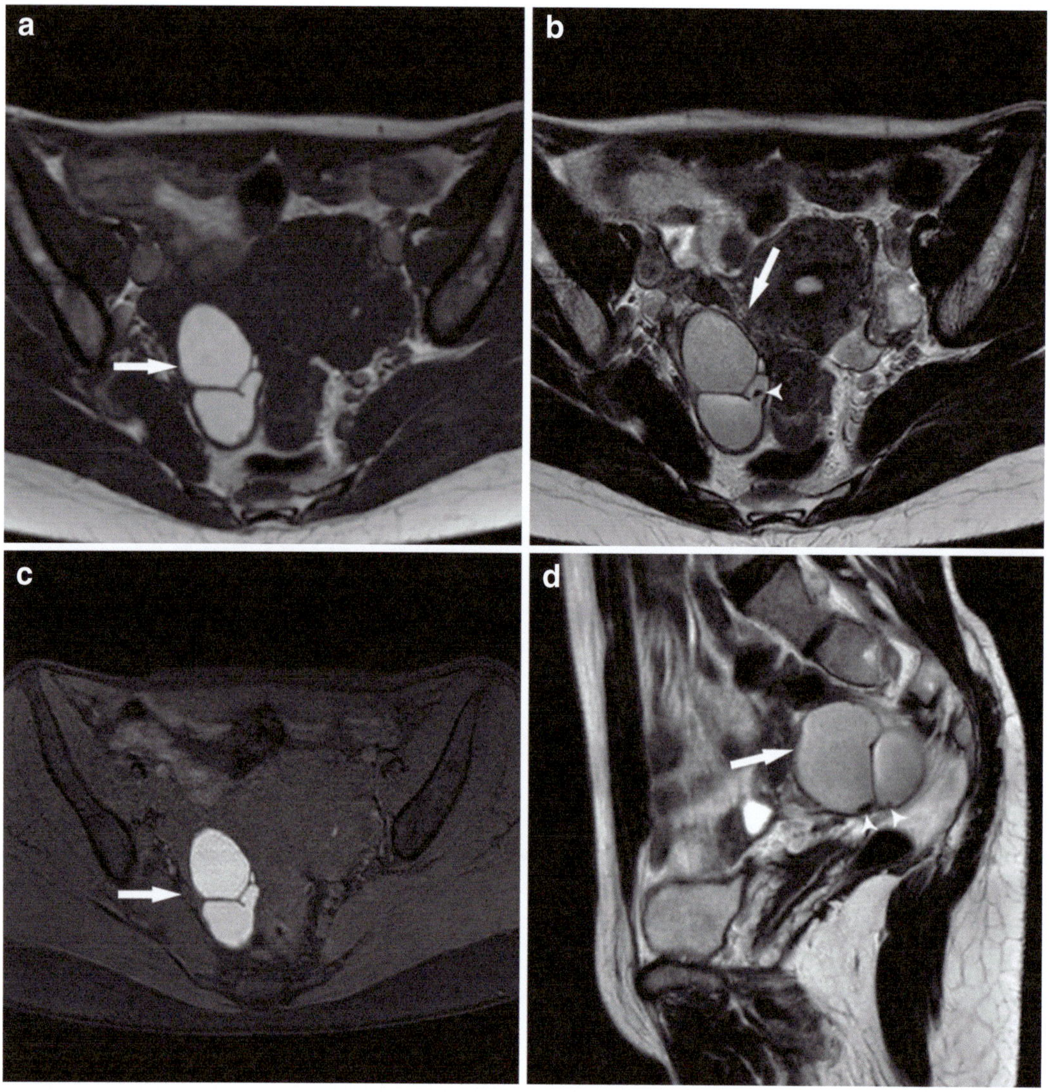

Fig. 15.1 *Endometriomas* in a 44-year-old woman with chronic pelvic pain and infertility. Axial T1-weighted (**a**), axial T2-weighted (**b**), axial T1-weighted with fat suppression (**c**) and sagittal T2-weighted MR images show in the right adnexa the presence endometriomas characterized by high signal in both T1-weighted sequences, with and without fat suppression, and T2-shading sign. Some low signal spot (arrowheads) are visible inside the cysts that correspond to chronic retracted blood clots containing a high concentration of protein and/or hemosiderin ("dark spot sign")

cystic teratomas, showed restricted diffusion [56]. However, as already mentioned in the previous paragraphs, Balaban et al. has demonstrated that endometrioma has lower ADC values, at all b values, compared with those of haemorrhagic ovarian cysts. Therefore, further studies are needed to clarify the role of DWI in evaluating these lesions.

In conclusion, the MR imaging criteria for the diagnosis of endometrioma are [20]:

- Multiple adnexal cysts with hyperintense signal on T1-weighted images
- One or more adnexal cysts with hyperintense signal on T1-weighted images and "shading sign" on T2-weighted images

Using these criteria, it has been demonstrated that MR imaging reaches a diagnostic accuracy of 91–96%, a sensitivity of 90–92% and a specificity of 91–98% in the diagnosis of endometrioma [53, 54, 57–59].

Routine follow-up is very important for endometriomas because of risk for many complications, in particular rupture.

15.2.4.2 Complications of Endometrioma

Usually, complications may occur in about 50% of patients with one or more endometriomas. The most frequent are:

Reduced Fertility: this complication involves about 30–50% of women affected by endometriosis. Many studies have reported a poorer pregnancy outcome in affected women probably due to the presence of adhesions involving the ovaries and the fallopian tubes, as well as anomalies of the endocrine and immune systems [27, 60].

Adhesions: extremely frequent. Adhesions appear as low signal stranding on both T1-weighted and T2-weighted images that mask organ interfaces; they could cause distortion of the normal pelvic anatomy. A characteristic diagnostic sign is the "kissing ovaries" characterized by the closing up of ovaries resulting in interovarian adhesions [20, 50, 51].

Acute Abdomen: this medical emergency is an uncommon complication of endometrioma. The rupture of endometriotic cyst, even very small in size, could lead to a hemoperitoneum with acute abdomen [27, 61].

Ovarian Torsion: uncommon. It represents a gynaecological emergency requiring urgent surgical treatment to prevent ovarian necrosis. In general, findings include an endometrioma within an enlarged oedematous ovary with multiple follicles located peripherally [14]. Twisting of the ovarian pedicle is the most specific feature of ovarian torsion, but it can be very difficult to detect.

Malignant Transformation: it represents a very rare complication, occurring in less than 1% of patients with the disease [62, 63]. MRI findings suspecting malignant degeneration include [49]:

- Presence of enhanced mural nodules (well detected on contrast-enhanced subtracted images)
- Loss of typical "T2-shading" sign on T2-weighted images
- Presence of mural nodule of more than 30 mm in size
- An interval increase in the size of the cyst

Enhanced mural nodules are the most sensitive feature on MR imaging of malignancies; others, however, are useful in suspecting neoplastic transformation but less reliable. It is important to evaluate the enhanced mural nodules with contrast-enhanced dynamic subtraction images since the haemorrhagic content of cysts (which is also hyperintense on T1-weighted images) may mask the enhancement of small nodules. Therefore, to better visualize areas of enhancement, it is mandatory to use contrast-enhanced subtracted images [20]. However, enhanced mural nodules represent a sensitive (97%) but not a specific (56%) feature for the diagnosis of endometrioma-associated cancer. In fact, a whole range of benign conditions (such as polypoid endometriosis, intracystic blood clots or decidualized endometriosis of pregnancy) should be considered in the differential diagnosis [27].

The loss of "T2-shading" sign seems to be due to tumour secretions that dilute blood degradation products [63, 64]. Cystic components appear hyperintense on both T1-weighted and T2-weighted images.

15.2.4.3 Differential Diagnosis

Typically, endometrioma appears as a cystic adnexal mass with hyperintensity signal on T1-weighted images with and without fat suppression, T2-shading sign, restricted diffusion (the most part of cases) and, on post-contrast sequences, an intense enhanced wall. However, some of these aspects may occur in other different adnexal cystic masses, with a consequent overlapping appearance. For instance, endometriomas are most commonly misdiagnosed as dermoid or haemorrhagic cysts. Hence, a whole range of differential diagnosis should be considered in order to make a correct evaluation.

General imaging differential considerations include:

Haemorrhagic cyst: it represents the most frequent and complex differential diagnosis of endometrioma. MRI findings depend on the age of haemorrhage. The haemorrhagic cyst is usually a solitary unilocular adnexal mass, lined by a thin wall. Like endometrioma, it appears hyperintense on T1-weighted sequences with and without fat suppression or shows a peripheral halo of signal hyperintensity on T1-weighted images. More frequently, it does not show the characteristic T2-shading sign, because there are not recurrent bleedings so that the viscosity and concentration of contents remain low; however sometimes the T2-shading sign can be present. The walls of the cyst do not show enhancement on post-contrast images.

Dermoid cysts and mature cystic ovarian teratomas: together with the haemorrhagic cysts, these lesions are one of the most frequent differential diagnoses of endometrioma. As fat-containing lesions, they appear hyperintense on T1-weighted images mimicking an endometrioma. They can be differentiated by chemical-selective T1-weighted fat-saturated sequences in which the loss of signal occurs only in these lesions and not in the endometrioma, because of the chemical shift artefact [49].

Multiple corpora lutea: this differential diagnosis must be considered in women who have been subjected to assisted conception treatments. After hormonal stimulation that induces ovulation, multiple corpora lutea frequently occur. In these cases, each corpus luteum cyst appears similar to endometrioma, but the patient's medical history of a recent oocyte retrieval helps in the diagnosis [33].

Tubo-ovarian abscess: it represents one of the late complications of pelvic inflammatory disease (PID). It consists of a pelvic inflammatory mass within both the ovary and the fallopian tube are not separately distinguished. Typically, the pelvic mass shows a thin wall and a fluid content that shows hypointense signal on T1-weighted images and heterogeneous or hyperintense signal on T2-weighted images.

Mucinous lesions and ovarian carcinoma: the most important ovarian mucinous masses to be considered in differential diagnosis are ovarian mucinous cystadenoma, ovarian borderline mucinous tumour and ovarian mucinous cystadenocarcinoma. In general, the degree of hyperintensity on T1-weighted images varies depending on the concentration of mucin; however, the signal intensity is still lower than that of fat or blood. In general, endometrioma has to be differentiated from almost all ovarian neoplasms.

Decidualized endometriosis in pregnant woman: it is a benign condition associated with ectopic endometrial tissue that undergone a decidual reaction during pregnancy. It may mimic an ovarian cancer in pregnancy. These benign nodules show the same signal intensity of the normal decidualized endometrium on T2-weighted images. In addition, in the postpartum or at the termination of a pregnancy, decidualized endometriosis resolve or regress to uncomplicated endometriomas [56].

15.2.5 Peritoneal Endometriosis (with or Without Adhesions)

Peritoneal endometriosis is characterized by the presence of endometrial implants on the surface of the pelvic peritoneum.

Small implants develop on the peritoneal surface and on the serosa of any abdominal and pelvic organ. In general, on MR imaging they appear as small solid masses or soft tissue thickening with irregular or stellate margins. Lesions show a low-to-intermediate signal on both T1-weighted and T2-weighted images; sometimes, they may have punctate areas of high signal on T1-weighted images with fat suppression which represent haemorrhagic foci [7]. A low signal stranding on both T1-weighted and T2-weighted images is the typical appearance of adhesions on MR imaging. Adhesions can occur between different pelvic structures, masking interfaces among them and causing, in the most advanced cases, distortion of the normal pelvic anatomy.

Unfortunately, the identification of these small peritoneal endometriosis lesions is very complex for both MRI and US. However, the presence of adhesions can be suspected in MRI by using *half-Fourier single shot turbo-spin-echo acquisition (HASTE)* sequences. As already mentioned, these sequences allow to evaluate the uterine peristalsis and the limited or absent motility between the pelvic organs.

15.2.6 Deep endometriosis

Deep endometriosis (DE), also known as deep pelvic endometriosis, is defined by the presence of endometrial implants infiltrating deeper at least 5 mm into the peritoneal surface, into the retroperitoneum or into the wall of other pelvic organs. It may occur in different fibromuscular pelvic structures, such as [8]:

- Rectovaginal septum and uterosacral ligaments (69.2%)
- Vagina (14.5%)
- Gastrointestinal tract (9.9%): usually rectosigmoid, small bowel, colon and appendix
- Urinary tract (6.4%): bladder and ureters, rarely urethra

DE is strongly associated with severe and debilitating symptoms, such as chronic pelvic pain, dyspareunia, dysmenorrhea and infertility. Of course, symptoms depend on the anatomical site affected by the disease. In case of rectosigmoid involvement, the symptomatology may consist of chronic deep pelvic pain (synchronized with menses) diarrhoea, constipation, abdominal bloating and even ascites; if the lesion infiltrates through the mucosa, rectal bleeding may also occur. In case of urinary tract involvement, DE can present with haematuria, dysuria, urgency or stress urinary incontinence and urinary tract infections [65, 66]. Often, however, symptoms are nonspecific, and this results in a delay in diagnosis, which obviously involves the need for more invasive surgical treatment.

When implants are composed of only endometrial stroma (without glands), the disease is known as “stromal endometriosis” [8, 14, 67]. The knowledge of histological aspects of endometriotic implants in DE is crucial, because it allows to better understand their appearance on MR imaging. In addition, as currently the standard treatment of DE is a complete excision of endometriotic implants, a proper MR imaging evaluation is needed to accurately understand the sites affected by the disease, the extent of implants and their degree of infiltration.

15.2.6.1 MRI Findings

Deep endometriotic implants have a characteristic infiltrative pattern of organ involvement on cross-sectional imaging. According to the presence of fibrotic tissue and hypertrophied smooth muscular cells, DE lesions appear as soft tissue thickening or solid irregular masses with low signal on T2-weighted sequences and intermediate signal on T1-weighted sequences. Nodules might have variable size and regular, irregular or indistinct margins; more often they show stellated margins due to the abundant fibrosis. Because of their typical low signal on T2 images, these solid masses are very difficult to detect and can be overlooked, as they are sited in close proximity to other pelvic structures that are normally hypointense on T2-weighted sequence. Unlike ovarian endometrioma, haemorrhagic foci within these lesions are rarely visible; if present, they appear as small areas of high signal on T1-weighted sequences (with and without fat suppression) within the nodules. Obviously, their signal intensity depends on the age of haematic content [34, 56]. Another uncommon feature is the presence of focal areas of increased T2 signal within the solid masses, which represent dilated endometrial glands [34, 56]. The appearance of lesions after administration of the contrast material, on enhanced sequences, is very variable; enhancement depends on how much inflammatory reaction and glandular and fibrous tissue there is in the lesion. So, the post-contrast appearance is neither specific nor sensitive for the diagnosis of DE [34, 56].

15.2.6.2 Anatomical Locations of Deep endometriosis

Many authors have subdivided the pelvis into three different compartments depending on the clinical and functional requirements: anterior, middle and posterior [68]. In the next paragraphs, we will analyse the common anatomical locations of solid nodules, considering the pelvic compartments classification used by Coutinho et al.

15.2.6.3 Anterior Compartment

The anterior compartment contains the urinary bladder and urethra. Furthermore, the terminal part of ureters is considered in this site. The bladder is separated from the vagina and the uterus through fat planes known as vesicovaginal septum and prevesical space. The vesicouterine pouch, or anterior cul-de-sac, is a peritoneum fold that lies between the bladder (anterior) and the uterus (posterior). The vesicouterine pouch is the most frequently affected site by endometriosis [68]. Implants into the vesicovaginal septum, bladder and ureters are less common.

An involvement of other pelvic structures has been reported in 50–75% of cases of urinary tract endometriosis involvement. Moreover, these patients have also a more advanced stage of disease than women without urinary tract involvement [69–71].

Lesions of the anterior cul-de-sac appear as nodules that adhere to the anterior uterine surface, with low signal intensity on T2-weighted sequences. Because of the tight adherence to the peritoneum of the bladder fold and the uterus, these lesions are associated to obliteration of the vesicouterine pouch and to anteflexion of the uterus [34] (Fig. 15.2 a, b).

Deep endometriosis that involves the vesicovaginal septum appears as a cystic lesion, with the same characteristics of an endometrioma [34].

MRI is considered the reference standard in urinary tract endometriosis diagnosis. According to some papers, if examination is performed on 3-T MRI system, the sensitivity reaches 88%, and specificity is higher than 98% [29, 33, 69, 72]. Recently, authors have compared three-dimensional colour Doppler US with MRI and cystoscopy in the diagnosis of bladder endometriosis; they have showed that US seems to be superior to cystoscopy and is at least as effective as MRI in diagnosing and planning the surgery for bladder endometriosis [73].

The urinary bladder is involved in about 0.3–12% of women with pelvic endometriosis, and the bladder is the most common affected site of the urinary system (80%) [74]. Bladder involvement may be extrinsic or intrinsic. Extrinsic involvement is more common and often asymptomatic; lesions are sited on the serosal surface. Usually lesions involve the posterior wall [34]. On MR examination, nodules appear as localized or diffuse thickening of the wall bladder, with low signal on T2-weighted sequences, which replace the normal signal of detrusor muscle. Sometimes it is possible to identify small foci with variable signal on T1 and high signal on T2-weighted sequences representing dilated endometrial glands. On contrast-enhanced sequences, there is a greater enhancement of lesions than normal detrusor muscle [75] (Fig. 15.2 c, d).

Endometriosis of the ureter is the second most common manifestation of urinary tract endometriosis. In extrinsic form, endometrial tissue invades only the outer layer of the ureter (the adventitia) and surrounding connective tissue, sometimes leading to obstruction of the ureter; lesions originate from adjacent disease of the ovary, broad ligaments or other uterosacral ligaments. Both forms may manifest with obstructive symptoms; cyclic haematuria is typical of the latter form [74]. On MRI examination, lesions appear as irregular nodules with low signal on T2-weighted sequences. Loss of the fat plane

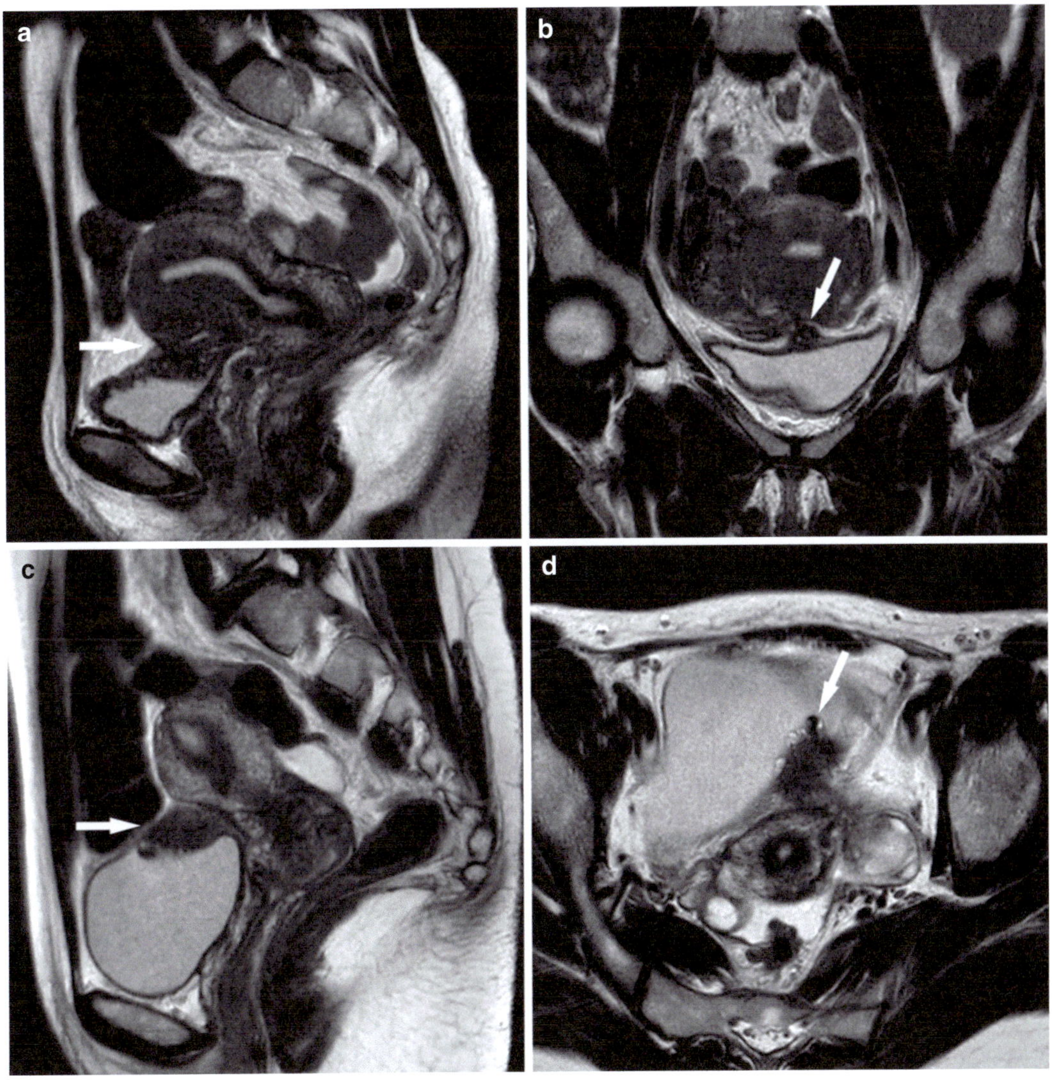

Fig. 15.2 *Anterior compartment.* (**a**, **b**) Endometriosis of the vesicouterine pouch in a 34-year-old woman with pelvic pain. Sagittal T2-weighted (**a**) and coronal T2-weighted (**b**) MR images show irregular hypointense nodular lesion that adheres to the anterior uterine surface and to the upper bladder wall surface. The lesion obliterates the vesicouterine recess. Anteflexion of the uterus is associated. (**c**, **d**) Endometriosis of the bladder in a 30-year-old woman with haematuria. Sagittal T2-weighted (**c**) and axial T2-weighted (**d**) MR images depict irregular focal thickening of the bladder wall, which contains small intermingled hyperintense foci that correspond to the dilated endometrial glands. The deep infiltrating endometriotic lesion does not adhere to the anterior uterine surface

between the ureter and nodule is highly suspicious of extrinsic involvement. Retractile adhesions may be present and appear as periureteral hypointense lines arranged in confluent angles [76]. If the nodule is obstructive, dilatation of the ureteral portion cranial to the lesion can be studied with MRI urography. Unfortunately, both MRI and other imaging techniques (US, Uro-CT, intravenous pyelogram, urography) have limited value in providing accurate information about the extent of the disease and the degree of tissue infiltration. Recently Sillou et al. demonstrated that MRI is more sensitive than surgery (91% vs. 82%) but less specific (59% vs. 67%) in diagnosing intrinsic involvement of ureteral endometriosis sites [74, 77].

15.2.6.4 Middle Compartment

The middle compartment of the pelvis includes the vagina, uterus, ovaries, fallopian tubes and uterine ligaments (broad ligaments and round ligaments). The broad ligaments are folds of peritoneum which reflect over the upper genital tract and connect the uterus and the lateral walls of the pelvis; they are part of the rectouterine and vesicouterine folds [68]. Every organ of this compartment may be involved by endometriosis.

Ovaries are the most frequently involved sites of the middle compartment. Endometriosis may manifest with one or more endometriotic cysts (endometrioma) or small implants which lead to scarring and adhesions with adjacent paraovarian structures [34] (Fig. 15.3 a, b).

Deep endometriosis of the uterus may appear as endometrial implants on the serosal surface, along with diffuse peritoneal enhancement on post-contrast T1-weighted sequence with fat suppression. Women with a retroflexed uterus are more likely to develop DE in the posterior compartment (while those with an anteflexed uterus are more likely to develop anterior compartment endometriosis) [34].

Concerning the fallopian tube, endometriosis is the main cause of peritubal adhesions in women of reproductive age. On MRI, it appears as a tortuous distension of the fallopian tube, filled with haemorrhagic fluid, with hyperintense signal in both T1- and T2-weighted sequences. Furthermore, it should be considered specific for pelvic endometriosis, and also it may be the only finding of the disease at MR imaging in some women [56, 78] (Fig. 15.3 c, d).

The involvement of uterine ligaments has a viable frequency, ranging from 0.3 to 14% for round ligaments. Round ligaments of the uterus (RLUs) course laterally from the uterus through the broad ligament, running along the pelvic sidewall and leaving the abdomen through the internal ring. They are divided into two portions: an intrapelvic and an extrapelvic (in the canal of Nuck). On MR images, normal RLUs appear as thin structures with low signal on both T1- and T2-weighted sequences. Several cases of endometriosis sited in the extrapelvic portion of RLUs are reported, while cases of intrapelvic localization are rarer. Endometriosis of round ligaments might manifest as thickening (usually more than 10 mm) or nodularity of these structures; RLUs may be shortened or irregular. Implant signal depends on the presence of stromal tissue, glands, haemorrhage or fibrosis. If lesions are made of fibrous tissue only, they show low signal on both T1- and T2-weighted images, while haemorrhagic foci are characterized by high signal on T1-weighted sequences with and without fat suppression. Moreover, if inflammatory reaction occurs, contrast enhancement is observed. According to Gui et al., the detection of free fluid around the RLUs on "anti-declive position" might be an indirect sign of endometriosis of the intrapelvic portion of the RLUs [79].

15.2.6.5 Posterior Compartment

The posterior compartments may be highly involved by deep endometriosis. It includes the rectovaginal septum, retrocervical area, posterior vaginal fornix, uterosacral ligaments, rectovaginal pouch (or posterior cul-de-sac or pouch of Douglas), the rectum and connective tissue that surrounds it. All these structures may be site of deep pelvic endometriosis. The rectal fascia represents the morphologic demarcation of this compartment; it appears as a thin structure with low signal that borders the perirectal compartment [34] (Fig. 15.4).

The rectovaginal is filled of fat and is visible on MRI; however, when interstitial fat is absent, the rectal and vaginal walls are not easily distinguishable. The use of rectal opacification with gel improves the visualization of this structure [54, 68]. Rectovaginal septum is rarely affected by DE. These lesions account only for 10% of retroperitoneal endometriotic lesions; they may involve the rectovaginal septum alone but frequently represent an extension from retrocervical or posterior vaginal implants. Nodules may be palpated at vaginal examination. On MR imaging, usually they appear as irregular hypointense solid masses, with low signal on T2-weighted sequences that fill the space between the walls of the two organs, retracting them. The most important thing to evaluate is whether the lesions have infiltrated the anterior rectal wall. The presence of a small

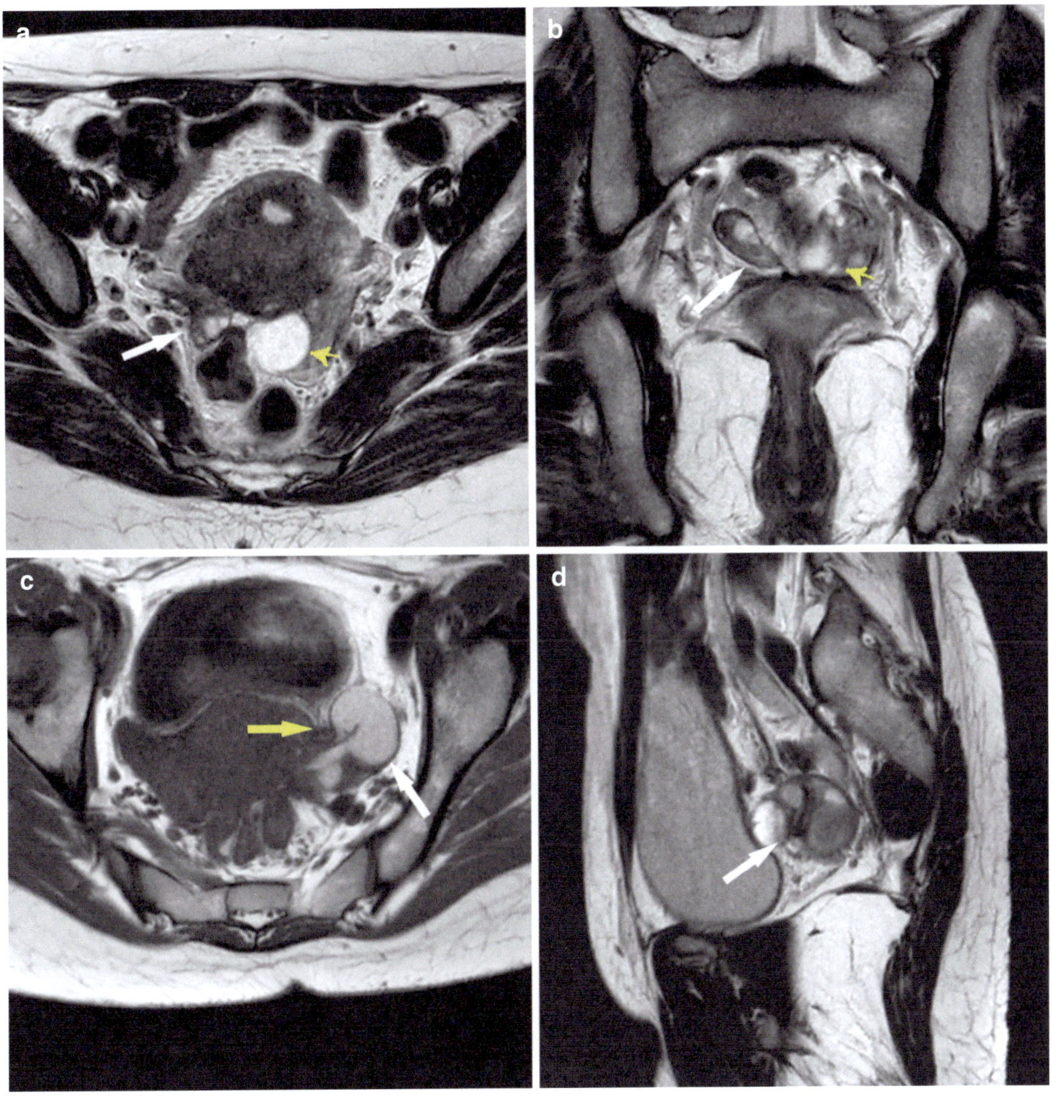

Fig. 15.3 *Adhesions*. (**a**, **b**) Endometriosis in a 37-year-old woman; axial T-weighted (**a**) and coronal T2-weighted (**b**) MR images show low signal stranding between the ovaries and between ovaries and uterus. The inter-ovarian adhesions cause the closing up of right adnexa (white arrow) and left adnexa (yellow arrow) with tethering to the uterus. (**c**, **d**) Haematosalpinx in a 36 year-old woman. Axial T1-weighted (**c**) and sagittal T2-weighted (**d**) MR images depict a tortuous distension of the left fallopian tube (white arrow) filled with haemorrhagic fluid, with high signal on T1-W sequences and low signal on T2-W. An implant is visible on the serosal surface of the fallopian tube (yellow arrow)

account of fluid in the rectovaginal pouch may facilitate the detection of peritoneal reaction. MR examination has an important role in the evaluation of these lesions because they are not readily accessible at endoscopic viewing [33].

The retrocervical area is a virtual region behind the cervix, above the rectovaginal septum, and it is commonly affected by DE. Implants often extent to the rectal wall posteriorly or to vaginal cuff inferiorly, in particular to vaginal fornices. The vaginal fornices are recesses into which the upper vagina is divided. These vault-like recesses (anterior, posterior and lateral fornices) are formed by the protrusion of the cervix into the vagina. The posterior fornix is the larger recess behind the cervix, close to the

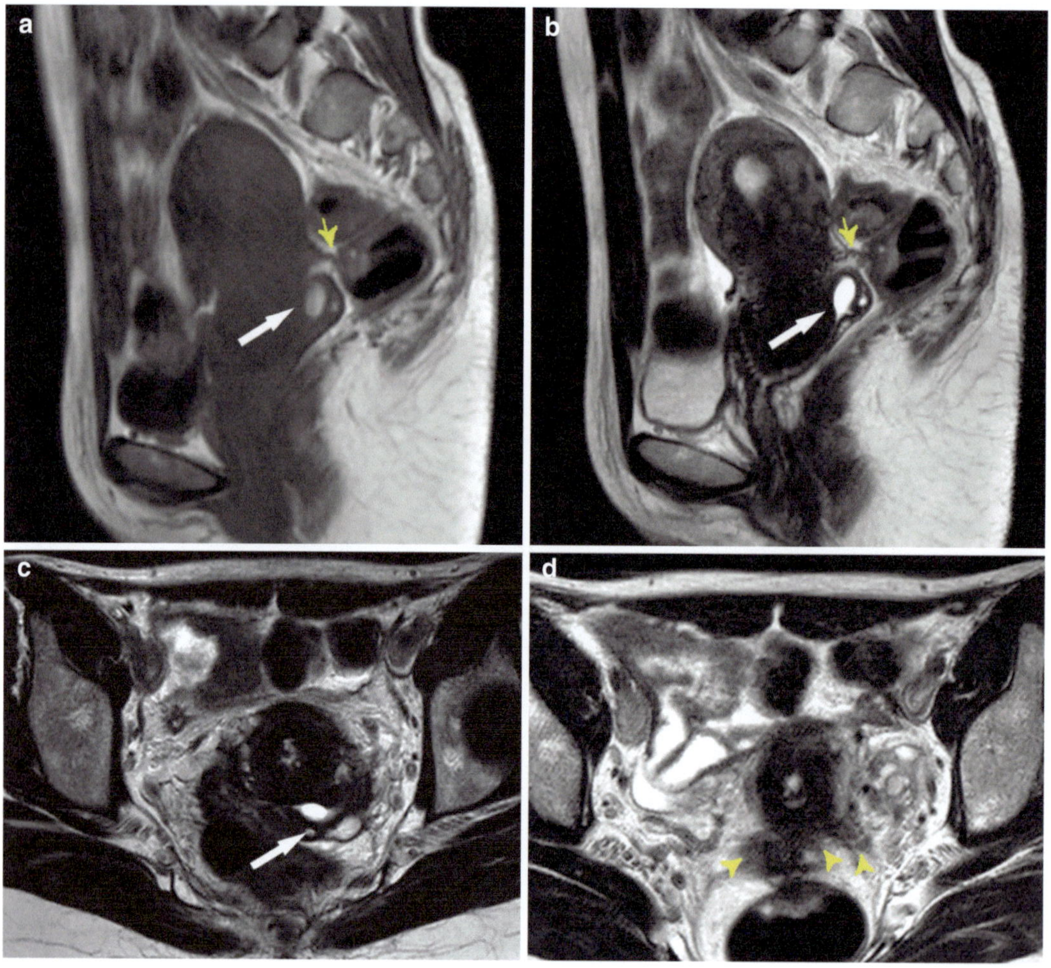

Fig. 15.4 *Posterior compartment* endometriosis in 45-year-old woman with a history of chronic pelvic pain and dyspareunia. Sagittal T1-weighted (**a**), sagittal T2-weighted (**b**) and axial T2-weighted MR images show a large solid nodular implant in the rectovaginal septum and retrocervical area (white arrow) with intermingled high signal foci due to bloody content. Sagittal T2-weighted images show low signal fibrotic thickening from the torus uterinus and lower uterine segment to the rectum (yellow arrow) associated to a solid nodular lesion sited in the anterior sigmoid wall. Involvement of the torus uterinus and of the USL is visible on axial T2-w images as a diffuse and irregular thickening within the ligaments (yellow arrowheads)

rectouterine pouch, more frequently involved by endometriosis [8, 33].

The rectouterine folds contain a considerable amount of nonstriated muscular fibres and fibrous tissue attached to the anterior surface of the sacrum; they form the uterosacral ligaments. Therefore, the uterosacral ligaments (USLs) are fibrous fascial band on each side of the uterus that passes along the lateral wall of the pelvis from the uterine cervix and the vaginal vault to the sacrum [54, 73]. The torus uterinus is anatomically defined as a transverse thickening that binds the insertion of USLs on the posterior wall of the cervix; usually it is visible only if it is thickened. When the torus uterinus is involved by endometriotic implants, they appear as a mass or thickening in the upper middle portion of the posterior cervix. Nodules may have regular or irregular margins. In many cases, the involvement may be unilateral. Often, associated findings might be uterine retroversion or angular rectal attraction, reflecting the fibrotic components [73].

USLs are considered the sites most frequently involved in deep endometriosis. Lesions may affect one or both of USLs; their proximal medial portion is the most commonly affected. On MR imaging, normal USLs appear as thin regular semi-circular structures with low signal. On the contrary, if they are involved by endometriosis, morphologic abnormalities may occur; they include diffuse or localized thickening and nodules with regular or irregular margin within the ligaments. Usually endometriotic implants show low signal on T2-weighted sequences; however, nodules can show cystic cavities with high signal on T2- and low signal on T1-weighted images or may have very small hyperintense foci on T1-weighted sequences, with and without fat suppression, due to haemorrhagic content. Considering their position and proximity to the rectum and vaginal walls, USLs lesions may extend to infiltrate these structures [33, 34]. Even in this case, rectal or vaginal opacification with sterile gel should allow a better detection of implants occurring in these structures.

The rectouterine pouch (called also posterior cul-de-sac or pouch of Douglas) represents the deepest point of the peritoneal cavity, sited between the bilateral rectouterine folds, behind the uterus and in front of the rectum. It extends till the middle third of the vagina in 93% of women [68]. The pouch of Douglas is another commonly involved site in DE. Sometimes solid infiltrative lesions of this region may be overlooked because of their extent and invasion of the posterior myometrium, mimicking adenomyosis [20]. Adenomyosis is a condition different, but closely related, to endometriosis. It represents a deep benign myometrial invasion of area of endometrial glands and stroma, with associated hyperplasia and hypertrophy of surrounding myometrium, that leads to uterine enlargement; it may form nodular lesions or be diffusely distributed [80]. DE implants appear as solid nodules of different size, with irregular margins that lead to a partial or complete obliteration of the rectouterine pouch, because of the strict adhesions. It is also possible to detect a lateralized fluid collection.

Finally, the rectosigmoid is the most common segment of bowel involved in endometriosis. It occurs in 12–37% of patients and is associated with severe DE in other pelvic structures (such as USLs, ovaries, vagina, bladder and pelvic sidewall) [81, 82]. Chapron et al. reported a high incidence of associated involvement of the ileocecal region: 12% of the lesions involve the ileum, 8% of the lesions involve the appendix and 6% of the lesion involves the cecum. Considering that the success of surgical treatment is related to the complete excision of endometriotic implants, MRI examination is fundamental to precisely assess the intestinal DE, in order to plan a proper surgical strategy [83]. DE intestinal implants have different morphological characteristics. They appear as nodular or plaque-like lesions. Plaque-like lesions have ill-defined margins and rectrative or infiltrative behaviour. Nodules are generally attached to the intestinal wall between the 10-o'clock and 2-o'clock position. They usually have a triangular shape with the base attached to the intestinal wall and the apex oriented towards the retrocervical region. Implants might be located on the serosal layer or infiltrate the deeper layers, causing thickening of the rectosigmoid colon wall with fibrosis. Nodules may be rectractile or nonretractile and may show regular or irregular margins with low signal on T2-weighted images [33, 83]. A specific finding of solid invasive endometriosis of the intestinal wall is the "mushroom cap" sign on T2-weighted images. The low- signal-intensity base of the mushroom represents the hypertrophy and fibrosis of the muscularis propria, while the high-signal-intensity cap is attributed to the mucosa and submucosa, displaced into the lumen [56] (Fig. 15.5). Further suspicious signs of DE intestinal involvement are the disappearance of the fat tissue plane between the uterus and the anterior rectosigmoid wall, the loss of the hypointense signal of the anterior intestinal wall on the T2-weighted images and the presence of a tissue mass extending on the anterior rectosigmoid colon wall showing contrast enhancement on T1-weighted images. Contrast enhancement is variable and depends on the degree of inflammation; moreover, inflammatory reaction causes distortions of the pelvic anatomy and leads to adhesion formation [33, 83]. Many authors report that both MRI and TVUS are limited in their ability to detect superficial endometriosis. According to Abrao et al., TVUS had a sensitivity and specificity of 98% and 100% while MRI of 83% and 98%, respectively, for detecting rectosigmoid endometriosis. More recently, Saba et al. has demonstrated that MRI and tenderness-guided TVUS have similar sensitivity and specificity in the identification of the rectosigmoid endometriosis (respectively, 73% and 90% for MRI and 73% and 86% for tenderness-guided TVUS) [84, 85]. In addition, MRI examination allows to evaluate the distance between the lesion and the anal junction, which is fundamental in presurgical planning, as well as the size and number of lesions, and also the depth of intestinal wall infiltration. All these information is essential for surgical planning.

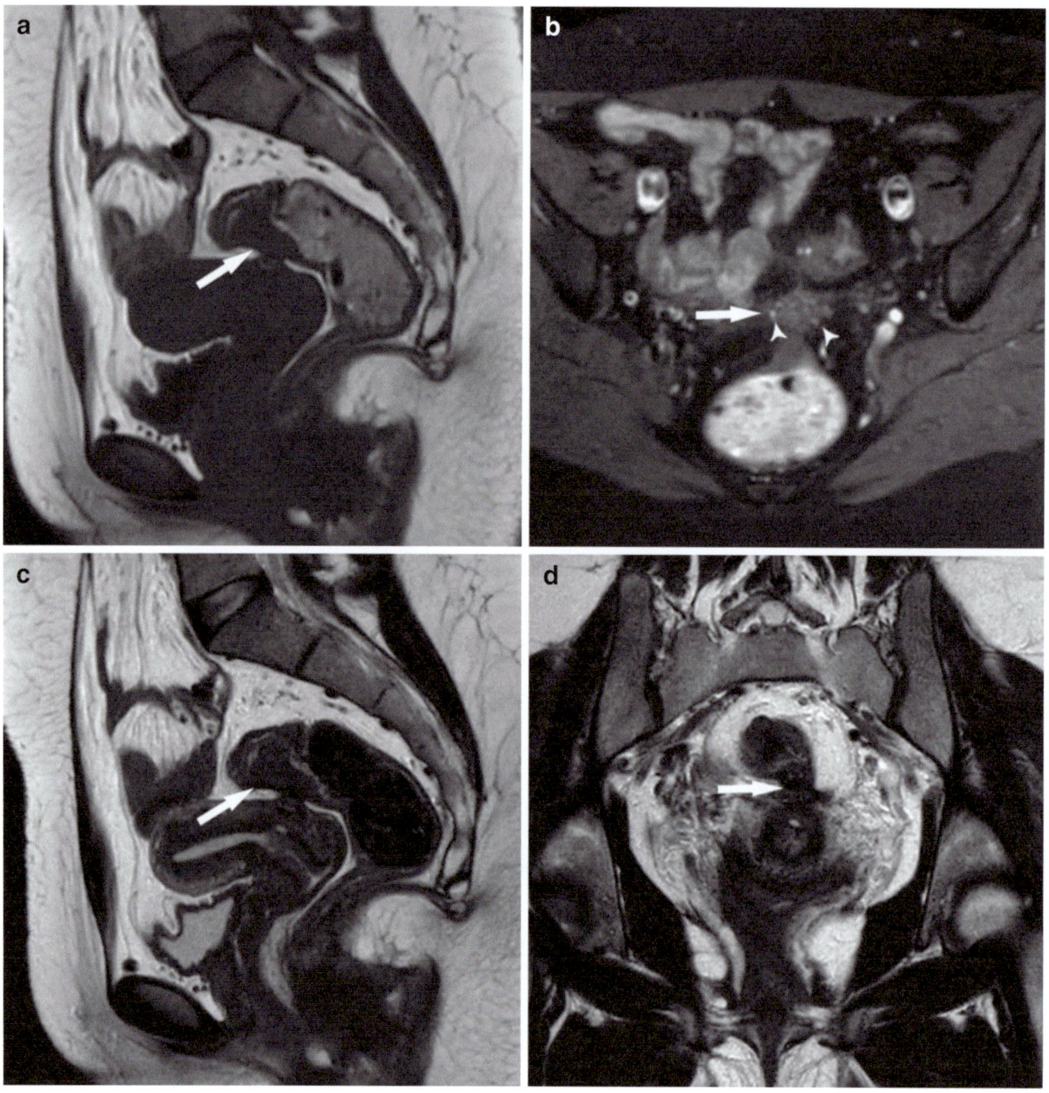

Fig. 15.5 *Rectosigmoid endometriosis* in a 34-year-old woman with pain during defecation and haematochezia synchronized with menses. Sagittal T1-weighted (**a**), axial T1-weighted with fat suppression (**b**), sagittal (**c**), and coronal (**d**) T2-weighted MR images show hypointense nodular thickening of the rectosigmoid wall that adheres to the posterior uterine surface. The "mushroom cap" sign is well visible on sagittal T2-w image (the low signal-intensity base of the mushroom represents the muscularis propria while the high-signal-intensity cap is attributed to the mucosa and submucosa, displaced into the lumen). Small intermingled hyperintense foci (arrowhead), due to bloody content, are detected on T1-weighted images with fat suppression

15.2.6.6 Atypical Sites of Implants

Terminal ileum and Appendix: Infiltrating endometriosis of the terminal ileum is infrequent, accounting for 4.1% of all intestinal endometriosis. More frequently, in two-third of cases, endometrial lesions (gland, stroma and haemorrhagic foci) involve the muscular and the seromuscolar layers, whereas in one-third of cases, they are sited solely on the serosal surface of the appendix. US is effective especially in the diagnosis of paediatric case; CT and less MRI are used in case of acute abdomen and appendix invagination. Preoperative diagnosis is a real challenge; however, this condition should be considered in the differential diagnosis of acute abdominal pain, especially in women with a medical history of endometriosis [86, 87].

Abdominal Wall: Endometriosis may occur in abdominal and pelvic wall scars, laparoscopy incision or caesarean delivery scars. The reported incidence of abdominal scar endometriosis following caesarean section is 0.03–0.6%. Nodules appear similar to solid endometriosis located in other pelvic sites; so, they demonstrate high signal both on T1-weighted and on T2-weighted images secondary to subacute haemorrhage [88, 89].

Chest: Endometriotic involvement of the chest was first described by Rokitansky in 1956, and many cases are reported in the literature. This condition is known as thoracic endometriosis syndrome (TES). It is always associated with coexistent pelvic endometriosis, but it manifests later (usually after 5 years after the diagnosis). Radiographic findings include pneumothorax, haemothorax, and lung nodules. CT or MR examination of the lung may show the endometrial lesions, but in many cases, they are not detectable with the exception of the occurrence of pneumothorax [12, 90].

Cutaneous Tissues: Cutaneous variant of endometriosis accounts for approximately 1% of all cases and is commonly associated with surgical scar. On MR imaging, the lesions showed heterogeneous mixed signal intensity on T1-weighted images, with several high signal foci presumed to be due to haemorrhage. For this reason, in case of detection of an infiltrative soft tissue mass in reproductive-age women, associated with pain synchronized with the menses, endometriosis must be suspected [91, 92].

Other: Even more rare is the involvement of the liver, the gall bladder, the pancreas and the breasts.

15.2.6.7 Complications

Adhesions represent the most common complication of extraovarian endometriosis. On MR imaging, they may appear as spiculated stranding with low signal intensity that obscure interfaces between the organs. Adhesions must be suspected in case of fixed pelvic organs (such as a fixed retroflexed uterus), posterior displacement of the uterus and ovaries, angulation of bowel loops, elevation of the posterior vaginal fornix, loculated fluid collections, hydrosalpinx and haematosalpinx [7]. Often laparoscopy is needed for definitive diagnosis because the evaluation of extent and severity of adhesions can be difficult to determine with imaging.

Unlike adhesions, *malignant transformation* of extraovarian endometriosis is a rare complication. While malignant transformation of endometrioma has been widely documented and explained, in the case of extraovarian endometriosis, it is still unclear. Approximately 25% of cases of the endometriosis-associated malignancies involve an endometriotic lesion located in an extraovarian site. Several histopathological types have been described, but endometrioid carcinoma and sarcomas are the most common. Rectovaginal and colorectal sites are the most frequently involved; the urinary bladder, vagina, ligaments, umbilicus, cervix and fallopian tube are less involved [62, 93–95]. On MR images neoplastic lesions appear as solid masses with intermediate signal both on T1- and T2-weighted sequences. Typically, they show contrast enhancement after administration of contrast material, and, moreover, they have restricted diffusion. The suspicion of malignant transformation should arise when a lesion with this MRI appearance is detected in a woman with a previous diagnosis of endometriosis or when a lesion with such MRI characteristics is seen along with other endometrial lesions [43, 96]. However, the definitive diagnosis is histologic. Obviously, these malignancies may spread by haematogenous and lymphatic routes or perineural spread. Differential diagnosis should consider primitive neoplasms that originate in different organs (such as colon cancer or vaginal squamous cell cancer) or, if the lesion occurs on a scar, with granuloma or dermoid tumours [49].

15.3 Technical Tips

For the assessment and evaluation of endometriosis:

- Use MRI as second-line approach, especially in symptomatic patients with negative US findings, and before surgery for preoperative workup.
- Fasting (3, 4 or 6 h), dietary preparation (low-residue regimen on the day before and the day of examination) and a moderately full urinary bladder are recommended; bowel preparation should be considered "best practice".
- Use antispasmodic agents in order to reduce motion artefacts caused by bowel and uterine peristalsis.
- Vaginal and rectal opacification may be used for a better visualization of anatomical structures that are close to each other; however, be aware to avoid the presence of small air bubbles that could be mistaken for nodular wall thickening.
- MRI protocol should be composed of:
  - 2D-T2-weighted sequences in the axial, sagittal and oblique plane
  - T1-weighted sequences with and without fat suppression
  - Half-Fourier single-shot turbo-spin-echo acquisition

Diffusion-weighted imaging and susceptibility-weighted imaging may lead to additional information.

- The use of contrast material is reserved for specific cases (especially in the suspicious of endometriosis-associated cancer) and therefore depends on the indication to MRI examination.
- MRI criteria for endometrioma:
  - Multiple adnexal cysts with hyperintense signal on T1-weighted images
  - One or more adnexal cysts with hyperintense signal on T1-weighted images and "shading sign" on T2-weighted images
- "T2 dark spots" finding seems to be highly specific for chronically haemorrhagic lesions; it could be considered a useful tool to differentiate ovarian endometriomas from functional haemorrhagic cysts.
- MRI findings suspecting malignant degeneration of endometrioma:
  - Enhanced mural nodules (well detected on contrast-enhanced subtracted images)
  - Loss of "T2-shading" sign on T2-weighted images
  - Mural nodule of more than 30 mm in size
  - Interval increase in the size of the cyst
- Deep endometriosis should be suspected in case of:
  - Haematosalpinx, as it may be the only finding in some women
  - Partial or complete obliteration of the rectouterine pouch with a lateralized fluid collection
  - Fixed pelvic organs (such as a fixed retroflexed uterus), posterior displacement of the uterus and ovaries, angulation of bowel loops and elevation of the posterior vaginal fornix

15.4 Future Perspectives

In the future, MRI will have a more important role in the assessment of endometriosis due to technical advances and improvement of software. With its great capacity to detect and characterize lesions, MRI has to be considered an important tool in staging endometriosis and planning adequate presurgical counselling and treatment. We postulate that it should reduce the need for diagnostic laparoscopy, even because the latter cannot detect lesions hidden by adhesions (and so not easily accessible at endoscopic viewing) or cannot even assess the depth of infiltration of peritoneal lesions. Diffusion weighted imaging (DWI) has greatly improved the diagnostic value of MR imaging, giving information that allow to differentiate between benign or malignant lesions. Indeed, DWI with ADC measurements could be useful tools in the differentiation between endometriosis and other pathologies, but more studies are needed in order to establish specific threshold in ADC values that allow to differentiate between them. Therefore, it is still necessary to prove DWI and ADC map usefulness in daily practice. Diffusion tensor imaging (DTI) studies are increasingly popular among researchers because of its ability to provide unique information about brain network; recently, even endometriosis become an important field of application. Indeed, DTI with tractography allow to detect changes and abnormalities in the structure of the sacral nerve roots, often site of endometriotic implants. Despite DTI is currently a promising tool to study nerves involvement, continuous studies are necessary to prove and validate its role.

References

1. Giudice LC, Kao LC. Endometriosis. Lancet. 2004;364(9447):1789–99. Review.
2. Shaw RW. Endometriosis. Current understanding and management. Oxford: Blackwell; 1995.
3. Venturini PL, Semino A, De Cecco L, editors. Endometriosi: Patofisiologia e Clinica. Carnforth: Parthenon; 1995.
4. Olive DL. Endometriosis. Obstet Gynecol Clin North Am. 1997;24:219–445.
5. Venturini PL, Prefumo F. Evers: Endometriosi: dalla Ricerca di Base alla Clinica. London: Parthenon; 1998.
6. Venturini P, Evers JLH. Endometriosis: basic research and clinical practice. London: The Parthenon Publishing Group; 1999.
7. Menni K, Facchetti L, Cabassa P. Extragenital endometriosis: assessment with MR imaging. A pictorial review. Br J Radiol. 2016;89(1060):20150672. https://doi.org/10.1259/bjr.20150672. Epub 2016 Feb 5. Review. PubMed PMID: 26846303; PubMed Central PMCID: PMC4846200.
8. Del Frate C, Girometti R, Pittino M, Del Frate G, Bazzocchi M, Zuiani C. Deep retroperitoneal pelvic endometriosis: MR imaging appearance with laparoscopic correlation. Radiographics. 2006;26(6):1705–18. Review. PubMed PMID:17102045.
9. Exacoustos C, Manganaro L, Zupi E. Imaging for the evaluation of endometriosis and adenomyosis. Best Pract Res Clin Obstet Gynaecol. 2014;28(5):655–81. https://doi.org/10.1016/j.bpobgyn.2014.04.010. Epub 2014 May 2. Review. PubMed PMID: 24861247.
10. Bulun SE. Endometriosis. N Engl J Med. 2009;360(3):268–79. https://doi.org/10.1056/NEJMra0804690. Review. PubMed PMID: 19144942.
11. Koninckx PR, Martin DC. Deep endometriosis: a consequence of infiltration or retraction or possibly adenomyosis externa? Fertil Steril. 1992;58(5):924–8. PubMed PMID: 1426377.
12. Woodward PJ, Sohaey MD, Mezzetti TP. From the archives of the AFIP. Endometriosis: radiologic-pathologic correlation. Radiographics. 2001;21:193–216.
13. Olive DL, Schwartz LB. Endometriosis. N Engl J Med. 1993;328(24):1759–69.
14. Gougoutas CA, Siegelman ES, Hunt J, Outwater EK. Pelvic endometriosis: various manifestations and MR imaging findings. AJR Am J Roentgenol. 2000;175(2):353–8.
15. Agarwal N, Subramanian A. Endometriosis—morphology, clinical presentations and molecular pathology. J Lab Physicians. 2010;2(1):1–9.
16. Schifrin BS, Erez S, Moore JG. Teen-age endometriosis. Am J Obstet Gynecol. 1973;116:973–80.
17. Gedgaudas-McClees RK. Gastrointestinal complications of gynecologic diseases. In: Textbook of gastrointestinal radiology. Philadelphia: Saunders; 1994. p. 2559–67.
18. Clement PB. Diseases of the peritoneum. In: Kurman RJ, editor. Blaustein's pathology of the female genital tract. 4th ed. New York: Springer; 1994. p. 660–80. 30.
19. Bianchi A, Pulido L, Espín F, Hidalgo LA, Heredia A, Fantova MJ, Muns R, Suñol J. [Intestinal endometriosis. Current status]. Cir Esp. 2007;81(4):170–6. Review. Spanish.
20. Brosens I, Puttemans P, Campo R, Gordts S, Kinkel K. Diagnosis of endometriosis: pelvic endoscopy and imaging techniques. Best Pract Res Clin Obstet Gynaecol. 2004;18(2):285–303.
21. de Venecia C, Ascher SM. Pelvic endometriosis: spectrum of magnetic resonance imaging findings. Semin Ultrasound CT MR. 2015;36(4):385–93.
22. Bazot M, Bharwani N, Huchon C, Kinkel K, Cunha TM, Guerra A, Manganaro L, Buñesch L, Kido A, Togashi K, Thomassin-Naggara I, Rockall AG. European society of urogenital radiology (ESUR) guidelines: MR imaging of pelvic endometriosis. Eur Radiol. 2017;27(7):2765–75. https://doi.org/10.1007/s00330-016-4673-z.
23. Suzuki S, Yasumoto M, Matsumoto R, Andoh A. MR findings of ruptured endometrial cyst: comparison with tubo-ovarian abscess. Eur J Radiol. 2012;81(11):3631–7. https://doi.org/10.1016/j.ejrad.2011.06.013.
24. Zanardi R, Del Frate C, Zuiani C, Bazzocchi M. Staging of pelvic endometriosis based on MRI findings versus laparoscopic classification according to the American Fertility Society. Abdom Imaging. 2003;28(5):733–42.
25. Carbognin G, Guarise A, Minelli L, Vitale I, Malagó R, Zamboni G, Procacci C. Pelvic endometriosis: US

and MRI features. Abdom Imaging. 2004;29(5):609–18. Epub 2004 May 27. Review.
26. Guerriero S, Ajossa S, Orozco R, Perniciano M, Jurado M, Melis GB, Alcazar JL. Accuracy of transvaginal ultrasound for diagnosis of deep endometriosis in the rectosigmoid: systematic review and meta-analysis. Ultrasound Obstet Gynecol. 2016;47(3):281–9. https://doi.org/10.1002/uog.15662. Epub 2015 Nov 4. Review. PubMed PMID: 26213903.
27. Guerriero S, Spiga S, Ajossa S, Peddes C, Perniciano M, Soggiu B, De Cecco CN, Laghi A, Melis GB, Saba L. Role of imaging in the management of endometriosis. Minerva Ginecol. 2013;65(2):143–66.
28. Hottat N, Larrousse C, Anaf V, Noël JC, Matos C, Absil J, Metens T. Endometriosis: contribution of 3.0-T pelvic MR imaging in preoperative assessment—initial results. Radiology. 2009;253(1):126–34. https://doi.org/10.1148/radiol.2531082113.
29. Manganaro L, Fierro F, Tomei A, Irimia D, Lodise P, Sergi ME, Vinci V, Sollazzo P, Porpora MG, Delfini R, Vittori G, Marini M. Feasibility of 3.0T pelvic MR imaging in the evaluation of endometriosis. Eur J Radiol. 2012;81(6):1381–7. https://doi.org/10.1016/j.ejrad.2011.03.049.
30. Rousset P, Peyron N, Charlot M, Chateau F, Golfier F, Raudrant D, Cotte E, Isaac S, Réty F, Valette PJ. Bowel endometriosis: preoperative diagnostic accuracy of 3.0-T MR enterography—initial results. Radiology. 2014;273(1):117–24. https://doi.org/10.1148/radiol.14132803.
31. Cornfeld D, Weinreb J. Simple changes to 1.5-T MRI abdomen and pelvis protocols to optimize results at 3 T. AJR Am J Roentgenol. 2008;190(2):W140–50. https://doi.org/10.2214/AJR.07.2903.
32. Schneider C, Oehmke F, Tinneberg HR, Krombach GA. MRI technique for the preoperative evaluation of deep infiltrating endometriosis: current status and protocol recommendation. Clin Radiol. 2016;71(3):179–94. https://doi.org/10.1016/j.crad.2015.09.014.
33. Chamié LP, Blasbalg R, Pereira RM, Warmbrand G, Serafini PC. Findings of pelvic endometriosis at transvaginal US, MR imaging, and laparoscopy. Radiographics. 2011;31(4):E77–100. https://doi.org/10.1148/rg.314105193.
34. Coutinho A Jr, Bittencourt LK, Pires CE, Junqueira F, Lima CM, Coutinho E, Domingues MA, Domingues RC, Marchiori E. MR imaging in deep pelvic endometriosis: a pictorial essay. Radiographics. 2011;31(2):549–67. https://doi.org/10.1148/rg.312105144.
35. Chamié LP, Blasbalg R, Gonçalves MO, Carvalho FM, Abrão MS, de Oliveira IS. Accuracy of magnetic resonance imaging for diagnosis and preoperative assessment of deeply infiltrating endometriosis. Int J Gynaecol Obstet. 2009;106(3):198–201. https://doi.org/10.1016/j.ijgo.2009.04.013.
36. Bazot M, Darai E, Hourani R, Thomassin I, Cortez A, Uzan S, Buy JN. Deep pelvic endometriosis: MR imaging for diagnosis and prediction of extension of disease. Radiology. 2004;232(2):379–89.
37. Bazot M, Gasner A, Ballester M, Daraï E. Value of thin-section oblique axial T2-weighted magnetic resonance images to assess uterosacral ligament endometriosis. Hum Reprod. 2011;26(2):346–53. https://doi.org/10.1093/humrep/deq336.
38. Bazot M, Jarboui L, Ballester M, Touboul C, Thomassin-Naggara I, Daraï E. The value of MRI in assessing parametrial involvement in endometriosis. Hum Reprod. 2012;27(8):2352–8. https://doi.org/10.1093/humrep/des211.
39. Kido A, Togashi K, Nishino M, Miyake K, Koyama T, Fujimoto R, Iwasaku K, Fujii S, Hayakawa K. Cine MR imaging of uterine peristalsis in patients with endometriosis. Eur Radiol. 2007;17(7):1813–9. Epub 2006 Nov 22.
40. Nakai A, Togashi K, Kosaka K, Kido A, Hiraga A, Fujiwara T, Koyama T, Fujii S. Uterine peristalsis: comparison of transvaginal ultrasound and two different sequences of cine MR imaging. J Magn Reson Imaging. 2004;20(3):463–9.
41. Leyendecker G, Kunz G, Wildt L, Beil D, Deininger H. Uterine hyperperistalsis and dysperistalsis as dysfunctions of the mechanism of rapid sperm transport in patients with endometriosis and infertility. Hum Reprod. 1996;11(7):1542–51.
42. Katayama M, Masui T, Kobayashi S, Ito T, Sakahara H, Nozaki A, Kabasawa H. Evaluation of pelvic adhesions using multiphase and multislice MR imaging with kinematic display. AJR Am J Roentgenol. 2001;177(1):107–10.
43. Coutinho AC Jr, Krishnaraj A, Pires CE, Bittencourt LK, Guimarães AR. Pelvic applications of diffusion magnetic resonance images. Magn Reson Imaging Clin N Am. 2011;19(1):133–57. https://doi.org/10.1016/j.mric.2010.10.003.
44. Balaban M, Idilman IS, Toprak H, Unal O, Ipek A, Kocakoc E. The utility of diffusion-weighted magnetic resonance imaging in differentiation of endometriomas from hemorrhagic ovarian cysts. Clin Imaging. 2015;39(5):830–3. https://doi.org/10.1016/j.clinimag.2015.05.003.
45. Manganaro L, Porpora MG, Vinci V, Bernardo S, Lodise P, Sollazzo P, Sergi ME, Saldari M, Pace G, Vittori G, Catalano C, Pantano P. Diffusion tensor imaging and tractography to evaluate sacral nerve root abnormalities in endometriosis-related pain: a pilot study. Eur Radiol. 2014;24(1):95–101. https://doi.org/10.1007/s00330-013-2981-0.
46. Solak A, Sahin N, Genç B, Sever AR, Genç M, Sivrikoz ON. Diagnostic value of susceptibility-weighted imaging of abdominal wall endometriomas during the cyclic menstrual changes: a preliminary study. Eur J Radiol. 2013;82(9):e411–6. https://doi.org/10.1016/j.ejrad.2013.04.030.
47. Takeuchi M, Matsuzaki K, Harada M. Susceptibility-weighted MRI of extra-ovarian endometriosis: preliminary results. Abdom Imaging. 2015;40(7):2512–6. https://doi.org/10.1007/s00261-015-0378-z.
48. Grammatikakis I, Evangelinakis N, Salamalekis G, Tziortzioti V, Samaras C, Chrelias C, Kassanos

D. Prevalence of severe pelvic inflammatory disease and endometriotic ovarian cysts: a 7-year retrospective study. Clin Exp Obstet Gynecol. 2009;36(4):235–6.
49. McDermott S, Oei TN, Iyer VR, Lee SI. MR imaging of malignancies arising in endometriomas and extraovarian endometriosis. Radiographics. 2012;32(3):845–63. https://doi.org/10.1148/rg.323115736.
50. Kobayashi H, Sumimoto K, Moniwa N, Imai M, Takakura K, Kuromaki T, Morioka E, Arisawa K, Terao T. Risk of developing ovarian cancer among women with ovarian endometrioma: a cohort study in Shizuoka, Japan. Int J Gynecol Cancer. 2007;17(1):37–43.
51. Kobayashi H, Sumimoto K, Kitanaka T, Yamada Y, Sado T, Sakata M, Yoshida S, Kawaguchi R, Kanayama S, Shigetomi H, Haruta S, Tsuji Y, Ueda S, Terao T. Ovarian endometrioma—risks factors of ovarian cancer development. Eur J Obstet Gynecol Reprod Biol. 2008;138(2):187–93. Epub 2007 Dec 26.
52. Takeuchi M, Matsuzaki K, Nishitani H. Susceptibility-weighted MRI of endometrioma: preliminary results. AJR Am J Roentgenol. 2008;191(5):1366–70. https://doi.org/10.2214/AJR.07.3974.
53. Togashi K, Nishimura K, Kimura I, Tsuda Y, Yamashita K, Shibata T, Nakano Y, Konishi J, Konishi I, Mori T. Endometrial cysts: diagnosis with MR imaging. Radiology. 1991;180(1):73–8.
54. Siegelman ES, Outwater EK. Tissue characterization in the female pelvis by means of MR imaging. Radiology. 1999;212(1):5–18.
55. Nishimura K, Togashi K, Itoh K, Fujisawa I, Noma S, Kawamura Y, Nakano Y, Itoh H, Torizuka K, Ozasa H. Endometrial cysts of the ovary: MR imaging. Radiology. 1987;162(2):315–8.
56. Corwin MT, Gerscovich EO, Lamba R, Wilson M, McGahan JP. Differentiation of ovarian endometriomas from hemorrhagic cysts at MR imaging: utility of the T2 dark spot sign. Radiology. 2014;271(1):126–32. https://doi.org/10.1148/radiol.13131394.
57. Siegelman ES, Oliver ER. MR imaging of endometriosis: ten imaging pearls. Radiographics. 2012;32(6):1675–91. https://doi.org/10.1148/rg.326125518.
58. Outwater EK, Dunton CJ. Imaging of the ovary and adnexa: clinical issues and applications of MR imaging. Radiology. 1995;194(1):1–18.
59. Sugimura K, Okizuka H, Imaoka I, Kaji Y, Takahashi K, Kitao M, Ishida T. Pelvic endometriosis: detection and diagnosis with chemical shift MR imaging. Radiology. 1993;188(2):435–8.
60. Brosens I. Endometriosis and the outcome of in vitro fertilization. Fertil Steril. 2004;81:1198–20.
61. Ueda Y, Enomoto T, Miyatake T, Fujita M, Yamamoto R, Kanagawa T, Shimizu H, Kimura T. A retrospective analysis of ovarian endometriosis during pregnancy. Fertil Steril. 2010;94(1):78–84. https://doi.org/10.1016/j.fertnstert.2009.02.092.
62. Benoit L, Arnould L, Cheynel N, Diane B, Causeret S, Machado A, Collin F, Fraisse J, Cuisenier J. Malignant extraovarian endometriosis: a review. Eur J Surg Oncol. 2006;32(1):6–11. Epub 2005 Nov 11.
63. SCOTT RB. Malignant changes in endometriosis. Obstet Gynecol. 1953;2(3):283–9. PubMed PMID: 13087921.
64. Tanaka YO, Okada S, Yagi T, Satoh T, Oki A, Tsunoda H, Yoshikawa H. MRI of endometriotic cysts in association with ovarian carcinoma. AJR Am J Roentgenol. 2010;194(2):355–61. https://doi.org/10.2214/AJR.09.2985.
65. Darvishzadeh A, McEachern W, Lee TK, Bhosale P, Shirkhoda A, Menias C, Lall C. Deep pelvic endometriosis: a radiologist's guide to key imaging features with clinical and histopathologic review. Abdom Radiol (NY). 2016;41(12):2380–400.
66. Turocy JM, Benacerraf BR. Transvaginal sonography in the diagnosis of deep infiltrating endometriosis: a review. J Clin Ultrasound. 2017;45(6):313–8. https://doi.org/10.1002/jcu.22483.
67. Choudhary S, Fasih N, Papadatos D, Surabhi VR. Unusual imaging appearances of endometriosis. AJR Am J Roentgenol. 2009;192(6):1632–44. https://doi.org/10.2214/AJR.08.1560.
68. Fritsch H. Clinical anatomy of the female pelvis. In: Hamm B, Forstner R, editors. MRI and CT of the female pelvis. New York: Springer; 2007. p. 1–24.
69. Balleyguier C, Chapron C, Dubuisson JB, Kinkel K, Fauconnier A, Vieira M, Hélénon O, Menu Y. Comparison of magnetic resonance imaging and transvaginal ultrasonography in diagnosing bladder endometriosis. J Am Assoc Gynecol Laparosc. 2002;9(1):15–23.
70. Le Tohic A, Chis C, Yazbeck C, Koskas M, Madelenat P, Panel P. [Bladder endometriosis: diagnosis and treatment. A series of 24 patients]. Gynecol Obstet Fertil. 2009;37(3):216–21. https://doi.org/10.1016/j.gyobfe.2009.01.018.
71. Fedele L, Bianchi S, Zanconato G, Bergamini V, Berlanda N, Carmignani L. Long-term follow-up after conservative surgery for bladder endometriosis. Fertil Steril. 2005;83(6):1729–33.
72. Saba L, Sulcis R, Melis GB, de Cecco CN, Laghi A, Piga M, Guerriero S. Endometriosis: the role of magnetic resonance imaging. Acta Radiol. 2015;56(3):355–67. https://doi.org/10.1177/0284185114526086.
73. Thonnon C, Philip CA, Fassi-Fehri H, Bisch C, Coulon A, de Saint-Hilaire P, Dubernard G. Three-dimensional ultrasound in the management of bladder endometriosis. J Minim Invasive Gynecol. 2015;22(3):403–9. https://doi.org/10.1016/j.jmig.2014.10.021.
74. Kołodziej A, Krajewski W, Dołowy Ł, Hirnle L. Urinary tract endometriosis. Urol J. 2015;12(4):2213–7.
75. Umaria N, Olliff JF. Imaging features of pelvic endometriosis. Br J Radiol. 2001;74(882):556–62. Review.
76. Balleyguier C, Roupret M, Nguyen T, Kinkel K, Helenon O, Chapron C. Ureteral endometriosis: the role of magnetic resonance imaging. J Am Assoc Gynecol Laparosc. 2004;11(4):530–6.

77. Sillou S, Poirée S, Millischer AE, Chapron C, Hélénon O. Urinary endometriosis: MR imaging appearance with surgical and histological correlations. Diagn Interv Imaging. 2015;96(4):373–81. https://doi.org/10.1016/j.diii.2014.11.010.
78. Foti PV, Ognibene N, Spadola S, Caltabiano R, Farina R, Palmucci S, Milone P, Ettorre GC. Non-neoplastic diseases of the fallopian tube: MR imaging with emphasis on diffusion-weighted imaging. Insights Imaging. 2016;7(3):311–27. https://doi.org/10.1007/s13244-016-0484-7.
79. Gui B, Valentini AL, Ninivaggi V, Marino M, Iacobucci M, Bonomo L. Deep pelvic endometriosis: don't forget round ligaments. Review of anatomy, clinical characteristics, and MR imaging features. Abdom Imaging. 2014;39(3):622–32. https://doi.org/10.1007/s00261-014-0091-3.
80. Struble J, Reid S, Bedaiwy MA. Adenomyosis: a clinical review of a challenging gynecologic condition. J Minim Invasive Gynecol. 2016;23(2):164–85. https://doi.org/10.1016/j.jmig.2015.09.018.
81. Chamié LP, Pereira RM, Zanatta A, Serafini PC. Transvaginal US after bowel preparation for deeply infiltrating endometriosis: protocol, imaging appearances, and laparoscopic correlation. Radiographics. 2010;30(5):1235–49. https://doi.org/10.1148/rg.305095221.
82. Chapron C, Fauconnier A, Vieira M, Barakat H, Dousset B, Pansini V, Vacher-Lavenu MC, Dubuisson JB. Anatomical distribution of deeply infiltrating endometriosis: surgical implications and proposition for a classification. Hum Reprod. 2003;18(1):157–61.
83. Trippia CH, Zomer MT, Terazaki CR, Martin RL, Ribeiro R, Kondo W. Relevance of imaging examinations in the surgical planning of patients with bowel endometriosis. Clin Med Insights Reprod Health. 2016;10:1–8. https://doi.org/10.4137/CMRH.S29472.
84. Abrao MS, Gonçalves MO, Dias JA Jr, Podgaec S, Chamie LP, Blasbalg R. Comparison between clinical examination, transvaginal sonography and magnetic resonance imaging for the diagnosis of deep endometriosis. Hum Reprod. 2007;22(12):3092–7.
85. Saba L, Guerriero S, Sulcis R, Pilloni M, Ajossa S, Melis G, Mallarini G. MRI and "tenderness guided" transvaginal ultrasonography in the diagnosis of recto-sigmoid endometriosis. J Magn Reson Imaging. 2012;35(2):352–60. https://doi.org/10.1002/jmri.22832.
86. Yoon J, Lee YS, Chang HS, Park CS. Endometriosis of the appendix. Ann Surg Treat Res. 2014;87(3):144–7. https://doi.org/10.4174/astr.2014.87.3.144.
87. Soylu L, Aydın OU, Aydın S, Özçay N. Invagination of the appendix due to endometriosis presenting as acute appendicitis. Ulus Cerrahi Derg. 2013;30(2):106–8. https://doi.org/10.5152/UCD.2013.19.
88. Hensen JH, Van Breda Vriesman AC, Puylaert JB. Abdominal wall endometriosis: clinical presentation and imaging features with emphasis on sonography. AJR Am J Roentgenol. 2006;186(3):616–20.
89. Barrow TA, Elsayed M, Liong SY, Sukumar SA. Complex abdominopelvic endometriosis: the radiologist's perspective. Abdom Imaging. 2015;40(7):2541–56. https://doi.org/10.1007/s00261-015-0413-0.
90. Badawy SZ, Shrestha P. Recurrent catamenial pneumothorax suggestive of pleural endometriosis. Case Rep Obstet Gynecol. 2014;2014:756040. https://doi.org/10.1155/2014/756040.
91. Pramanik SR, Mondal S, Paul S, Joycerani D. Primary umbilical endometriosis: a rarity. J Hum Reprod Sci. 2014;7(4):269–71. https://doi.org/10.4103/0974-1208.147495.
92. Ding Y, Gibbs J, Xiong G, Guo S, Raj S, Bui MM. Endometriosis mimicking soft-tissue neoplasms: a potential diagnostic pitfall. Cancer Control. 2017;24(1):83–8.
93. Heaps JM, Nieberg RK, Berek JS. Malignant neoplasms arising in endometriosis. Obstet Gynecol. 1990;75(6):1023–8.
94. Modesitt SC, Tortolero-Luna G, Robinson JB, Gershenson DM, Wolf JK. Ovarian and extraovarian endometriosis-associated cancer. Obstet Gynecol. 2002;100(4):788–95.
95. Brooks JJ, Wheeler JE. Malignancy arising in extragonadal endometriosis: a case report and summary of the world literature. Cancer. 1977;40(6):3065–73.
96. Sala E, Rockall A, Rangarajan D, Kubik-Huch RA. The role of dynamic contrast-enhanced and diffusion weighted magnetic resonance imaging in the female pelvis. Eur J Radiol. 2010;76(3):367–85. https://doi.org/10.1016/j.ejrad.2010.01.026.

Biomarkers in Endometriosis

16

Vicki Nisenblat and M. Louise Hull

16.1 Introduction

Although there are no data to show that early treatment of endometriosis prevents progression of the disease, untreated endometriosis is linked with reduced quality of life and outcomes such as depression, inability to work, sexual dysfunction, and missed opportunity for motherhood [1, 2].

The accuracy of diagnosing endometriosis based on symptoms alone is low due to the varied and nonspecific nature of the clinical presentation of disease. Furthermore, there is a poor association between the presenting symptoms and severity of the disease [3]. A recent multicenter study, which included 1396 women in 19 hospitals in 13 countries, assessed the accuracy of a variety of features in a woman's history that best predicted endometriosis and revealed that a symptom-based model had insufficient diagnostic accuracy to be relied on in a clinical setting [4]. While examination findings can help to improve the accuracy of diagnosis, the majority of women with laparoscopically proven endometriosis have a normal pelvic examination [5].

Laparoscopic visualization of lesions in the peritoneal cavity is the only test sufficiently accurate to be accepted as the diagnostic "gold standard" in clinical care. However, diagnosis using this method is limited by the experience of the surgeon and histological confirmation by the expertise of the pathologist. A systematic review of four studies of the diagnostic test accuracy of laparoscopic visualization showed it had 94% sensitivity and 79% specificity when compared to histological confirmation of endometriosis in excised lesions [6]. Surgery also confers a risk of infection, bleeding, and damage to other structures in the pelvis, anesthetic risks, and a small risk of mortality. Even though the major complications of laparoscopy are rare, it is difficult to determine the exact incidence of complications associated with long-term morbidity.

The high cost of surgery restricts access to diagnosis particularly for women in developing countries, in low socioeconomic groups, and in rural and remote locations. Additionally, some women with pelvic pain prefer to avoid surgery opting for empirical medical treatment which is an approach that has widespread acceptance [7]. An accurate noninvasive diagnostic test for endometriosis would afford these groups of women an opportunity to validate their symptoms and to reduce anxiety related to diagnostic uncertainty regardless of their reasons for not undertaking surgery.

Consensus groups are increasingly recognizing the need for more accurate noninvasive diagnostics and recommending that nonsurgical diagnosis should be considered before embarking on an operative procedure [8, 9]. A simple and

V. Nisenblat (✉) · M. L. Hull
Discipline of Obstetrics and Gynaecology, School of Medicine, Robinson Research Institute, The University of Adelaide, Adelaide, SA, Australia

S. Guerriero et al. (eds.), *How to Perform Ultrasonography in Endometriosis*,
https://doi.org/10.1007/978-3-319-71138-6_16

reliable low-invasive test for endometriosis is expected to minimize surgical risks, reduce diagnostic delay, and provide an opportunity for earlier interventions with potential to improve patient outcomes and to decrease healthcare-related costs. Furthermore, the ability to assess the progression of endometriosis in a noninvasive way would advance clinical research in endometriosis, including development of new effective therapeutic and preventive strategies.

The literature on low-invasive peripheral and endometrial biomarkers and on imaging diagnostic tests for endometriosis is growing, with a steady stream of new reports on accurate diagnostic tests. Although none of the proposed tests have been considered sufficiently accurate to legitimately replace laparoscopy in everyday practice, imaging tests are being increasingly employed as a diagnostic adjunct to surgery, and their use is being progressively explored.

This chapter provides a synthesis of the up-to-date research evidence on diagnostic accuracy of low-invasive tests for endometriosis. It aims to answer the question whether any low-invasive diagnostic tests, either individually or in combination, may be considered sufficiently accurate to either replace laparoscopy as a diagnostic test for endometriosis or be used as a triage test to improve selection of women for a diagnostic surgery. In addition, this chapter evaluates the applicability of the presented findings to clinical practice and provides insight regarding future research in the field.

16.2 Quantifying Performance of the Diagnostic Tests for Endometriosis

To discuss diagnostic test accuracy studies in a meaningful way, the tests need to be interpreted in an appropriate clinical and methodological framework. Diagnostic test accuracy refers to the degree of agreement between the diagnostic performance of the test under study (index test) and that of a clinical gold standard (reference test). The ideal diagnostic test classifies all individuals as either diseased or non-diseased 100% of the time. In practice, false-positive and false-negative tests create a misclassification of some individuals in the non-diseased and diseased groups. The basic measures of how well a test discriminates between disease and non-disease states include sensitivity, defined as the proportion of all patients with the disease who indeed have a positive test result, and specificity, defined as the proportion of all patients without the disease who have a negative test result. Sensitivity and specificity are independent of the prevalence of the disease and are commonly used in the diagnostic studies to evaluate and compare the performance of different tests. A trade-off exists between the sensitivity and specificity of index test as their values vary inversely in relation to the cutoff point chosen to define a positive or negative result.

The purpose of the test and the clinical consequences of under- and overdiagnosis of the condition determines the level of diagnostic performance required for a clinically useful test. In endometriosis, a noninvasive test could be used as (1) a replacement test which replaces diagnostic laparoscopy as it has similar or better accuracy and (2) a triage test, used to identify the individuals who likely to benefit from laparoscopy, which may alter the number of those who are offered a surgical intervention [10]. A replacement test is expected to have high sensitivity and specificity, while triage tests could be highly sensitive but less specific or vice versa. A high sensitivity triage test rules out the condition if the test is negative, but a positive result has little diagnostic value (SnOUT test). Alternatively, a high specificity triage test rules conditions "in" if the test is positive but is less informative if the result is negative (SpIN test). Both types of triage test are clinically useful and can be implemented in sequential manner to optimize a diagnostic algorithm (Fig. 16.1).

To assist with the interpretation of the diagnostic estimates and to put the results into clinical context, a series of Cochrane Library diagnostic test reviews proposed the cutoff values for the potentially clinically significant diagnostic estimates. The diagnostic threshold for a replacement test for endometriosis was determined as a sensitivity ≥0.94 and a specificity ≥0.79, which is the same diagnostic accuracy conferred by a diagnostic laparoscopy [6]. It was assumed that a 5% error in the correct diagnosis was statistically and clinically acceptable for a triage test, whereas diagnostic uncertainty should be limited to less than 50% of individuals. Therefore, the criteria for triage tests were set as a sensitivity ≥0.95 and a specificity ≥0.50 for a SnOUT test and a sensitivity ≥0.50 and a specificity ≥0.95 for a SpIN test [10].

Highly diagnostic accuracy on its own is not sufficient to determine that a test is clinically useful, and the value of diagnostic tests ultimately lies in their effect on patient outcomes. Evaluation of the diagnostic test to advance the markers from benchtop to clinically relevant products usually comprises a series of sequential steps to assess clinical, financial, psychological, and societal consequences of the test [11]. Diagnostic performance of the test is an important initial step in the pipeline of test evaluation and thus has to rely on high-quality reproducible evidence.

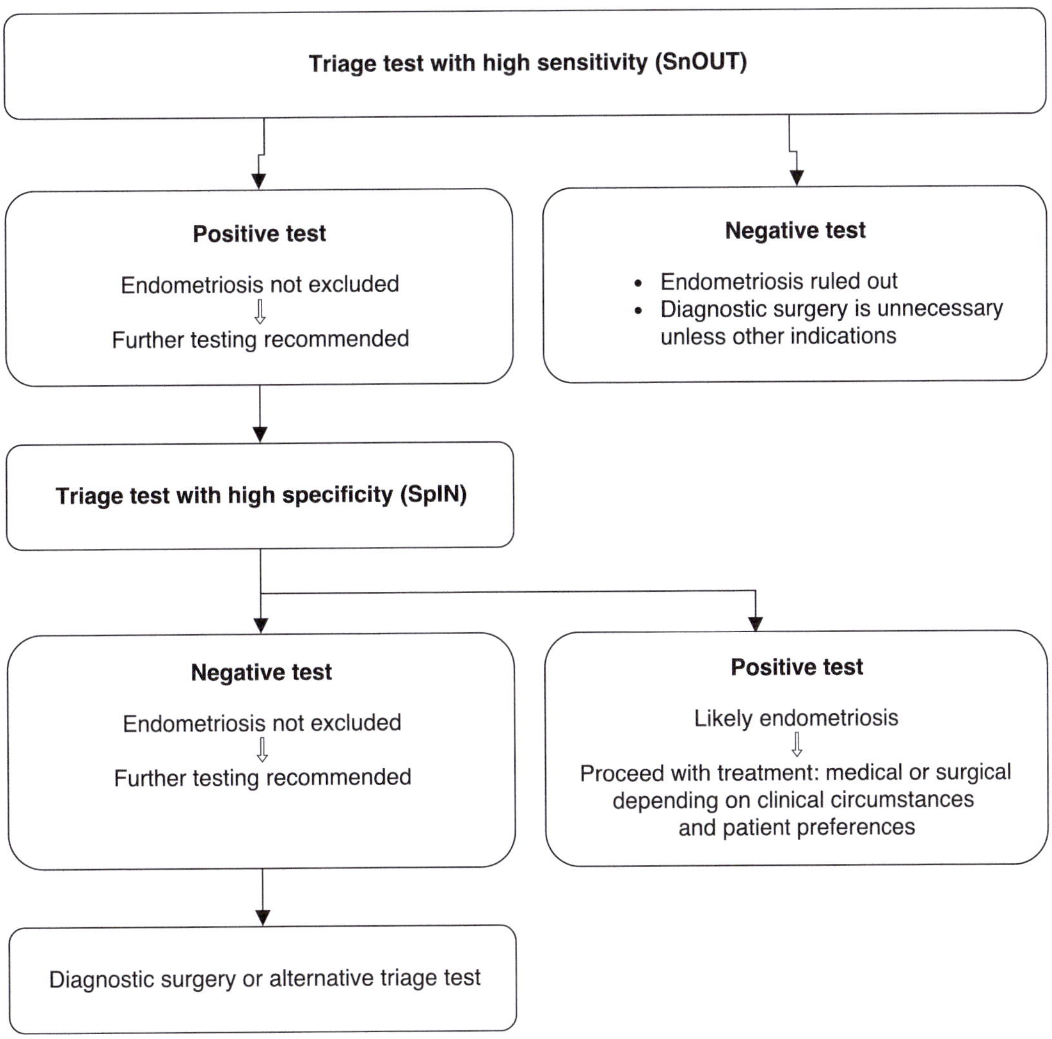

Fig. 16.1 Sequential approach to non-invasive testing of endometriosis

16.3 Biomarkers for Endometriosis

16.3.1 Peripheral Biomarkers

Hormonal dysregulation, immune dysfunction, and inflammation are features of endometriosis, which is increasingly recognized as a systemic condition rather than localized pelvic disease [12, 13]. Identification of the cellular and molecular systemic hallmarks of endometriosis has prompted the evaluation of their potential as diagnostic tools. Peripheral biomarkers for endometriosis have been extensively explored in the blood and urine and were appraised in several recent systematic reviews [10, 14, 15].

The diagnostic test accuracy of 122 biomarkers measured in serum, plasma, or whole blood was evaluated in a Cochrane Library systematic review [10]. Diagnostic estimates (sensitivity and specificity) were reported for 47 biomarker-based tests, which included angiogenesis/growth factors, apoptosis markers, cell adhesion molecules, high-throughput markers, hormonal markers, immune system/inflammatory markers, oxidative stress markers, microRNAs, tumor markers, and other proteins. The majority of index tests were assessed in small individual studies, often using different cutoff thresholds and diverse laboratory methods. Meta-analysis was only possible for four tests (anti-endometrial antibodies, interleukin-6 (IL-6), cancer antigen-19.9 (CA-19.9), and CA-125), and there was substantial heterogeneity in diagnostic estimates between the studies in every meta-analysis. None of the meta-analyses revealed a test which met the criteria for consideration as a replacement or triage test for pelvic endometriosis.

CA-125 is the most studied biomarker in endometriosis. Its diagnostic role has been explored for several decades since its first publications in the early 1980s. The first systematic review that assessed the performance of CA-125 in endometriosis in 22 studies with a total of 2866 women revealed that while CA-125 has limited performance in endometriosis, it performs better in advanced disease and hence may be of clinical value in selected subsets of patients [16]. Over the years, considerable number of studies demonstrated high specificity but low sensitivity of the test but explored different cutoff levels and showed substantial heterogeneity in the obtained diagnostic estimates. Two recent systematic reviews reached different conclusions regarding the optimal diagnostic cutoff level of CA-125. The Cochrane Database systematic review that included 45 studies with a total of 5534 women demonstrated that although none of the evaluated cutoffs showed adequate diagnostic performance, CA-125 > 16.0–17.6 U/ml was the best performing test for pelvic endometriosis, with a mean sensitivity of 0.56 (95% CI 0.24, 0.88) and mean specificity of 0.91 (95% CI 0.75, 1.00) [10]. The test approached the criteria for a SpIN triage test, being able to confirm the diagnosis if positive result, but remained nonconclusive for the levels below the cutoff point. CA-125 seemed to perform better for ovarian endometriosis compared with the other forms of the disease, but there were no sufficient data for formal comparison, and valid conclusions could not be made. A systematic review of 14 studies, with a total of 2920 participants, solely focused on CA-125 > 30 U/ml and demonstrated higher diagnostic estimates for this threshold than those presented in the Cochrane review [17]. The authors suggested using a cutoff >30 U/ml to rule the disease in, and this was supported by more recent well-designed prospective study in 58 consecutive women, which demonstrated a sensitivity of 0.57 (95% CI 0.37, 0.75) and a specificity of 0.96 (95% CI 0.82, 1.00%) for detecting endometriosis using CA-125 at a cutoff of ≥30 U/ml [18]. Earlier studies have also suggested a role of CA-125 as a marker for the recurrence of endometriosis and for monitoring the response medical therapy but did not reach firm conclusions. While some showed progressive reduction in CA-125 levels in women treated with postoperative danazol of GnRH agonists with posttreatment rebound [19, 20], others revealed that 50% of patients with clinical improvement showed no change in serum CA-125 levels [21]. Moreover, second-look laparoscopy in small subset of treated patients demonstrated persistent endometriosis despite normal CA-125 levels [19].

Furthermore, there is no consensus on optimal timing of the test in relation to phase of the menstrual cycle. Koninckx was the first to show that plasma concentrations of CA-125 were higher during menses than during follicular or midluteal phase in both control and endometriosis groups and observed more pronounced differences in mild forms of the disease [22]. Since then, the literature on inter-cycle differences of CA-125 remains inconsistent, and there is substantial variation between the studies with regard to timing of the test in menstrual cycle. Overall, biases in study design and limitations in reporting in most studies contributed to low quality of current evidence. The diagnostic role of CA-125 in endometriosis, either as a single test or when integrated in more complex diagnostic algorithms, remains elusive and needs to be established in patients with different clinical phenotypes.

A number of biomarkers demonstrated high diagnostic estimates for pelvic endometriosis or endometrioma in individual studies (Table 16.1). Future research needs to confirm their diagnostic value and in endometriosis using high-quality diagnostic test accuracy methodologies in large cohorts of well-characterized patients. The list of blood-derived biomarkers continues to expand as high-throughput profiling of the metabolome [23–25], proteome [26–29], and miRNAs, the posttranscriptional regulators of gene expression [30–33], becomes increasingly accessible.

The high-throughput platforms carry great potential, since they enable comprehensive coverage of molecules of interest in small amount of biological material. However, the identification and characterization of metabolic and proteomic fingerprint molecules is a challenging task, and methodology is still under development. Unstandardized approach to sample processing and data handling and variation in analytical techniques across studies invariably limit translational application of the "omics" science. High-throughput experiments have limited reproducibility and are rarely validated in large independent cohorts. For example, several research groups have examined potential use of circulating miRNA as diagnostic marker for endometriosis and identified miRNA panels with high diagnostic estimates [30–33]. Each study, however, reported different set of miRNA biomarkers, and the results could not be replicated by others (personal communication). It becomes increasingly evident that emerging advances in technology and bioinformatics provide a unique opportunity for elucidating biological pathways and discovering clinical biomarkers. Optimization and standardization of the laboratory and analytical methods with a focus on reproducible research are important to advance the preliminary discoveries into clinical applications.

A limited number of urinary tests have been assessed for their potential to diagnose endometriosis. A Cochrane Library diagnostic test accuracy review of 8 studies with a total of 646 participants evaluated 6 tests: enolase 1 (NNE), vitamin D binding protein (VDBP), cytokeratin 19 (CK 19 or CYFRA 21-1), vascular endothelial growth factor (VEGF), tumor necrosis factor-alpha (TNF-α), and urinary proteome [15]. Most were evaluated in small individual studies and meta-analyses could not be performed. Of these, NNE, VDBP, and cytoskeleton molecule CK-19 showed low diagnostic estimates, whereas VEGF and TNF-α did not distinguish women with and without endometriosis and their diagnostic accuracy was not assessed.

Matrix-enhanced laser desorption/ionization time-of-flight mass spectrometry (MALDI-TOF-MS) was used to identify the urinary proteome in two studies with some variation in methodology between studies and some inconsistencies with regard to the identified peptide markers. In one study, a test that included five urinary peptides of 1433.9 Da, 1599.4 Da, 2085.6 Da, 6798.0 Da, and 3217.2 Da had a sensitivity of 0.91 [95%CI 0.59, 1.00] and a specificity of 0.93 [95%CI 0.66, 1.00] [34]. Although clinically attractive, these findings require replication using similar technical and analytical approaches before their value in clinical practice can be established. Recent reports indicated that nuclear magnetic resonance (NMR) spectroscopy can be used to reveal the metabolome of women with endometriosis in urine samples, but the diagnostic validity of the test is yet to be established [35].

Table 16.1 Peripheral and endometrial biomarkers of endometriosis that require further validation [14, 17, 44]

Blood biomarkers	Angiogenesis and growth markers	• Vascular endothelial growth factor (VEGF) >680 pg/ml and >236 pg/ml • Brain-derived neurotrophic factor (BDNF)
	High-throughput markers	• Metabolome signatures • Proteome signatures
	Immune system and inflammatory markers	• Interleukin-6 (IL-6) >12.2 pg/ml
	Oxidative stress markers	• Paraoxonase-1 (PON-1) <141.5 U/l • Carbonyls <14.9 µM
	Post-transcriptional regulators of gene expression (miRNAs)	• miR-9* • miR-141* • miR-145* • miR-20a • miR-22 • miR-532-3p
	Tumor markers	• CA-125 (cut-off value > 43 U/ml)
	Combination of several blood tests	• Interleukin-6 (IL-6) >12.2 pg/ml + Tumor necrosis factor-α (TNF-α) > 12.45 pg/ml • IL-6 > 12.2 pg/ml + C-reactive protein (CRP) >438 µg/ml • TNF-α > 12.45 pg/ml + CRP > 438 µg/ml • CA-125 + Syntaxin-5 (STX-5) + Laminin-1 (LN-1) • IL-6 > 12.2 pg/ml + TNF-α > 12.45 pg/ml + CRP > 438 µg/ml • CA-125 > 17.6 IU/ml + VEGF > 236 pg/ml • CA-125 + CA-19-9 + Survivin • CA-125 > 50 IU/ml + C-C motif receptor-1(CCR1) > 1.16 + Monocyte chemotactic protein-1 (MCP-1) > 140 pg/ml • CA-125 > 20 IU/ml + MCP-1 > 152.744 pg/ml + leptin > 3.14 ng/ml • CA-125 + IL-8 + TNF-α • CA-125 + CA-19.9 + IL-6 + IL-8 + TNF-α + CRP • miR-199a + miR-542-3p • miR-199a + miR-122 + miR-145* + miR-542-3p
	Tests that differentiate endometrioma from other benign ovarian cysts	• Urocortin > 29 pg/ml • Urocortin > 33 pg/ml • Follistatin > 1433 pg/ml • CA-125 > 30 U/ml and >36 U/ml • CA-125 ≥ 25 U/ml + CA-19.9 ≥ 22 U/ml
Urinary biomarkers	High-throughput markers	• Proteome signatures
Endometrial biomarkers	High-throughput markers	• Proteome signatures
	Hormonal markers	• 17-β hydroxysteroid dehydrogenase type 2 gene (17βHSD2)
	Immune system and inflammatory markers	• Interleukin-1 receptor type II gene (IL-1R2)
	Myogenic markers	• Caldesmon
	Neural and nerve sheath markers	• Protein gene product 9.5 (PGP 9.5) • Vasoactive intestinal polypeptide (VIP) • Calcitonin gene-related protein (CGRP) • Substance P (SP) • Neuropeptide Y (NPY) • Combined test (VIP + PGP 9.5 + SP)

16.3.2 Endometrial Biomarkers

Many studies have demonstrated biological differences when endometrium from endometriosis patients is compared to that from disease-free women. The eutopic endometrium from women with endometriosis had an aberrant responsiveness to ovarian hormones characterized by progesterone resistance and incomplete transition from proliferative to luteal phase of menstrual cycle, which was associated with decreased endometrial receptivity [36–38]. Dysregulated gene expression profiles and changes in hormone-responsive, gene regulatory pathways were also identified in eutopic endometrium from endometriosis [39]. An analysis of the DNA methylome in endometrium from women with endometriosis and disease-free individuals revealed different methylation patterns that fluctuated across the phases of the menstrual cycle indicative of aberrant epigenetic regulation of the endometrium in endometriosis [40].

The inflammatory and hypoxic peritoneal environment identified in endometriosis was linked to an aberrant expression of chemokines, cytokines, growth factors, and immune cells in eutopic endometrium that are involved in immune response, proliferation, cell migration, and neovascularization [10]. Secretomic approaches have characterized protein composition of the endometrial secretions and revealed the presence of cytokines, growth factors, ions, carbohydrates, and steroids, in human uterine fluid [41]. Taken together, these observations support the premise that eutopic endometrium and aspirated uterine fluid could contain diagnostic biomarkers relevant to endometriosis.

A Cochrane Library diagnostic test accuracy review explored 95 endometriosis-associated biomarkers in eutopic endometrium and menstrual fluid [42]. Included were angiogenesis factor prokineticin 1 (PROK-1), cell adhesion molecules (integrins α3β1, α4β1, β1, and α6), DNA repair molecule human telomerase reverse transcriptase (hTERT), endometrial and mitochondrial proteome, tumor marker (CA-125), inflammatory marker interleukin-1 receptor type II (IL-1R2), and myogenic marker caldesmon (CALD-1). Other hormonal markers (aromatase cytochrome P450 (CYP19), 17β-hydroxysteroid dehydrogenase type 2 (17βHSD2), and estrogen receptors (ER-α, ER-β)) and neural markers (protein gene product 9.5 (PGP 9.5), vasoactive intestinal polypeptide (VIP), calcitonin gene-related protein (CGRP), substance P (SP), neuropeptide Y (NPY), and neurofilament (NF)) were also assessed.

The only markers with sufficient data for a meta-analysis were PGP 9.5 and CYP19 as the other biomarkers were assessed in single studies and could not be statistically evaluated in any meaningful way. CYP19 (8 studies, 444 women) had a mean sensitivity of 0.77 (95% CI 0.70, 0.85) and a specificity of 0.74 (95% CI 0.65, 84). PGP 9.5 (7 studies, 361 women) showed a mean sensitivity of 0.96 (95% CI 0.91, 1.00) and a specificity of 0.86 (95% CI 0.70, 1.00). While the pooled estimates for PGP 9.5 suggest it could replace surgical diagnosis, there was significant diversity in the diagnostic estimates between the studies. It has been noted that PGP 9.5 expression is highly sensitive to variation in endometrial sampling and a narrow full-thickness biopsy with an adequate amount of stroma is critical to its detection. PGP 9.5 expression is also influenced by the microscopy method used and optimization of the assay as studies that utilized conventional light microscopy showed lower diagnostic estimates [43] and some immunohistochemical assays did not demonstrate a difference in PGP 9.5 staining between groups [44]. Thus, while the data for PGP 9.5 are encouraging, this biomarker needs further validation in large independent high-quality studies using standardized endometrial sampling and laboratory methods.

Several additional biomarkers assessed in individual studies displayed high diagnostic potential (Table 16.1). Additional work to comprehensively assess these biomarkers would be important to confirm their diagnostic role. Overall, most studies had major methodological flaws, and the data should be interpreted with caution.

Nonstandard methods of sample collection and processing, sampling at different phases of the menstrual cycle, and inconsistency in phenotyping the samples across studies lead to heterogeneity in papers that report the diagnostic accuracy of endometrial biomarkers. The method of obtaining endometrial sample appeared to influence the results of PGP 9.5, and this may be an issue for other biomarkers. Furthermore, different uterine or pelvic pathologies such as such as leiomyoma or adenomyosis could engender overlapping endometrial aberrations.

Uterine fluid has been increasingly explored using proteomic and metabolomics methods to try and identify biomarkers of endometriosis. To date there are no identified biomarkers in menstrual fluid that distinguish women with and without endometriosis with an acceptable sensitivity and specificity.

16.3.3 Concluding Remarks on Biomarkers for Endometriosis

In summary, none of the peripheral or endometrial biomarkers can be used in clinical practice outside a research setting. CA-125, the most studied biomarker, could serve as a rule in triage test (SpIN) , but the quality of CA-125 literature had not sufficiently improved in over several decades. The questions regarding its adequate cutoff levels and optimal test timing and contribution to clinical decision-making remain unanswered. While the majority of the investigated biomarkers were not diagnostically useful for endometriosis, for those markers that showed adequate diagnostic estimates, the evidence remains either conflicting or insufficient for meaningful recommendations. Low-quality heterogeneous studies and unstandardized research methods undermine the reliability of the presented results. There were no diagnostic studies that focused on the downstream value of the test in terms of health or behavioral consequences. Likewise, except for early low-quality reports on CA-125, no studies specifically assessed the role of the biomarkers in monitoring disease progression or recurrence.

16.4 Imaging Tests as a Diagnostic Tool for Endometriosis

While clinical presentations of endometriosis vary, morphological characteristics of endometriotic lesions appear to be consistent across different patient phenotypes and, if visualized with imaging methods, serve as basis for radiological markers of the disease. In addition, distorted pelvic anatomies such as retroverted uterus and decreased pelvic organ mobility indicate the presence of endometriosis in specific clinical context.

In addition to their ability to identify endometriosis lesions in a noninvasive way, imaging tests carry substantial advantages in preoperative assessment of women with clinically suspected deep endometriosis. In severe forms of the disease, proper pelvic visualization at laparoscopy can be obscured by adhesions, while preoperative lesion mapping can assist with completeness of surgical treatment. Furthermore, identifying deep infiltrating lesions of the bowel, bladder, or ureter can improve preoperative planning and patient counseling, which allows to establish appropriate referral pathways and to utilize multidisciplinary team approach in more effective way.

Over the years, large number of studies attempted to define diagnostic performance of different imaging tests in endometriosis, integrating emerging technologies and modifications to more traditional methods. In ultrasound field, modified methods include transvaginal ultrasound with bowel preparation (TVUS-BP), instillation of contrast medium transrectally (RWC-TVUS) or transvaginally (sonovaginography), and "tenderness-guided" approach with particular attention to the tender points evoked during examination and 3-D technology. In MRI, 3.0Tesla Magnetom system (3.0 T MRI); introduction of ultrasonographic gel into the vagina, rectum, or rectosigmoid (MRI jelly method); or utilization of three-dimensional coronal single-slab MRI (3D Cube) have been used in addition to more traditional systems.

The Cochrane Library systematic review assessed all the available imaging methods in one coherent document and demonstrated that transvaginal ultrasound (TVUS) and magnetic resonance imaging (MRI) were the most studied modalities [45]. In studies that did not specify type of endometriosis and presumably looked at the overall pelvic endometriosis, no imaging method met the diagnostic criteria for a replacement test or a triage test (Table 16.2). TVUS was the best performing method and had sensitivity of 0.79 (95% CI 0.36, 1.00) and specificity of 0.91 (95% CI 0.74, 1.00), although there was

Table 16.2 Diagnostic performance of different imaging methods for the diagnosis of endometriosis: a meta-analysis [47]

	Test	No. of studies; No. of participants	Pooled sensitivity (95% CI)	Pooled specificity (95% CI)	Comments
Pelvic endometriosis	TVUS	5; 1222	0.79 (0.36, 1.00)	0.91 (0.74, 1.00)	1 outlier study was excluded[a]
	MRI	7; 303	0.79 (0.70, 0.88)	0.72 (0.51, 0.92)	3.0T MRI (2 studies) showed the highest diagnostic accuracy
Ovarian endometriosis	TVUS	8; 765	0.93 (0.87, 0.99)	0.96 (0.92, 0.99)	Studies published after 2006 (4 studies) showed the highest diagnostic accuracy
	TRUS	1; 92	0.89 (0.74, 0.97)	0.77 (0.64, 0.87)	Meta-analysis was not possible
	MRI	3; 179	0.95 (0.90, 1.00)	0.91 (0.86, 0.97	3.0T MRI (2 studies) showed the highest diagnostic accuracy
Deep endometriosis (DE)	TVUS	9; 934	0.79 (0.69, 0.89)	0.94 (0.88, 1.00)	TVUS-BP (1 study) showed the highest diagnostic accuracy
	MRI	6; 266	0.94 (0.90, 0.97)	0.77 (0.44, 1.00)	3.0T MRI (2 studies) and MRI jelly method (1 study) showed the highest diagnostic accuracy
	DCBE	1; 69	0.36 (0.24, 0.48)	1.00 (0.16, 1.00)	Meta-analysis was not possible

DCBE double-contrast barium enema, *MRI* magnetic resonance imaging, *TRUS* transrectal ultrasound, *TVUS* transvaginal ultrasound, *TVUS-BP* transvaginal ultrasound with bowel preparation

[a]The excluded study utilized a sole single marker of endometriosis (kissing ovaries), in contrast to the other four studies that surveyed pelvic anatomy

substantial diversity in diagnostic estimates between the studies. Integration of TVUS with history of dysmenorrhea or dyspareunia and vaginal examination for the presence of pelvic tenderness, fixed retroverted uterus, or deeply infiltrating nodules resulted in improved sensitivity of 0.92 (95% CI 0.78, 0.98) but lower specificity of 0.61 (95% CI 0.48, 0.72) in a single study that included 106 women and did not present direct comparative data with TVUS alone [46].

For ovarian endometriosis, MRI met the criteria for a replacement test and TVUS approached these criteria and could qualify as a rule in (SpIN) triage test (Table 16.2). Overall, the studies published after 2006 demonstrated higher sensitivity for diagnosing endometrioma with ultrasound. Combination with CA-125 and CA-19.9 at different cutoff levels did not improve diagnostic performance of TVUS for detecting endometrioma, as demonstrated in one study in a total of 118 women [47], and there were no studies on other diagnostic combinations of imaging tests for endometrioma. One small study that performed direct head-to-head comparison between MRI, TVUS, and transrectal ultrasound (TRUS) showed that both MRI and TVUS provided comparable estimates in diagnosing ovarian endometriosis, while TRUS had lower diagnostic values [48].

For DE, MRI approached the criteria for a replacement test, and TVUS approached the criteria for a rule in (SpIN) triage test (Table 16.2). The direct comparison performed in one small study demonstrated that MRI performed better than 3D-TVUS in the diagnosis of DE, and there were no comparisons between MRI and other ultrasound methods [49]. Double-contrast barium enema (DCBE) was inferior to the other diagnostic methods for detecting DE.

Notably, tenderness-guided TVUS and TVUS-BP seemed to be the most accurate in detecting ovarian and deep endometriosis. Tenderness-guided TVUS (one study in 50 women) showed sensitivity of 1.00 (95% CI 0.66, 1.00) and specificity of 1.00 (95% CI 0.91, 1.00) in detecting ovarian endometrioma and sensitivity of 0.90 (95% CI 0.74, 0.98) with specificity of 0.95 (95% CI 0.74, 1.00) in detecting DE [50]. TVUS-BP (one study in 57 women) demonstrated sensitivity of 0.97 (95% CI 0.83, 1.00) with specificity of 1.00 (95% CI 0.87, 1.00) for endometrioma and sensitivity of 0.94 (95% CI 0.81, 0.99) with specificity of 1.00 (95% CI 0.85, 1.00) for DE [51], and the findings were replicated by another group in 85 women with endometrioma [52]. 3.0 T MRI showed higher sensitivity and specificity for diagnosing pelvic, ovarian, or deep endometriosis compared to other conventional MRI methods. However, there were no sufficient data for formal comparative analysis between different modified methods.

Substantial number of studies focused on mapping deep endometriotic lesions at specific anatomical sites, the approach which does not have primary diagnostic role but is important for planning surgical strategy (Table 16.3). For rectosigmoid endometriosis, which was evaluated in the largest number of studies, TVUS, TRUS, and MRI reached the criteria for a SpIN triage, indicating that positive findings could confirm rectosigmoid involvement, whereas negative imaging result was nonconclusive. Multi-detector computerized tomography enema (MDCT-e) appeared to be the best performing modality for rectosigmoid and other bowel endometriosis, showing sensitivity of 0.98 (95% CI 0.94, 1.00) with specificity of 0.99 (95% CI 0.97, 1.00) and sensitivity of 0.98 (95% CI 0.92, 1.00) with specificity of 1.00 (95% CI 1.00, 1.00), respectively.

For other anatomical locations, TVUS met the criteria for a rule in SpIN triage test in mapping DE to USL, rectovaginal septum (RVS), vaginal wall, and POD, which is consistent with the previous reports [53–55]. Combination of vaginal examination with TVUS much improved diagnostic accuracy for detecting DE in RVS, vaginal wall, POD, and rectum, but this was demonstrated in only one well-designed study in 200 women [56]. Modified ultrasound methods such as TVUS-BP and RWC-TVS showed the highest diagnostic accuracy for the evaluated anatomical locations of endometriosis. MRI could qualify as a SpIN triage test only for POD and vaginal wall endometriosis with overall better performance of 3.0 T MRI and MRI jelly methods. TRUS could not be adequately assessed for any of these sites due to paucity of the data. For the detection of bladder endometriosis (not evaluated in the Cochrane review), both TVUS and MRI could qualify as a SpIN triage test [54, 57]. Formal comparative analyses between TVUS and MRI methods were not possible due to paucity of the data.

Collectively, the meta-analysis revealed that although MRI was superior to TVUS in detecting endometrioma and DE, both methods showed comparable high diagnostic estimates when modified techniques were applied. Recently, MRI was promoted as the noninvasive imaging technique of choice for the detection and classification of endometriosis [58], although major advantages of MRI over TVUS were not consistently demonstrated. Both TVUS and MRI could accurately detect ovarian and deep endometriosis, which is consistently reported by most systematic reviews on the topic [53–57, 59]. TRUS does not appear to be superior to TVUS for any type or site of endometriosis, which questions clinical application of this method considering the discomfort experienced by women during transrectal examination. That said, TRUS remains a valid alternative for the subgroup of patients for whom transvaginal examination is not possible or not applicable.

Several factors limit translation of the above findings into clinical practice. Firstly, diagnostic efficacy was largely reported by small, uncontrolled studies lacking comparative data. Most tests showed considerable heterogeneity of the diagnostic estimates, which could be explained by variation in study design, populations studied, and surgical criteria applied. It is also possible that advances in technology make it difficult to compare earlier studies with more recent ones. Importantly, there is no consistency between the testing protocols and radiological diagnostic criteria across the studies, particularly for the ultrasound methods. Finally, most studies were conducted at the specialized centers for endometriosis with a high level of expertise in gynecological imaging, which is likely to result in higher diagnostic accuracy, and the method may not perform that well in more general setting. It has been reported that competency in performing ultrasound for DE can be achieved within 40 procedures [52, 60]. Thus, wide implementation of training programs by the centers of excellence in

Table 16.3 Imaging methods for surgical mapping of endometriosis to specific anatomical sites: a meta-analysis [47]

	Test	No. of studies; No. of participants	Pooled sensitivity (95% CI)	Pooled specificity (95% CI)	Comments
USL endometriosis	TVUS	7; 751	0.64 (0.50, 0.79)	0.97 (0.93, 1.00)	TVUS-BP (1 study) showed the highest diagnostic accuracy
	TRUS	2; 232	0.52 (0.29, 0.74)	0.94 (0.86, 1.00)	
	MRI	4; 199	0.86 (0.80, 0.92)	0.84 (0.68, 1.00)	3.0T MRI (1 study) showed the highest diagnostic accuracy
RVS endometriosis	TVUS	10; 983	0.88 (0.82, 0.94)	1.00 (0.98, 1.00)	TVUS-BP (3 studies) and RWC-TVS (1 study) showed the highest diagnostic accuracy
	TRUS	2; 232	0.78 (0.51, 1.00)	0.96 (0.89, 1.00)	
	MRI	3; 288	0.81 (0.70, 0.93)	0.86 (0.78, 0.95)	
Vaginal wall endometriosis	TVUS	6; 679	0.57 (0.21, 0.94)	0.99 (0.96, 1.00)	tg-TVUS (1 study) showed the highest diagnostic accuracy
	TRUS	2; 232	0.39 (0.08, 0.70)	1.00 (1.00, 1.00)	3.0T MRI (1 study) showed the highest diagnostic accuracy
	MRI	4; 248	0.77 (0.67, 0.88)	0.97 (0.92, 1.00)	3.0T MRI (1 study) showed the highest diagnostic accuracy
POD obliteration	TVUS	6; 755	0.83 (0.77, 0.88)	0.97 (0.95, 0.99)	TVUS-BP (2 studies) showed the highest diagnostic accuracy
	MRI	5; 154	0.90 (0.76, 1.00)	0.98 (0.89, 1.00)	3.0T MRI (3 studies) showed the highest diagnostic accuracy
Rectosigmoid endometriosis	TVUS	14; 1616	0.90 (0.82, 0.97)	0.96 (0.94, 0.99)	TVUS-BP (2 studies) and RWC-TVS (2 studies) showed the highest diagnostic accuracy
	TRUS	4; 330	0.91 (0.85, 0.98)	0.96 (0.91, 1.00)	
	MRI	6; 612	0.92 (0.86, 0.99)	0.96 (0.93, 0.98)	MRI jelly method (1 study) and 3.0T MRI (1 study) showed the highest diagnostic accuracy
	MDCT-e	3; 389	0.98 (0.94, 1.00)	0.98 (0.94, 1.00)	
	DCBE	2; 106	0.56 (0.32, 0.80)	0.77 (0.41, 1.00)	
Bowel (ileum-rectum) endometriosis	TVUS	3; 314	0.89 (0.81, 0.97)	0.96 (0.91, 1.00)	
	TRUS	1; 134	0.96 (0.89, 0.99)	1.00 (0.94, 1.00)	Meta-analysis was not possible
	MDCT-e	2; 194	0.98 (0.92, 1.00)	1.00 (1.00, 1.00)	

DCBE double-contrast barium enema, *MDCT-e* multi-detector computerized tomography enema, *MRI* magnetic resonance imaging, *RWC-TVS* rectal water contrast transvaginal ultrasonography, *TRUS* transrectal ultrasound, *TVUS* transvaginal ultrasound, *TVUS-BP* transvaginal ultrasound with bowel preparation, *tg-TVUS* tenderness-guided TVUS, *USL* utero-sacral ligament, *RVS* recto-vaginal septum, *POD* pouch of Douglas

endometriosis ultrasound is an important prerequisite for successful implementation of the method in general practice.

History and vaginal examination seem to improve the detection of overall pelvic and deep endometriosis, but these findings require further validation. Little data is available on combination of imaging tests with biomarkers and on incorporation of such tests in clinical decision pathways.

There is an ongoing debate regarding the significance of detecting superficial peritoneal implants, and some investigators suggest considering only the ovarian and deep forms as "definite disease" [8]. To resolve the controversy, noninvasive classification of different types of endometriosis would enable large population studies on natural history and clinical outcomes of surgical versus medical treatment in women with superficial peritoneal disease. As there are no diagnostic studies that applied modified, presumably more sensitive, techniques to detect superficial peritoneal lesions, the role of imaging in detecting this form of endometriosis remains unclear. Until new data emerge, the statement that superficial endometriosis cannot be readily seen with imaging methods continues to hold true.

16.5 Future Perspectives

The search for a noninvasive test for endometriosis has been an ongoing and challenging issue. Despite substantial research efforts, there is no rigorous scientific evidence to support the use of any of the evaluated biomarkers in everyday practice. Imaging tests are being increasingly employed as a diagnostic adjunct to surgery, but the evidence on their clinical efficacy and contribution to patient management remains elusive. There is an increasing demand on researches to reduce the effect of bias and to demonstrate clinical value of the tests in future evaluations.

It is important that future authors focus on clinically relevant population comprising the individuals who would benefit from the test in clinical practice [61]. Adherence to the standards for reporting of the diagnostic studies [62, 63], bio-specimen handling [64, 65], and laparoscopy [66] would result in more reliable assessment of test performance. We still don't have universally adopted criteria for any of the radiological methods in endometriosis, and these are urgently needed to standardize practice.

Applying testing to different clinical phenotypes rather than to rASRM staging and accounting for confounding effect of comorbidities is expected to refine a personalized approach to diagnosis [67]. Combining several tests in diagnostic algorithms is more likely to capture complex underlying mechanisms of endometriosis and may improve diagnostic performance [68, 69].

Reproducible research involves replication of the results by independent groups to improve validation of promising discoveries and relies on refined radiological protocols and standardized laboratory methods. Moreover, publishing negative findings, although less scientifically attractive, is important to guide clinically relevant experimental work [70].

The value of diagnostic test expands beyond its diagnostic accuracy, and there is a growing awareness that test should show clear evidence that it improves patient's health. Patient outcome studies that correlate test result with clinical outcomes [71] and test-treatment trials that inform on patient outcomes following treatment based on test results are essential within test evaluation framework [11]. Meaningful economic evaluations require high-quality data to rely on and should be carried out once the clinical performance of the test is demonstrated [71].

Finally, the authors of the original and review papers should shift from the standard "more studies needed" to more constructive topic-specific suggestions for future work. This will contribute to the collaborative effort to strengthen the clinically relevant diagnostic research in endometriosis.

References

1. Matsuzaki S, Canis M, Pouly JL, Rabischong B, Botchorishvili R, Mage G. Relationship between delay of surgical diagnosis and severity of disease in patients with symptomatic deep infiltrating endometriosis. Fertil Steril. 2006;86:1314–6.
2. Gao X, Yeh YC, Outley J, Simon J, Botteman M, Spalding J. Health-related quality of life burden of women with endometriosis: a literature review. Curr Med Res Opin. 2006;22:1787–97.
3. Ballard KD, Seaman HE, de Vries CS, Wright JT. Can symptomatology help in the diagnosis of endometriosis? Findings from a national case-control study - Part 1. BJOG. 2008;115(11):1382–91.
4. Nnoaham KE, Hummelshoj L, Kennedy SH, Jenkinson C, Zondervan KT, World Endometriosis Research Foundation Women's Health Symptom Survey Consortium. Developing symptom-based pre-

dictive models of endometriosis as a clinical screening tool: results from a multicenter study. Fertil Steril. 2012;98:692–701.

5. Eskenazi B, Warner M, Bonsignore L, Olive D, Samuels S, Vercellini P. Validation study of nonsurgical diagnosis of endometriosis. Fertil Steril. 2001;76(5):929–35.
6. Wykes CB, Clark TJ, Khan KS. Accuracy of laparoscopy in the diagnosis of endometriosis: a systematic quantitative review. BJOG. 2004;111:1204–12.
7. Johnson NP, Hummelshoj L, Consortium WESM. Consensus on current management of endometriosis. Hum Reprod. 2013;28:1552–68.
8. Vercellini P, Giudice LC, Evers JL, Abrao M. Reducing low-value care in endometriosis between limited evidence and unresolved issues: a proposal. Hum Reprod. 2015;30:1996–2004.
9. Johnson NP, Hummelshoj L, Adamson GD, Keckstein J, Taylor HS, Abrao MS, Bush D, Kiesel L, Tamimi R, Sharpe-Timms KL, Rombauts L. World Endometriosis Society consensus on the classification of endometriosis. Hum Reprod. 2017;32:315–24.
10. Nisenblat V, Bossuyt PMM, Shaikh R, Arora D, Farquhar C, Jordan V, Scheffers CS, Mol BWJ, Johnson N, Hull ML. Blood biomarkers for the non invasive diagnosis of endometriosis. Cochrane Database Syst Rev. 2016;(5):CD012179. doi:https://doi.org/10.1002/14651858.
11. Bossuyt PMM, Reitsma JB, Linnet K, Moons KGM. Beyond diagnostic accuracy: the clinical utility of diagnostic tests. Clin Chem. 2012;58(12):1636–43.
12. Giudice LC, Kao LC. Endometriosis. Lancet. 2004;364:1789–99.
13. Burney RO. The genetics and biochemistry of endometriosis. Curr Opin Obstet Gynecol. 2013;25(4):280–6.
14. May KE, Conduit-Hulbert SA, Villar J, Kirtley S, Kennedy SH, Becker CM. Peripheral biomarkers of endometriosis: a systematic review. Hum Reprod Update. 2010;16:651–74.
15. Liu E, Nisenblat V, Farquhar C, Fraser I, Bossuyt PMM, Johnson N, Hull ML. Urinary biomarkers for the non invasive diagnosis of endometriosis. Cochrane Database Syst Rev. 2015;(12):CD012019. doi: https://doi.org/10.1002/14651858.
16. Mol BW, Bayram N, Lijmer JG, Wiegerinck MA, Bongers MY, van der Veen F, Bossuyt PM. The performance of CA-125 measurement in the detection of endometriosis: a meta-analysis. Fertil Steril. 1998;70(6):1101–8.
17. Hirsch M, Duffy J, Davis CJ, Nieves Plana M, Khan KS. Diagnostic accuracy of cancer antigen 125 for endometriosis: a systematic review and meta-analysis. BJOG. 2016;123(11):1761–8.
18. Hirsch M, Duffy JMN, Deguara CS, Davis CJ, Khan KS. Diagnostic accuracy of Cancer Antigen 125 (CA125) for endometriosis in symptomatic women: a multi-center study. Eur J Obstet Gynecol Reprod Biol. 2017;210:102–7.
19. Chen FP, Soong YK, Lee N, Lo SK. The use of serum CA-125 as a marker for endometriosis in patients with dysmenorrhea for monitoring therapy and for recurrence of endometriosis. Acta Obstet Gynecol Scand. 1998;77(6):665–70.
20. Agic A, Djalali S, Wolfler MM, Halis G, Diedrich K, Hornung D. Combination of CCR1 mRNA, MCP1, and CA125 measurements in peripheral blood as a diagnostic test for endometriosis. Reprod Sci. 2008;15(9):906–11.
21. Lanzone A, Marana R, Muscatello R, Fulghesu AM, Dellacqua S, Caruso A, Mancuso S. Serum Ca-125 levels in the diagnosis and management of endometriosis. J Reprod Med. 1991;36(8):603–7.
22. Vouk K, Hevir N, Ribic-Pucelj M, Haarpaintner G, Scherb H, Osredkar J, et al. Discovery of phosphatidylcholines and sphingomyelins as biomarkers for ovarian endometriosis. Hum Reprod. 2012;27(10):2955–65.
23. Koninckx PR, Meuleman C, Oosterlynck D, Cornillie FJ. Diagnosis of deep endometriosis by clinical examination during menstruation and plasma CA-125 concentration. Fertil Steril. 1996;65(2):280–7.
24. Vicente-Muñoz S, Morcillo I, Puchades-Carrasco L, Payá V, Pellicer A, Pineda-Lucena A. Pathophysiologic processes have an impact on the plasma metabolomic signature of endometriosis patients. Fertil Steril. 2016;106(7):1733–41.
25. Letsiou S, Peterse DP, Fassbender A, Hendriks MM, van den Broek NJ, Berger R, O DF, Vanhie A, Vodolazkaia A, Van Langendonckt A, Donnez J, Harms AC, Vreeken RJ, Groothuis PG, Dolmans MM, Brenkman AB, D'Hooghe TM. Endometriosis is associated with aberrant metabolite profiles in plasma. Fertil Steril. 2017;107(3):699–706.
26. Liu HY, Zheng YH, Zhang JZ, Leng JH, Sun DW, Liu ZF, et al. Establishment of endometriosis diagnostic model using plasma protein profiling. Chung-Hua Fu Chan Ko Tsa Chih [Chinese J Obstet Gynecol]. 2009;44(8):601–4.
27. Seeber B, Sammel MD, Fan X, Gerton GL, Shaunik A, Chittams J, et al. Proteomic analysis of serum yields six candidate proteins that are differentially regulated in a subset of women with endometriosis. Fertil Steril. 2010;93(7):2137–44.
28. Fassbender A, Waelkens E, Verbeeck N, Kyama CM, Bokor A, Vodolazkaia A, et al. Proteomics analysis of plasma for early diagnosis of endometriosis. Obstet Gynecol. 2012;119(2 Pt 1):276–85.
29. Wolfler MM, Schwamborn K, Otten D, Hornung D, Liu HY, Rath W. Mass spectrometry and serum pattern profiling for analyzing the individual risk for endometriosis: promising insights? Fertil Steril. 2009;91(6):2331–7.
30. Jia SZ, Yang Y, Lang J, Sun P, Leng J. Plasma miR-17-5p, miR-20a and miR-22 are down-regulated in women with endometriosis. Hum Reprod. 2013;28(2):322–30.
31. Wang WT, Zhao YN, Han BW, Hong SJ, Chen YQ, Wang X, et al. Circulating microRNAs identified in a genome-wide serum microRNA expression analysis as noninvasive biomarkers for endometriosis

[Study on polymorphism of human leukocyte antigen I in patients with endometriosis]. J Clin Endocrinol Metab. 2013;98(1):281–9.
32. Cosar E, Mamillapalli R, Ersoy GS, Cho S, Seifer B, Taylor HS. Serum microRNAs as diagnostic markers of endometriosis: a comprehensive array-based analysis. Fertil Steril. 2016;106(2):402–9.
33. Cho S, Mutlu L, Grechukhina O, Taylor HS. Circulating microRNAs as potential biomarkers for endometriosis. Fertil Steril. 2015;103(5): 1252–60.
34. Wang L, Liu HY, Shi HH, Lang JH, Sun W. Urine peptide patterns for non-invasive diagnosis of endometriosis:a preliminary prospective study. Eur J Obstet Gynecol Reprod Biol. 2014;177:23–8.
35. Vicente-Muñoz S, Morcillo I, Puchades-Carrasco L, Payá V, Pellicer A, Pineda-Lucena A. Nuclear magnetic resonance metabolomic profiling of urine provides a noninvasive alternative to the identification of biomarkers associated with endometriosis. Fertil Steril. 2015;104(5):1202–9.
36. Burney RO, Talbi S, Hamilton AE, Kim CV, Nyegaard M, Nezhat CR, et al. Gene expression analysis of endometrium reveals progesterone resistance and candidate susceptibility genes in women with endometriosis. Endocrinology. 2007;148:3814–26.
37. Kim JJ, Taylor HS, Lu Z, Ladhani O, Hastings JM, Jackson KS, et al. Altered expression of HOXA10 in endometriosis: potential role in decidualization. Mol Hum Reprod. 2007;13:323–32.
38. Brosens I, Brosens JJ, Benagiano G. The eutopic endometrium in endometriosis: are the changes of clinical significance? Reprod Biomed Online. 2012;24:496–502.
39. Guo SW. Epigenetics of endometriosis. Mol Hum Reprod. 2009;15:587–607.
40. Houshdaran S, Nezhat CR, Vo KC, Zelenko Z, Irwin JC, Giudice LC. Aberrant endometrial DNA methylome and associated gene expression in endometriosis. Biol Reprod. 2016;95(5):93.
41. Bhusane K, Bhutada S, Chaudhari U, Savardekar L, Katkam R, Sachdeva G. Secrets of endometrial receptivity: some are hidden in uterine secretome. Am J Reprod Immunol. 2016;75:226–36.
42. Gupta D, Hull ML, Fraser I, Miller L, Bossuyt PMM, Johnson N, Farquhar C, Nisenblat V. Endometrial biomarkers for the non invasive diagnosis of endometriosis. Cochrane Database Syst Rev. 2016;(4):CD012165. doi:https://doi.org/10.1002/14651858.
43. Leslie C, Ma T, McElhinney B, Leake R, Stewart CJ. Is the detection of endometrial nerve fibers useful in the diagnosis of endometriosis? Int J Gynecol Pathol. 2013;32(2):149–55.
44. Cetin C, Serdaroglu H, Tuzali S. The importance of endometrial nerve fibres and macrophage cell count in the diagnosis of endometriosis. Iran J Reprod Med. 2013;11(5):405–14.
45. Nisenblat V, Bossuyt PMM, Farquhar C, Johnson N, Hull ML. Imaging modalities for the non invasive diagnosis of endometriosis. Cochrane Database Syst Rev. 2016;4:CD009591. doi:https://doi.org/10.1002/14651858.
46. Marasinghe J, Senanayake H, Saravanabhava N, Arambepola C, Condous G, Greenwood P. History, pelvic examination findings and mobility of ovaries as a sonographic marker to detect pelvic adhesions with fixed ovaries. J Obstet Gynaecol Res. 2014;40(3):785–90.
47. Guerriero S, Ajossa S, Paoletti AM, Mais V, Angiolucci M, Melis GB. Tumour marker and transvaginal ultrasonography in the diagnosis of endometrioma. Obstet Gynaecol. 1996;88(3):403–7.
48. Bazot M, Lafont C, Rouzier R, Roseau G, Thomassin-Naggara I, Darai E. Diagnostic accuracy of physical examination, transvaginal sonography, rectal endoscopic sonography, and magnetic resonance imaging to diagnose deep infiltrating endometriosis. Fertil Steril. 2009;92(6):1825–33.
49. Grasso RF, Di Giacomo V, Sedati P, Sizzi O, Florio G, Faiella E, et al. Diagnosis of deep infiltrating endometriosis: accuracy of magnetic resonance imaging and transvaginal 3D ultrasonography. Abdom Imaging. 2010;35(6):716–25.
50. Guerriero S, Ajossa S, Gerada M, D'Aquila M, Piras B, Melis GB. "Tenderness-guided" transvaginal ultrasonography: a new method for the detection of deep endometriosis in patients with chronic pelvic pain. Fertil Steril. 2007;88:1293–7.
51. Scarella AC, Devoto LC, Villarroel CQ, Inzunza NP, Quilodrán FR, Sovino HS. Transvaginal ultrasound for preoperative detection of deep endometriosis in patients with chronic pelvic pain [Ultrasonido transvaginal para la detección preoperatoria de endometriosis profunda en pacientes con dolor pélvico crónico]. Rev Chil Obstet Ginecol. 2013;78(2):114–8.
52. Piessens S, Healey M, Maher P, Tsaltas J, Rombauts L. Can anyone screen for deep infiltrating endometriosis with transvaginal ultrasound? Aust N Z J Obstet Gynaecol. 2014;54(5):462–8.
53. Hudelist G, English J, Thomas AE, Tinelli A, Singer CF, Keckstein J. Diagnostic accuracy of transvaginal ultrasound for non-invasive diagnosis of bowel endometriosis: systematic review and meta-analysis. Ultrasound Obstet Gynecol. 2011;37(3):257–63.
54. Guerriero S, Ajossa S, Minguez JA, Jurado M, Mais V, Melis GB, Alcazar JL. Accuracy of transvaginal ultrasound for diagnosis of deep endometriosis in uterosacral ligaments, rectovaginal septum, vagina and bladder: systematic review and meta-analysis. Ultrasound Obstet Gynecol. 2015;46:534–45.
55. Guerriero S, Ajossa S, Orozco R, Perniciano M, Jurado M, Melis GB, Alcazar JL. Accuracy of transvaginal ultrasound for diagnosis of deep endometriosis in the rectosigmoid: systematic review and meta-analysis. Ultrasound Obstet Gynecol. 2016;47(3):281–9.
56. Hudelist G, Oberwinkler KH, Singer CF, Tuttlies F, Rauter G, Ritter O, et al. Combination of transvaginal sonography and clinical examination for preoperative diagnosis of pelvic endometriosis. Hum Reprod. 2009;24(5):1018–24.

57. Medeiros LR, Rosa MI, Silva BR, Reis ME, Simon CS, Dondossola ER, da Cunha Filho JS. Accuracy of magnetic resonance in deeply infiltrating endometriosis: a systematic review and meta-analysis. Arch Gynecol Obstet. 2015;291(3):611–21.
58. Saba L, Sulcis R, Melis GB, de Cecco CN, Laghi A, Piga M, et al. Endometriosis: the role of magnetic resonance imaging. Acta Radiol. 2014, 56(3):355–67.
59. Moore J, Copley S, Morris J, LIndsell D, Golding S, Kennedy S. A systematic review of the accuracy of ultrasound in the diagnosis of endometriosis. Ultrasound Obstet Gynecol. 2002;20:630–4.
60. Tammaa A, Fritzer N, Strunk G, Krell A, Salzer H, Hudelist G. Learning curve for the detection of pouch of Douglas obliteration and deep infiltrating endometriosis of the rectum. Hum Reprod. 2014;29(6):1199–204.
61. Rutjes AWS, Reitsma JB, Vandenbroucke JP, Glas AS, Bossuyt PMM. Case–control and two-gate designs in diagnostic accuracy studies. Clin Chem. 2005;51(8):1335–41.
62. Bossuyt PM, Reitsma JB, Bruns DE, Gatsonis CA, Glasziou PP, Irwig LM, et al. Towards complete and accurate reporting of studies of diagnostic accuracy: the STARD initiative. BMJ. 2003;326(7379):41–4.
63. Whiting PF, Rutjes AW, Westwood ME, Mallett S, Deeks JJ, Reitsma JB, et al., the QUADAS-2 Group. QUADAS-2: a revised tool for the quality assessment of diagnostic accuracy studies. Ann Intern Med. 2011;155(8):529–36.
64. Fassbender A, Rahmioglu N, Vitonis AF, Vigano P, Giudice LC, D'Hooghe TM, Hummelshoj L, Adamson GD, Becker CM, Missmer SA, Zondervan KT. World Endometriosis Research Foundation Endometriosis Phenome and biobanking harmonization project: IV. Tissue collection, processing, and storage in endometriosis research. Fertil Steril. 2014;102(5):1244–53.
65. Rahmioglu N, Fassbender A, Vitonis AF, Tworoger SS, Hummelshoj L, D'Hooghe TM, Adamson GD, Giudice LC, Becker CM, Zondervan KR, Missmer SA. World Endometriosis Research Foundation Endometriosis Phenome and biobanking harmonization project: III. Fluid biospecimen collection, processing, and storage in endometriosis research. Fertil Steril. 2014;102(5):1233–43.
66. Becker CM, Laufer MR, Stratton P, Hummelshoj L, Missmer SA, Zondervan KT, Adamson GD. World Endometriosis Research Foundation Endometriosis Phenome and biobanking harmonization project: I. Surgical phenotype data collection in endometriosis research. Fertil Steril. 2014;102(5):1213–22.
67. Vitonis AF, Vincent K, Rahmioglu N, Fassbender A, Buck Louis G, Hummelshoj L, Giudice L, Stratton P, Adamson GD, Becker CM, Zondervan KR, Missmer SA. World Endometriosis Research Foundation Endometriosis Phenome and biobanking harmonization project: II. Clinical and covariate phenotype data collection in endometriosis research. Fertil Steril. 2014;102(5):1223–32.
68. Ahn SH, Singh V, Tayade C. Biomarkers in endometriosis: challenges and opportunities. Fertil Steril. 2017;107(3):523–32.
69. Nisenblat V, Prentice L, Bossuyt PMM, Farquhar C, Hull ML, Johnson N. Combination of the non-invasive tests for the diagnosis of endometriosis. Cochrane Database Syst Rev. 2016;7:CD012281.doi:https://doi.org/10.1002/14651858.
70. Pusztai L, Hatzis C, Andre F. Nat Rev Clin Oncol. 2013;10:720–4.
71. Horvath AR, Lord SJ, StJohn A, Sandberg S, Cobbaert CM, Lorenz S, Monaghan PJ, Verhagen-Kamerbeek WD, Ebert C, Bossuyt PM, Test Evaluation Working Group of the European Federation of Clinical Chemistry Laboratory Medicine. From biomarkers to medical tests: the changing landscape of test evaluation. Clin Chim Acta. 2014;427:49–57.

17 Clinical Cases and Videos

Mauricio León, Hugo Sovino, and Juan Luis Alcazar

17.1 Introduction

The diagnosis of deep endometriosis (DE) using transvaginal ultrasound (TVS) is an operator-dependent technique. For this method to be optimized, it must be done in a standardized way by an experienced operator. This standard approach in obtaining and analyzing the images has been recently published by a group of world experts, the International Deep Endometriosis Analysis (IDEA) group, and this consensus statement is reviewed in detail in Chap. 3 [1].

This chapter aims to show some of examples of different clinical scenarios in women with different types of DE lesions diagnosed using TVS. Each case will also discuss the subsequent management implemented.

Electronic Supplementary Material The online version of this chapter (https://doi.org/10.1007/978-3-319-71138-6_17) contains supplementary material, which is available to authorized users.

M. León (✉)
Ultrasound Unit, Department of Gynaecology and Obstetrics, Clinica INDISA, Santiago, Chile

H. Sovino
Department of Obstetrics and Gynecology, Human Reproduction Unit, Clìnica INDISA, Santiago, Chile

J. L. Alcazar
Department of Obstetrics and Gynecology, Clínica Universidad de Navarra School of Medicine, University of Navarra, Pamplona, Spain
e-mail: jlalcazar@unav.es

17.2 Clinical Case Number 1

AGE: 28 years.
Ethnic Origin: Latina.
Surgical Antecedents: no.
Family History of Endometriosis: no.

History

Nulligravida, with past history of using contraceptive pills in the context of severe dysmenorrhea of 4 years of evolution. Dyspareunia (+); dyschezia (+); without hematuria, hematochezia, or dysuria; with chronic pelvic pain since 2 years ago.

Currently under study for infertility.

Vaginal Examination

Presence of palpable nodule in the posterior vaginal fornix of 2 cm in diameter. In addition, it can be observed a vagina with complete longitudinal septum and, in the bottom of it, can be observed two cervices.

Video

Explanation (video): complete septate uterus, rectovaginal nodule with involvement of vaginal posterior wall, uterosacral ligaments, and anterior rectum wall (diabolo-like nodule).

S. Guerriero et al. (eds.), *How to Perform Ultrasonography in Endometriosis*,
https://doi.org/10.1007/978-3-319-71138-6_17

Management

Laparoscopy and hysteroscopy were done in the same surgery. Resection of the uterus septum was done. Rectovaginal nodule was confirmed during surgery, and only was necessary a shaving rectal procedure. Evolution: satisfactory.

17.3 Clinical Case Number 2

AGE: 30 years.
Ethnic Origin: Latina.
Surgical Antecedents: no.
Family History of Endometriosis: no.

History

Nulligravida, with history of using contraceptive pills in the context of polycystic ovary syndrome. After leaving contraceptives, the patient had severe dysmenorrhea for 1 year. Dyspareunia (+), dyschezia (+), without hematuria, hematochezia, or dysuria. No infertility.

Vaginal Examination

Palpable nodule in the posterior vaginal fornix of 1.5 cm in diameter and involvement of uterosacral ligament insertion.

Video

Explanation (video): Presence of negative sliding sign in the anterior compartment (obliteration of uterovesical region). Also can be observed a uterovesical region nodule of 12 × 10 × 12 mm.

In the posterior compartment, it is possible to observe a nodule of 16 × 9 × 12 mm with involvement of left uterosacral ligament insertion.

Management

Laparoscopy was done. In this procedure, deep endometriosis (DE) was found. Left uterosacral ligament resection was necessary due to presence of nodule in these site of 2 comes .anuterovesical region nodule of 3 cm was also confirmed and resected.

17.4 Clinical Case Number 3

AGE: 41 years.
Ethnic Origin: Latina.
Surgical Antecedents: ovarian cystectomy for endometriosis (2010).
Family History of Endometriosis: no.

History

Multiparous of two vaginal births, with past history of dysmenorrhea for 7 years and use of contraceptive pills, diverse analgesics, and anti-inflammatories. Dysmenorrhea (+), dyspareunia (+), dyschezia (+), without hematuria, hematochezia, or dysuria.

Vaginal Examination

Palpable nodule in the posterior vaginal fornix of 3 cm in diameter.

Video

Explanation (video): Presence of fixed ovaries, right atypical endometrioma with solid component without vascularization. Corpus luteum in the left ovary and presence of two anterior rectal wall nodules of 12 × 11 × 8 mm and 13 × 7 × 9 mm, respectively (multifocal lesions). Also, it can be observed another lesion of 14 × 10 × 11 mm in between both rectal lesions. Negative sliding sign in the posterior compartment.

Management

Multidisciplinary equipment was used. Diagnostic and surgical laparoscopy was done. In this procedure, extensive DIE was found, and the findings visualized in the transvaginal ultrasound were confirmed. Hysterectomy was performed, and a discoidal resection was necessary to remove the rectal lesion.

17.5 Clinical Case Number 4

AGE: 32 years.
Ethnic Origin: Latina.
Surgical Antecedents: no.
Family History of Endometriosis: no.

History

Nulligravida, with antecedents of using contraceptive pills for 2 years, with infertility history and failed treatment. Also since 6 months ago, the patient refers progressive dysmenorrhea, with dyspareunia and dyschezia, without hematuria, hematochezia, or dysuria.

Vaginal Examination

Palpable nodule in the posterior vaginal fornix and pouch of Douglas of 3 cm in diameter.

Video

Explanation (video): Multifocal compromise of rectosigmoid with anterior rectal wall nodules with complete septate uterus. In addition, you can observe another lesion with compromise of the left uterosacral ligament and posterior vaginal wall.

Management

Multidisciplinary equipment was used. In laparoscopic surgery, an anterior rectal nodule of 4 cm with uterosacral ligament and vaginal involvement was found. A discoidal resection and termino-terminal resection were necessary to remove the rectal lesion completely.

17.6 Clinical Case Number 5

AGE: 35 years.
Ethnic Origin: Latina.
Surgical Antecedents: LIE I surgery.
Family History of Endometriosis: no.

History

Nulligravida, with antecedents of the use of contraceptive pills during 1 year. She refers progressive dysmenorrhea, with dyspareunia and dyschezia, without hematuria, hematochezia, or dysuria.

Vaginal Examination

Palpable rectovaginal nodule of 2.5 cm of higher diameter, painful on palpation.

Video

Explanation (video): The measurement of anterior rectal wall nodule was 22 × 9 × 14 mm, without involvement of submucosa. Another lesion of 14 × 9 × 10 mm, fixed to the previous one, involving the uterosacral ligaments was found.

Management

Multidisciplinary equipment was used. In laparoscopic surgery was found an anterior rectal nodule of 2 cm in diameter with uterosacral ligament involvement. A shaving resection was necessary to remove the rectal lesion.

17.7 Clinical Case Number 6

AGE: 37 years.
Ethnic Origin: Latina.
Surgical Antecedents: no.
Family History of Endometriosis: no.

History

Multiparous of one vaginal birth, with antecedents of 1 year with left lumbar pain associated to dysmenorrhea and occasional dysuria, without dyspareunia, dyschezia, hematuria, or hematochezia.

Vaginal Examination

Vaginal examination: normal.

Video

Explanation (video): Bladder dome nodule of 10 × 7 × 10 mm.
Ureteral intravesical segment nodule (extrinsic compromise) of 18 × 9 × 10 mm.

Management

Multidisciplinary equipment was used (urologist-gynecologist). In laparoscopic surgery, the findings visualized in the transvaginal ultrasound were confirmed. A laparoscopic resection of both lesions was realized. A ureteral neo-implant was required.

17.8 Clinical Case Number 7

AGE: 28 years.
Ethnic Origin: Latina-Amerindian.
Surgical Antecedents: NO.
Family History of Endometriosis: no.

History

Nulligravida, with antecedents of 2 years with progressive dysmenorrhea accompanied by dysuria, without dyspareunia, dyschezia, hematuria, or hematochezia.

Vaginal Examination

A painful nodule of 1.5 cm behind the cervix was palpated.

Video

Explanation (video): Bladder base intramural nodule of 19 × 20 × 21 mm, without compromise of intravesical ureters. Also can be observed a right uterosacral ligament nodule of 9 × 6 × 7 mm, fixed to the posterior vaginal wall.

Management

Multidisciplinary equipment was used (urologist-gynecologist). In laparoscopic surgery was resected a bladder base nodule of 4 cm of higher diameter, without mucosa involvement. A right uterosacral ligament nodule of 1 cm was resected.

17.9 Clinical Case Number 8

AGE: 31 years.
Ethnic Origin: Latina.
Surgical Antecedents: no.
Family History of Endometriosis: no.

History

Nulligravida, referring with dysmenorrhea, dyspareunia, dyschezia, and anal catamenial pain, without hematochezia, hematuria, or dysuria, for 2 years.

Vaginal Examination

Palpable nodule in the posterior vaginal fornix and pouch of Douglas of 2.5 cm in diameter.

Video

Explanation (video): A rectosigmoid anterior rectal wall nodule of 43 × 13 × 14 mm with involvement of vagina and uterosacral ligament. In addition, you can observe another lesion of 16 × 16 × 11 mm.

Management

Multidisciplinary equipment was used. In laparoscopic surgery was found an anterior rectal nodule of 4 cm in diameter with uterosacral ligament and vaginal involvement. A discoidal resection and termino-terminal resection were necessary to remove the rectal lesion completely.

17.10 Clinical Case Number 9

AGE: 39 years.
Ethnic Origin: Latina.
Surgical Antecedents: left nephrectomy secondary to chronic urinary obstruction.
Family History of Endometriosis: no.

History

Multiparous of one vaginal birth, with antecedents of one missed abortion. A clinical history of chronic pelvic pain (7 years of evolution) with severe dysmenorrhea, dyspareunia (+), dyschezia (+), without hematochezia, hematuria, or dysuria.

Vaginal Examination

Very difficult vaginal examination due to severe pain.

Video

Explanation (video): At seven centimeters from the anal verge, it can be seen a rectosigmoid anterior rectal wall nodule with involvement of vagina and uterosacral ligaments of 42 × 7 × 19 mm. Also you can observe vaginal lesion of 17 × 8 × 12 mm.

Management

Multidisciplinary equipment was used (proctologist-gynecologist). In laparoscopic surgery was found an anterior rectal nodule of 4 cm of higher diameter with uterosacral ligament and vaginal involvement. A vaginal shaving was performed, and termino-terminal resection of the rectosigmoid lesion (with immediate reanastomosis) was necessary to remove the rectal lesion completely.

17.11 Clinical Case Number 10

AGE: 30 years.
Ethnic Origin: Latina.
Surgical Antecedents: no.
Family History of Endometriosis: no.

History

Nulligravida, with history of 3 years of infertility and of 3 years with progressive and severe dysmenorrhea, which has worsened in the last 4 months. Dyspareunia (+), dyschezia (+), hematochezia (+), without hematuria, or dysuria.

Vaginal Examination

Very difficult vaginal examination due to severe pain.

Video

Explanation (video): Retroverted uterus. A rectosigmoid anterior rectal wall nodule with transmural compromise with involvement of submucosa of 30 × 10 × 22 mm. It can be observed a lesion involving the uterosacral ligaments with superficial vaginal involvement.

Management

Multidisciplinary equipment was used (proctologist-gynecologist). In laparoscopic surgery was found an anterior rectal nodule of 2 cm of higher diameter (with involvement of submucosa) with uterosacral ligament and vaginal involvement. A rectal shaving was performed, and termino-terminal resection of the rectosigmoid lesion (with immediate reanastomosis) was necessary to remove the rectal lesion totally.

Reference

1. Guerriero S, Condous G, van den Bosch T, Valentin L, Leone FP, Van Schoubroeck D, Exacoustos C, Installé AJ, Martins WP, Abrao MS, Hudelist G, Bazot M, Alcazar JL, Gonçalves MO, Pascual MA, Ajossa S, Savelli L, Dunham R, Reid S, Menakaya U, Bourne T, Ferrero S, Leon M, Bignardi T, Holland T, Jurkovic D, Benacerraf B, Osuga Y, Somigliana E, Timmerman D. Systematic approach to sonographic evaluation of the pelvis in women with suspected endometriosis, including terms, definitions and measurements: a consensus opinion from the International Deep Endometriosis Analysis (IDEA) group. Ultrasound Obstet Gynecol. 2016;48(3):318–32. https://doi.org/10.1002/uog.15955. Epub 2016 Jun 28. PubMed PMID: 27349699.

Index

A

Abdominal wall endometriosis
- appendiceal endometriosis, 126
- causes, 122
- definition, 121
- evaluation of localization, 127
- hepatic endometriosis, 126
- HIFU ablation, 128
- inguinal endometriosis, 122, 125
- intra-abdominal endometriosis, 125
- MRI, 128
- oral contraceptives, 126
- rectus abdominis endometriosis, 125, 126, 130
- scar endometriosis, 122–124, 128, 129
- symptoms of, 122
- technical guidelines, 127, 128
- 3D sonography, 128
- transabdominal sonography, 127
- ultrasonographic findings, 127
- Villar's nodule, 122, 124, 129

Acoustic streaming, 51
Add-back therapy, 16
Adenomyosis, 37–45, 161
Allodynia, 3, 4
Anterior compartment endometriosis, *see* Urinary tract endometriosis (UTE)
Antiangiogenic agents, 17–18
Appendiceal endometriosis, 126
Aromatase inhibitors, 17
Asymptomatic ovarian endometrioma, 47
Atypical endometriomas, 50
Avascular pelvic spaces, 7

B

Benign endometriomas, 51
Biomarkers
- endometrial biomarkers, 174–176
- peripheral biomarkers, 172–174

Bladder endometriosis, 19, 68–70
Bladder endometriotic nodule, 69–74
Bowel endometriosis, 9–10, 33

C

CA-125, 172, 173, 176
Cabergoline, 18
Canal of nuck endometriosis, *see* Inguinal endometriosis
Case studies, 185–189
Chocolate cyst, 47
Chocolate cysts, *see* Ovarian endometrioma
Cochrane Library diagnostic test review, 170, 172, 173, 175, 176
Color score, 41, 42
Combined technique, 18
Computed tomography (CT), 148, 163
CYP19 biomarker, 175
Cystic lesion, 47, 48
Cystoscopy, 69
Cytokeratin 19 (CK 19 or CYFRA 21-1), 173

D

Danazol, 16
Decidualized endometriosis, 51, 54, 153, 154
Deep endometriosis, 28, 57, 67
- anatomical locations, 156
- anterior compartment, 156
- anterior pelvic compartment (*see* Urinary badder endometriosis)
- bladder involvement, 156
- clinical and functional requirements, 156
- contrast enhancement, 161
- cyclic haematuria, 156
- endometrial tissue, 156
- endometriotic implants, 155, 161
- fibrous tissue, 160
- inflammatory reaction, 161
- intestinal wall infiltration, 162
- middle compartment, 158
- MRI, 155, 156
- nonstriated muscular fibres, 160
- posterior compartments, 158, 160
- pouch of Douglas, 161
- presurgical planning, 162
- rectal opacification, 158

S. Guerriero et al. (eds.), *How to Perform Ultrasonography in Endometriosis*,
https://doi.org/10.1007/978-3-319-71138-6

Deep infiltrating endometriosis (*cont.*)
    rectosigmoid, 161
    rectouterine pouch, 161
    retractile adhesions, 157
    retrocervical area, 159
    symptoms, 155
    torus uterinus, 160
    treatment, 155
    of uterus, 158
    vesicovaginal septum, 156
Deep intestinal endometriosis
    computerized tomography, 104
    cul-de-sac block blockage, 114, 115
    definition, 103
    differential diagnoses, 116
    double discoid resection, 114
    exam time, 116
    false positives, 116
    MRI, 104
    multifocal bowel lesions, 103
    noninvasive diagnosis, 104
    pain reduction factors, 117, 118
    rectosigmoidectomy, 114
    right iliac fossa examination, 112
    slow development curve, 115
    suprapubic examination, 112, 113
    symptoms, 103
    3D equipment, 118
    three-dimensional transducers, 113
    transvaginal transducer, 113, 115
    treatment, 104
    TVUS examination
        anal verge, 109–111
        bowel circumference, 106–108
        bowel layers, 105, 106
        deep lesions, 105–107
        distal segment of colon, 104, 105
        infiltrated intestinal layer, 109, 110
        learning process, 118
        lesion size, 106, 108
        number of lesions, 106, 108
        rectal and sigmoid lesions, 110
        stenosis, 109
    ultrasound examination, 110–112
Deep pelvic endometriosis, *see* Deep infiltrating endometriosis
Dermoid cysts, 154
Diagnosis
    imaging, 6
    limitations, 1, 2
    triage patients, 4
Diagnostic test for endometriosis, 172, 176–178
    biomarkers (*see* Biomarkers)
    future perspectives, 180
    laparoscopic visualization, 169
    quantifying performance, 170–171
    tenderness-guided TVUS, 177
    TVUS and MRI
        DIE, 177, 178
        ovarian endometriosis, 177
        pelvic endometriosis, 176, 177
Dichorionic-diamniotic twin pregnancies, 48
Doppler mapping, 52
Double-contrast barium enema (DCBE), 177

E

Echogenic bands, 49
Echogenic rim, 41
Edge shadows, 40
Endometrial biomarkers, 174–176
Endometrioma decidualization, 51
Endometriosis, 147
    clinical assessment, 4
    definition, 1
    examination, 3
    family history, 2
    forms, 28
    prevalence, 1
    signs and symptoms, 2
Endometriotic involvement
    in abdominal and pelvic wall scars, 163
    chest, 163
    cutaneous variants, 163
Endometriotic nodules, 31
Enolase 1 (NNE), 173
Extra-abdominal bladder, 68, 69
Extraovarian endometriosis, 163, 164
Extrapelvic endometriosis, 2, 121

F

Fallopian tubes, 28, 29
Fan-shaped shadowing, 40
Fibroids, 37–39, 42, 45
Forniceal-vaginal deep endometriosis
    classification, 89, 90
    gel sonovaginography, 94
    histologic findings, 89
    location, 89
    tenderness-guided ultrasound examination, 93
    TVS
        diabolo-like nodule, 92, 93
        forniceal nodule, 91–93
        3D TVS, 93, 94

G

Gastrointestinal stromal tumor (GIST), 116
Gel sonovaginography, 80, 81
Gonadotropin-releasing hormone analogues, 16
Ground-glass echogenicity, 47, 48, 51, 54

H

Haematocrit effect, 151
Haemorrhagic cyst, 152, 154
Hematuria, 67
Hepatic endometriosis, 126
Hidden disease, 6

High-intensity-focused ultrasound (HIFU) ablation, 128
Hormone replacement treatment (HRT), 16
Hydronephrosis, 68, 74
Hydroureteronephrosis, 30
Hyperalgesia, 3, 4
Hyperechogenic islands, 41
Hypoestrogenizing drugs, 14

I
Ill-defined lesions, 37–40
Infiltrating endometriosis of the terminal ileum, 163
Inguinal endometriosis, 122, 125
Inner lesion-free margin (IFM), 39
Internal shadows, 40
International Deep Endometriosis Analysis (IDEA), 28, 30, 34, 57, 66, 89, 90, 94, 99
Intra-abdominal endometriosis, 125

J
Junctional zone (JZ)/inner myometrium, 41

K
Kissing ovaries, 29, 51, 151, 153

L
Lambda sign, 50
Lambda sing, 48
Latzko's space, 8
Letrozole, 17
Levonorgestrel-releasing intrauterine device (LNG-IUD), 15, 16
Low-invasive tests for endometriosis, 170

M
Magnetic resonance imaging
  antispasmodic agents, 149
  bladder distension, 149
  bowel preparation, 149
  diffusion-weighted imaging, 150
  endovaginal coil, 149
  half-Fourier single-shot turbo-spin-echo acquisition, 150
  indications, 148
  intravenous contrast-enhanced MRI, 150–151
  1.5-T magnet, 149
  patient positioning, 149
  patient preparation, 149
  pelvic phased-array coils, 149
  susceptibility-weighted imaging, 150
  3.0-T magnet, 149
  timing of, 149
  2D-T2-weighted sequences, 150
  vaginal/rectal opacification, 150
Matrix-enhanced laser desorption/ionization time-of-flight mass spectrometry (MALDI-TOF-MS), 173
Mature cystic ovarian teratomas, 154
Mature cystic teratoma, 152
Mean gray value (MGV), 53
Medical management
  antiangiogenic agents, 17, 18
  aromatase inhibitors, 17
  GnRH analogues, 16
  NSAIDs, 16, 17
  oral contraceptives, 14, 15
  progestins, 15–16
  risk and side effects, 13
  SERMs, 17
  vs. surgical treatment, 14
Medroxyprogesterone acetate (MPA), 15
miRNA biomarkers, 173
Modified SVG technique, 135
Morphological Uterus Sonographic Assessment (MUSA) consensus, 28
MRI jelly method, 176, 178
Mucinous lesions, 154
Multi-detector computerized tomography enema (MDCT-e), 178
Multiple corpora lutea, 154
Multiple endometriomas, 48
Muscularis propria, 161
Myometrial cysts, 39–41
Myometrial lesions, MUSA
  adenomyosis cyst, 40, 41
  circumferential flow, 42, 43
  color score, 41, 42
  cyst, 41
  echogenicity, 37, 40
  future perspectives, 45
  IFM, 39
  ill-defined lesion, 39, 40
  junctional zone/inner myometrium, 41, 44
  location, 39
  myometrial walls, 37
  OFM, 39
  radial vessels, 44
  shadowing, 40
  sliding sign, 43
  3D acquisition, 43
  uterine corpus, 43
  uterus total length, 43
  vessel morphology, 42
  well-defined lesions, 39

N
Neoangiogenesis, 17
Non-menstrual pelvic pain (NMPP), 2
Nonsteroidal anti-inflammatory drugs (NSAIDs), 16
Norethindrone acetate (NETA), 15
Norethisterone acetate, 17

O
Obliterated cul-de-sac fibroids, 5
Okabayashi's space, 8
Oral contraceptives, 14, 15

Outer lesion-free margin (OFM), 39
Ovarian carcinoma, 154
Ovarian endometrioma, 18–19
  acute abdomen, 153
  ADC values, 153
  adhesions, 153, 159
  chemical-selective T1-weighted fat-saturated sequences, 151–152
  complications, 153
  description, 151
  differential diagnosis, 154
  DWI imaging, 152
  malignant transformation, 153
  menstrual cycles, 151
  MR imaging, 151, 153
  multiple cysts, 151
  mural nodules enhancement, 153
  ovarian torsion, 153
  reduced fertility, 153
  restricted diffusion, 153
  short-tau inversion recovery sequences, 152
Ovarian endometriosis
  depth, 53
  diagnosis, 52
  Doppler ultrasound, 52
  future research, 54
  incidence, 47
  machine settings, 54
  pathogenesis, 47
  sonographic spectrum
    anechoic cyst, 48, 49
    atypical endometrioma, 50
    benign endometriomas, 51
    echogenic bands, 48, 49
    endometrioma decidualization, 51
    hyperechoic foci, 50
    kissing ovaries, 51
    low-level echogenicity, 48, 49
    multilocular endometrioma, 48, 49
    multiple endometriomas, 48, 50
    ovarian parenchyma, 49
    septate endometrioma, 48, 50
    unilocular cyst, 48
  symptoms, 47
  3D ultrasound, 52, 53
  transvaginal ultrasound, 48
Ovarian mobility, 28, 29, 57–58

P

Pain mapping, 73
Pararectal space, 8
Pelvic endometriosis, 7, 156
Pelvic floor hypertonicity, 3
Pelvic sidewall anatomy, 8–9
Pelvic spaces, 7–8
Peripheral biomarkers, 172–174
Peristalsis, 71–74
Peritoneal endometriosis, 154, 155
PGP 9.5 biomarker, 175
Pouch of Douglas (POD), 29, 30, 34
  description, 63
  future perspectives, 65, 66
  rectal/rectosigmoid deep endometriosis, 63
  technical guidelines, 65
  TVS, 63, 64
  uterine sliding sign, 65
  in women, 63
Presacral space/retrorectal space, 8
Prevesical space, 7, 8
Progestins, 15–16

Q

Quinagolide, 18

R

rASRM classification, 58
Rectal endoscopic sonography (RES), 98
Rectal hypoechoic endometriotic nodule, 141
Rectal water contrast transvaginal ultrasonography (RWC-TVS), 137–142
Rectosigmoid endometriosis, 162
Rectovaginal septum (RVS) endometriosis, 32
  anatomy, 97, 98
  DE nodules, 100
  definition, 97
  drawing, 99
  four-step systematic approach, 99
  future perspective, 101, 102
  prevalence, 98
  TVS
    hyperechogenic layer, 100
    RES, 98
    sensitivity rates, 98, 99
    3D, 98
    visualization of, 100
  vaginal examination, 98, 99
Rectovaginal space, 8
Rectus abdominis endometriosis, 125, 126, 130
Retrocervical endometriosis, 97
Retroperitoneal/retrocervical lesion, 89, 90
Retropubic space, 7
Retzius, *see* Retropubic space
Round ligaments of the uterus (RLUs), 158

S

Saline contrast sonography, 98
Scar endometriosis, 122–124, 128, 129
Selective estrogen receptor modulators (SERMs), 17
Septate endometrioma, 50
Shadowing, 40
Site-specific tenderness (SST), 28, 29, 58
Sliding sign technique, 29, 30, 43, 44, 63–66
SnOUT test, 170, 171
Soft marker, TVS, 28
  ovarian mobility, 57–59
  SST, 58, 59

technical tips, 59, 60
UBESS, 60
usefulness, 60
Sonovaginography (SVG), 80, 81, 134–137
SpIN triage test, 170–172, 176–178
Standoff technique, 93
Stromal endometriosis, 155
Subendometrial echogenic lines and buds, 41
Surgical layers, 8, 9
Surgical management
bladder endometriosis, 19
bowel endometriosis, 20, 21
vs. medical therapies, 14
ovarian endometrioma, 18–19
ureteral endometriosis, 19, 20
urinary tract endometriosis, 19
uterosacral endometriosis, 20
Symptomatic endometrioma, 47

T
Tenderness-guided transvaginal ultrasonography (tg-TVS), 133, 134, 177
Three-dimensional rectosonography (3D-RSG), 142
Three-stage technique, 18
3.0Tesla Magnetom system (3.0 T MRI), 176
Tomographic ultrasound imaging (TUI), 82
Transrectal sonography, 81
Transvaginal ultrasound (TVS), 27
Transvaginal ultrasound with bowel preparation (TVUS-BP), 105–108, 110, 112, 115, 116, 118, 176–179
Tubo-ovarian abscess, 154
Tumor necrosis factor-a (TNF-a), 17

U
Ultrasound-based endometriosis staging system (UBESS), 60
Umbilical endometriosis, *see* Villar's nodule
Ureteral endometriosis, 19, 20, 68, 70–73
Ureteral jet, 71
Ureteroneocystostomy, 19, 20
Urinary badder endometriosis, 68–70
Urinary tract endometriosis (UTE), 156
bladder endometriosis, 68–70
incidence, 67
pathogenesis, 67
surgical management, 19
technical guidelines, 73
ureteral endometriosis, 70–73
Uterine abnormalities, 28
Uterine corpus, 43
Uterine fibroids, 39
Uterine fluid, 175
Uterosacral ligament (USL) endometriosis
clinical history, 77
clinical pelvic examination, 77
future perspectives, 82
preoperative diagnosis, 77
sonovaginography with saline/gel, 80, 81
3D-transvaginal sonography, 81, 82
transrectal sonography, 81
2D-TVS, 77–80
Uterosacral ligaments (USL), 57

V
Vaginal and rectal opacification, 164
Vaginal fornix, 33
Vaginal nodule, 3, 4
Vaginal/rectal opacification, 150
Vesicovaginal space, 8
Villar's nodule, 124, 129
Virtual organ computer-aided analysis (VOCAL) mode, 53, 142
Vitamin D binding protein (VDBP), 173
Volume contrast imaging (VCI), 82
Volume rendering analysis, 82

MIX
Papier aus verantwortungsvollen Quellen
Paper from responsible sources
FSC® C105338

If you have any concerns about our products,
you can contact us on
ProductSafety@springernature.com

In case Publisher is established outside the EU,
the EU authorized representative is:
Springer Nature Customer Service Center GmbH
Europaplatz 3, 69115 Heidelberg, Germany

Printed by Libri Plureos GmbH
in Hamburg, Germany